Complementary and Alternative Medicine: Evidence-Based Approach

Complementary and Alternative Medicine: Evidence-Based Approach

Editor: Brendon Gould

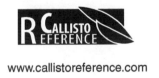

www.callistoreference.com

Callisto Reference,
118-35 Queens Blvd., Suite 400,
Forest Hills, NY 11375, USA

Visit us on the World Wide Web at:
www.callistoreference.com

ISBN: 978-1-63239-883-3 (Hardback)

The publisher's policy is to use permanent paper from mills that operate a sustainable forestry policy. Furthermore, the publisher ensures that the text paper and cover boards used have met acceptable environmental accreditation standards.

Trademark Notice: Registered trademark of products or corporate names are used only for explanation and identification without intent to infringe.

Printed in the United States of America.

Cataloging-in-Publication Data

Complementary and alternative medicine : evidence-based approach / edited by Brendon Gould.
   p. cm.
Includes bibliographical references and index.
ISBN 978-1-63239-883-3
1. Alternative medicine. 2. Medicine. 3. Integrative medicine. 4. Therapeutics. I. Gould, Brendon.
R733 .C66 2017
615.5--dc23

Table of Contents

Preface... VII

Chapter 1   **Antibacterial and Antimetastatic Potential of *Diospyros lycioides* Extract on Cervical Cancer Cells and Associated Pathogens**... 1
V. P. Bagla, V. Z. Lubisi, T. Ndiitwani, M. P. Mokgotho, L. Mampuru,
V. Mbazima

Chapter 2   **Immune Signatures in Patients with Psoriasis Vulgaris of Blood-Heat Syndrome**.. 11
Xin Li, Qing-qing Xiao, Fu-lun Li, Rong Xu, Bin Fan, Min-feng Wu, Min Zhou,
Su Li, Jie Chen, Shi-guang Peng, Bin Li

Chapter 3   **Veratri Nigri Rhizoma et Radix (*Veratrum nigrum* L.) and its Constituent Jervine Prevent Adipogenesis via Activation of the LKB1-AMPKα-ACC Axis *In Vivo* and *In Vitro***.. 22
Jinbong Park, Yong-Deok Jeon, Hye-Lin Kim, Dae-Seung Kim, Yo-Han Han,
Yunu Jung, Dong-Hyun Youn, Jong Wook Kang, Daeyeon Yoon, Mi-Young Jeong,
Jong- Hyun Lee, Seung-Heon Hong, Junhee Lee, Jae-Young Um

Chapter 4   **Systems Pharmacology Uncovers the Multiple Mechanisms of Xijiao Dihuang Decoction for the Treatment of Viral Hemorrhagic Fever**.................... 34
Jianling Liu, Tianli Pei, Jiexin Mu, Chunli Zheng, Xuetong Chen, Chao Huang,
Yingxue Fu, Zongsuo Liang, Yonghua Wang

Chapter 5   **Electroacupuncture Attenuates Cerebral Ischemia and Reperfusion Injury in Middle Cerebral Artery Occlusion of Rat via Modulation of Apoptosis, Inflammation, Oxidative Stress, and Excitotoxicity**.. 51
Mei-hong Shen, Chun-bing Zhang, Jia-hui Zhang, Peng-fei Li

Chapter 6   **Garlic Attenuates Plasma and Kidney ACE-1 and AngII Modulations in Early Streptozotocin-Induced Diabetic Rats: Renal Clearance and Blood Pressure Implications**.. 66
Khaled K. Al-Qattan, Martha Thomson, Divya Jayasree, Muslim Ali

Chapter 7   **Stress and Fatigue Management using Balneotherapy in a Short-Time Randomized Controlled Trial**... 77
Lolita Rapolienė, Artūras Razbadauskas, Jonas Sąlyga, Arvydas Martinkėnas

Chapter 8   **The Effects of Xiangqing Anodyne Spray on Treating Acute Soft-Tissue Injury Mainly Depend on Suppressing Activations of AKT and p38 Pathways**.. 87
ShudongWang, Tao Li, Wei Qu, Xin Li, Shaoxin Ma, Zheng Wang, Wenya Liu,
Shanshan Hou, Jihua Fu

Chapter 9   **Influence of the *Melissa officinalis* Leaf Extract on Long-Term Memory in Scopolamine Animal Model with Assessment of Mechanism of Action**...................................... 98
Marcin Ozarowski, Przemyslaw L. Mikolajczak, Anna Piasecka, Piotr Kachlicki, Radoslaw Kujawski, Anna Bogacz, Joanna Bartkowiak-Wieczorek, Michal Szulc, Ewa Kaminska, Malgorzata Kujawska, Jadwiga Jodynis-Liebert, Agnieszka Gryszczynska, Bogna Opala, Zdzislaw Lowicki, Agnieszka Seremak-Mrozikiewicz, Boguslaw Czerny

Chapter 10   **Berberine Inhibition of Fibrogenesis in a Rat Model of Liver Fibrosis and in Hepatic Stellate Cells**..115
Ning Wang, Qihe Xu, Hor Yue Tan, Ming Hong, Sha Li, Man-Fung Yuen, Yibin Feng

Chapter 11   **The Relieving Effects of BrainPower Advanced, a Dietary Supplement, in Older Adults with Subjective Memory Complaints**.. 126
Jingfen Zhu, Rong Shi, Su Chen, Lihua Dai, Tian Shen, Yi Feng, Pingping Gu, Mina Shariff, Tuong Nguyen, Yeats Ye, Jianyu Rao, Guoqiang Xing

Chapter 12   **Antiobesity Effects of the Combined Plant Extracts Varying the Combination Ratio of *Phyllostachys pubescens* Leaf Extract and *Scutellaria baicalensis* Root Extract**..142
Dong-Seon Kim, Seung-Hyung Kim, Jimin Cha

Chapter 13   **Therapeutic Effects of Traditional Chinese Medicine on Spinal Cord Injury: A Promising Supplementary Treatment in Future**..153
Qian Zhang, Hao Yang, Jing An, Rui Zhang, Bo Chen, Ding-Jun Hao

Chapter 14   **Untargeted Metabolomics Reveals Intervention Effects of Total Turmeric Extract in a Rat Model of Nonalcoholic Fatty Liver Disease**..171
Ya Wang, Ming Niu, Ge-liu-chang Jia, Rui-sheng Li, Ya-ming Zhang, Cong-en Zhang, Ya-kun Meng, He-rong Cui, Zhi-jie Ma, Dong-hui Li, Jia-bo Wang, Xiao-he Xiao

Chapter 15   **Identification of "Multiple Components-Multiple Targets-Multiple Pathways" Associated with Naoxintong Capsule in the Treatment of Heart Diseases using UPLC/Q-TOF-MS and Network Pharmacology**.. 183
Xianghui Ma, Bin Lv, Pan Li, Xiaoqing Jiang, Qian Zhou, Xiaoying Wang, Xiumei Gao

Chapter 16   **Ligustrazine for the Treatment of Unstable Angina**.. 198
Suman Cao, Wenli Zhao, Huaien Bu, Ye Zhao, Chunquan Yu

Permissions

List of Contributors

Index

Preface

This book on complementary and alternative medicine discusses topics related to energy harnessing and nutritional value that is related to alternative medical practices. Alternative medical diagnosis and medication consider the overall well-being and fitness of a patient while treating disease. This book discusses the fundamentals as well as modern approaches of this field. It consists of contributions made by international experts. It strives to provide a fair idea about this discipline and to help develop a better understanding of the latest advances within this field. In this book, using case studies and examples, constant effort has been made to make the understanding of the difficult concepts of alternative medicine as easy and informative as possible, for the readers.

This book has been the outcome of endless efforts put in by authors and researchers on various issues and topics within the field. The book is a comprehensive collection of significant researches that are addressed in a variety of chapters. It will surely enhance the knowledge of the field among readers across the globe.

It gives us an immense pleasure to thank our researchers and authors for their efforts to submit their piece of writing before the deadlines. Finally in the end, I would like to thank my family and colleagues who have been a great source of inspiration and support.

Editor

Antibacterial and Antimetastatic Potential of *Diospyros lycioides* Extract on Cervical Cancer Cells and Associated Pathogens

V. P. Bagla, V. Z. Lubisi, T. Ndiitwani, M. P. Mokgotho, L. Mampuru, and V. Mbazima

Department of Biochemistry, Microbiology and Biotechnology, Faculty of Science and Agriculture,
University of Limpopo, Turfloop Campus, Private Bag X1106, Sovenga, Limpopo 0727, South Africa

Correspondence should be addressed to V. P. Bagla; drvictorb@yahoo.com

Academic Editor: Daniela Rigano

Cervical cancer is among the most prevalent forms of cancer in women worldwide. *Diospyros lycioides* was extracted using hexane, ethyl acetate, acetone, and methanol and finger print profiles were determined. The leaf material was tested for the presence of flavonoids, tannins, saponins, terpenoids, and cardiac glycosides using standard chemical methods and the presence of flavonoids and phenolics using thin layer chromatography. The total phenolic content was determined using Folin-Ciocalteu procedure. The four extracts were tested for antibacterial activity using bioautography against *Staphylococcus aureus*, *Enterococcus faecalis*, *Pseudomonas aeruginosa*, and *Escherichia coli*. The acetone extract with the highest number of antibacterial and antioxidant compounds was assessed for its cytotoxicity on BUD-8 cells using the real-time xCELLigence system and its potential effects on metastatic cervical cancer (HeLa) cell migration and invasion were assessed using wound healing migration and invasion assays. The leaf extract tested positive for flavonoids, tannins, and terpenoids while the four different extracts tested in the antimicrobial assay contained constituents active against one or more of the organisms tested, except *E. coli*. The cytotoxicity of the acetone extract in real-time was concentration-dependent with potent ability to suppress the migration and invasion of HeLa cells. The finding demonstrates the acetone extract to contain constituents with antibacterial and antimetastatic effects on cervical cancer cells.

1. Introduction

Medicinal plants act as one of nature's primary reservoirs since time immemorial as a source of potent pharmacological constituents for the treatment of various diseases. Multidrug resistance to antibacterial agents and the high incidences of various cancers on the other hand have grown at an alarming rate in recent years. Cervical cancer is the second leading form of cancer in South African women after breast cancer. It affects young women with resultant adverse effects such as infertility and impaired sexual quality [1].

The causative agent of cervical cancer is the Human Papilloma Virus (HPV) which is transmitted sexually, while *Staphylococcus aureus* and *Escherichia coli* are amongst the most common bacteria incriminated in vaginitis and associated cellular changes of the cervix [2]. Several other bacteria have also been implicated in chronic infections or are capable of producing toxins that influence the cell cycle resulting in altered cell growth [3], with a resultant DNA damage similar to that observed in apoptosis induced by carcinogens.

In South Africa, the bark and root decoctions of *Diospyros lycioides* are administered as treatment for bloody faeces and dysentery [4], while in Namibia the plant is used as a chewing stick [5]. Extract of this plant is also taken as a remedy for infertility in women [6], an associated problem in women with cervical cancer. Investigations of the antimicrobial activity of this plant have demonstrated the methanolic extract, from the twigs, to possess activity against common oral pathogens including *Streptococcus mutans* and *Porphyromonas gingivalis*, while isolated compounds have been found to possess marginal growth inhibitory activity against *Streptococcus sanguinis* and *S. mutans* [7].

Diospyros lycioides is known to contain some naphthoquinone constituents, including 7-methyljuglone, diospyrin, and isodisopyrin [8, 9]. Both 7-methyljuglone and diospyrin are reported to have a variety of pharmacological activities including anticancer activity [10, 11]. Evaluation of this plant in a recent study for its antiproliferative activity against MCF-7 breast cancer cells from our research group revealed the acetone leaf extract to induce apoptosis in a p53-dependent manner. The extract was also shown to upregulate Bax and downregulate Bcl-2 mRNA expression levels in MCF-7 breast cancer cells [12]. The current study was therefore aimed at investigating the antimetastatic effect of this plant on cervical cancer cells and the antibacterial activity against the pathogens that have been implicated in the condition. The extracts were also tested for the presence of selected phytochemical constituents.

2. Materials and Methods

2.1. Collection of Plant Material. The leaves of *D. lycioides* were collected from *Bolahlakgomo* area (*Lepelle-Nkumpi* Municipality, Limpopo Province, South Africa) and voucher specimen number UNIN 111076 is deposited at the Larry Leach Herbarium of the University of Limpopo. Leaves were separated from the stem and air-dried at room temperature in the dark. Dried plant material was ground into fine powder using a commercial blender.

2.2. Extraction of Plant Materials. The finely ground leaf material of *D. lycioides* (4 g) was serially extracted using 40 mL of each solvent, namely, hexane, acetone, ethyl acetate, and methanol for 3 h, 3 h, and 1 h at room temperature on a shaker (series 25 incubator shaker) set at 200 rpm. The extracts were filtered using Whatman filter paper number 3 into preweighed Erlenmeyer flasks, dried under a stream of air and masses obtained.

2.3. Phytochemical Screening

2.3.1. Flavonoids. Dilute ammonia (5 mL) was added to a portion of an aqueous filtrate of the plant material. Concentrated sulphuric acid (1 mL) was added. A yellow colouration that disappears on standing indicates the presence of flavonoids [13].

2.3.2. Tannins. About 0.5 g of the plant material was boiled in 10 mL of water in a test tube and filtered. A few drops of 0.1% of ferric chloride solution were added. A blue-black colouration indicated the presence of tannins [13].

2.3.3. Saponins. To a 0.5 g of plant material, 5 mL of distilled water was added in a test tube. The solution was shaken vigorously and observed for a stable persistent froth [13].

2.3.4. Terpenoids. To a 0.5 g of plant material, 2 mL of chloroform was added. Concentrated sulphuric acid (3 mL) was carefully added to form a layer. A reddish brown colouration at the interface indicated the presence of terpenoids [13].

2.3.5. Cardiac Glycosides. To a 0.5 g of plant material dissolved in 5 mL of water, 2 mL of glacial acetic acid containing one drop of ferric chloride solution was added. About 1 mL of concentrated sulphuric acid was also added and a brown ring at the interface was observed for the presence of cardiac glycosides [13].

2.4. TLC Fingerprint Profile of D. lycioides Extracts. Thin layer chromatographic profile of the hexane, ethyl acetate, acetone, and methanol leaf extracts dissolved in acetone was analysed on an aluminium backed thin layer chromatography (TLC) plates (Fluka, silica gel F25). Stock solutions of 10 mg/mL each were made and 10 μL of the extracts was spotted on TLC plates. TLC plates were developed in a saturated chamber using three mobile phases of different polarities, namely, benzene/ethanol/ammonia hydroxide [BEA, 5 : 4 : 1] (nonpolar/basic), chloroform/ethyl acetate/formic acid [CEF, 5 : 4 : 1] (intermediate polarity/acidic), and ethyl acetate/methanol/water [EMW, 4 : 1 : 5] (polar/neutral). TLC plates were sprayed with vanillin-sulphuric acid [0.1 g vanillin (Sigma®), 28 methanol, and 1 mL sulphuric acid] and heated at 110°C for optimal colour development [14]. For visualization of phenolic compounds, plates were sprayed with FeCl$_3$ (2% in ethanol) and aromatics were viewed by spraying with iodine vapour.

2.5. Qualitative DPPH Assay on TLC Plates (Antioxidant Activity). The TLC plates were prepared as described in methods for TLC finger print profile. All plates were dried in the fume hood before visualization. To detect compounds with antioxidant activity, the chromatographs were sprayed with 0.1% of 2,2-diphenyl-1-picrylhydrazyl (DPPH) (Sigma). The presence of yellow spots against purple background indicates the presence of antioxidant constituent [15].

2.6. Qualitative Detection of Phenolic Compounds Using TLC. TLC plates were prepared and eluted in the eluent systems as described methods for TLC finger print profile. Eluted plates were prayed with FeCl$_3$. Grey or black bands indicate the presence of phenolic compounds.

2.7. Quantitative Detection of Flavonoids Using TLC. TLC plates were prepared and eluted in the eluent systems as described methods for TLC finger print profile. The flavonoid constituents were visualized using 10% antimony (III) chloride in chloroform. Yellow bands indicate the presence of flavonoids.

2.8. Detection of Starch and Glycogen Using TLC. TLC plates were prepared and eluted in the eluent systems as described methods for TLC finger print profile. Starch and glycogen constituents were visualized using iodine vapour indicated by the presence of blue bands.

2.9. Total Phenolic Content Assay. The total phenolic contents of *D. lycioides* extracts were determined by using the Folin-Ciocalteu assay. Hexane, ethyl acetate, acetone, and methanol extracts or standard solution of gallic acid (0.02, 0.04, 0.06, 0.08, and 0.10 mg/mL) was added to a 25 mL test tube, containing 9 mL of distilled water. The blank was prepared using water. One millilitre of Folin-Ciocalteu's phenol reagent was added to the mixture and shaken. After 5 min, 10 mL of

7% Na_2CO_3 solution was added to the mixture. The mixture was adjusted with water to a final volume of 25 mL. After incubation for 90 min at room temperature, the absorbance was read at 750 nm. Total phenolic content was expressed as mg/mL [16].

2.10. Bioautography. The TLC plates were prepared as described in Section 2.4 without spraying with vanillin-sulphuric acid and dried for 7 days under a stream of air to remove residual solvents. Plates were sprayed with 50 mL of concentrated suspension of fresh bacteria cultures, namely, *Staphylococcus aureus* (ATCC 29213), *Enterococcus faecalis* (ATCC 29212), and *Pseudomonas aeruginosa* (ATCC 27853), and incubated overnight at 37°C at 100% relative humidity. After incubation, plates were sprayed with 2 mg/mL solution of *p*-iodonitrotetrazolium chloride (INT) (Sigma). Retardation factor (R_f) values of inhibitory zones, depicted as white areas [17], where reduction of INT to formazan did not occur, were recorded.

2.11. Cytotoxicity Assay Using xCELLigence System. BUD-8 cells were grown in Dulbecco's modified Eagle's medium (DMEM) (Gibco®) containing 10% fetal bovine serum (FBS) (Gibco) until about 75% confluent. Cells (100 μL) at a density of 4000 cells/mL were seeded in each well of the E-plate 96 and incubated overnight. The cells were then exposed to various concentrations (5, 10, 100, 500, and 1000 μg/mL) of *D. lycioides* acetone extract. Acetone extract was chosen for toxicity studies due to the presence of high number of antioxidant and antibacterial compounds active against tested pathogens. Controls received either 7.4 μg/mL curcumin (positive control) or DMSO (negative control) at a final concentration of 0.05%. All experiments were run for 24 h.

2.12. Wound Healing Assay. The effect of the noncytotoxic concentration (150 and 300 μg/mL) of the acetone extract of *D. lycioides* on mobility of HeLa cells was assayed using the wound healing assay. Cells suspended in DMEM containing 10% FBS were seeded in 12-well plates and incubated at 37°C for 24 h for cells to attain 90% confluence. A sterile plastic pipette tip was later used to create a linear wound across the centre of the cell monolayers. Cells were then washed twice with DMEM to remove detached cells and debris. The cell monolayers were then exposed to extracts at varying concentrations (0, 150, and 300 μg/mL). Curcumin (7.4 μg/mL) was used as positive control. Wound closure was monitored at 0, 6, and 24 h by photographing the monolayers under an inverted phase-contrast microscope (Nikon Eclipse, Ti series, USA) at 10x magnification.

2.13. Invasion Assay. Invasion assay was employed to determine the effect of the noncytotoxic concentrations of acetone extract of *D. lycioides* on HeLa cell invasion. Cells were treated with different concentrations of the extract (0, 150, and 300 μg/mL) in serum-free DMEM. The cells were then seeded in cell culture inserts (8 μm pore size) coated with 1 mg/mL of matrigel (BD Biosciences, USA). The inserts were then placed in 24-well plates filled with DMEM supplemented with 10%

FBS (chemoattractant). The plates were incubated at 37°C for 24 and 48 h. Nonmigrating cells were wiped with a cotton-tipped swab, and invading cells were fixed with 80% methanol and stained with 0.5% crystal violet and photographed with a phase-contrast microscope at 10x magnification.

3. Results

3.1. TLC-Fingerprints of Extracts of D. lycioides. TLC profile of extracts from *D. lycioides* leaves showing different compounds that were separated using different mobile phases is presented in Figure 1. The TLC plates were developed using vanillin/H_2SO_4 and heated at 110°C. The movement of compound from the base of the TLC plates was dependent on the polarity of the solvent system used. More bands reacted with vanillin/H_2SO_4 with most of the separated constituents having a purple colour. With vanillin/H_2SO_4 spray, steroids, higher alcohols, phenols, and essential oils are likely to be detected which is suggestive of the presence of these groups of compounds in the extracts. Only few bands on reaction with the reagent did not produce coloured bands in all the mobile phases. Ethyl acetate (EA), acetone (AC), and methanol (MeOH) extracts showed the presence of almost similar compounds in all three mobile phases (Figures 1(a), 1(b), and 1(c)). Hexane extract showed a good separation of compounds only in the nonpolar (BEA) mobile phase (Figure 1(a)). Intermediate mobile phase (Figure 1(b)) showed more compounds compared to the other two systems, possibly because of the type of compounds that were well separated in the polar and acidic eluent system [18].

3.2. Test for the Presence of Antioxidant Constituents on TLC. A representative TLC profile of different extracts of *D. lycioides* leaves eluted in CEF showing different constituents with antioxidant activity is presented in Figure 2(b). Chromatographs were sprayed with 0.1% DPPH solution. The yellow bands against a purple background indicate the presence of constituents with antioxidant activity. All extracts showed the presence of antioxidant constituents after spraying the chromatogram with DPPH. Hexane extract showed the least antioxidant active compounds while ethyl acetate and acetone showed more active compounds, especially in the intermediate mobile system. Most of the antioxidant compounds in ethyl acetate, acetone, and methanol could not move from the base of TLC plates when eluted in BEA solvent system, suggestive of the high polar nature of the constituent compounds.

The R_f values of constituents with antioxidant activity are presented in Table 1. With the hexane extract, antioxidant compounds migrated the most in the nonpolar and intermediate mobile phases, while acetone extract had more active compounds with R_f values ranging from 0 to 0.93 in both intermediate and polar mobile phases.

The phenolic constituents were visualized by spraying the eluted plates with $FeCl_3$. Grey or black bands indicated the presence of phenolic compounds (Figure 2(c)). The compounds that tested positive for phenolics were consistent with those detected on qualitative analysis of antioxidant activity using DPPH on TLC, signifying that the antioxidant

TABLE 1: R_f values and number bands with antioxidant activity.

Extracts	BEA		CEF		EMW	
	Number of bands	R_f values	Number of bands	R_f values	Number of bands	R_f values
Hexane	1	0.9	1	0.94	0	—
Ethyl acetate	1	0.96	4	0.06; 0.12; 0.79; 0.93	2	0.55; 0.90
Acetone	1	0.94	6	0.06; 0.12; 0.6; 0.8; 0.93	4	0.54; 0.60; 0.83; 0.89
Methanol	1	0.94	4	0; 0.06; 0.12; 0.93	2	0.38; 0.53

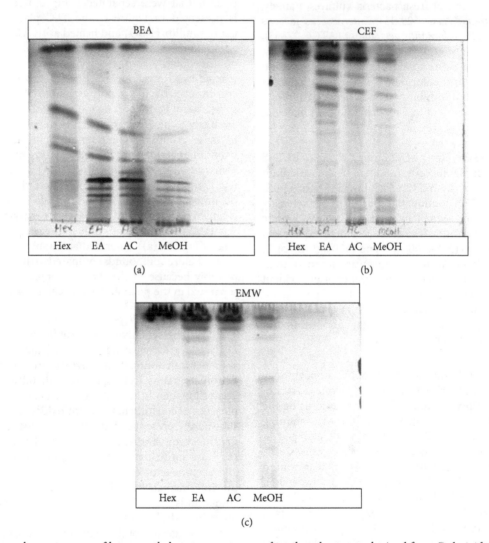

(a)

(b)

(c)

FIGURE 1: Thin layer chromatograms of hexane, ethyl acetate, acetone, and methanol extracts obtained from *D. lycioides* eluted in BEA (a), CEF (b), and EMW (c) mobile phases. The chromatograms were sprayed with vanillin/H_2SO_4 and heated at 110°C for colour development. Hex: hexane, EA: ethyl acetate, AC: acetone, and MeOH: methanol.

constituents in these extracts are generally phenolics. Flavonoid constituents on the other hand were visualized using 10% antimony (III) chloride in chloroform. Yellow bands indicated the presence of flavonoids (Figure 2(d)).

3.3. Evaluation of Total Phenolic Content in the Different Extracts. The phenolic content in the different extracts increased with increasing polarity of the extractant (Figure 3). Methanol extract showed the highest amount of phenolics followed by acetone. In hexane and ethyl acetate extracts, the difference was not significant. The amounts of phenolics did not correlate well with the presence of phenolics in the TLC-qualitative assay where acetone showed more bands compared to methanol.

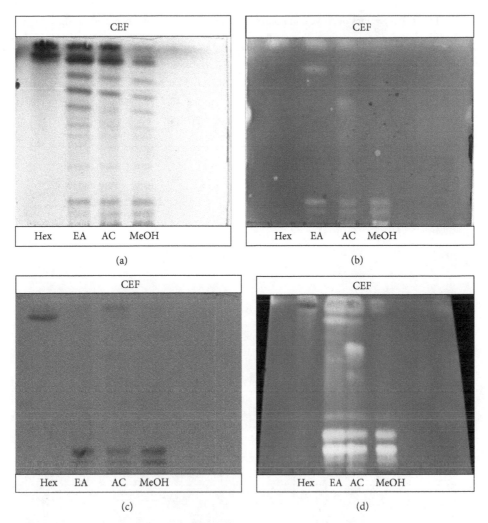

FIGURE 2: TLC finger print profiles (a), presence of antioxidant constituents (b), presence of phenolic compounds (c), and presence of flavonoids (d) eluted in CEF. Hex: hexane, EA: ethyl acetate, AC: acetone, and MeOH: methanol.

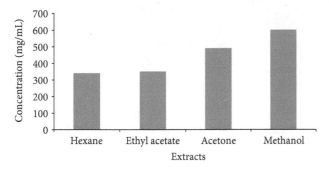

FIGURE 3: Phenolic content of *D. lycioides* leaves extracted from hexane, ethyl acetate, acetone, and methanol.

3.4. Classes of Secondary Metabolite Contained in Extract.

Test for the presence of phytochemical constituents in *D. lycioides* revealed the presence of tannins, terpenoids, flavonoids, and steroids and absence of saponins and cardiac glycosides. The presence of tannins and flavonoids has also been detected in this plant by other authors [19]. Flavonoids

have been reported to have strong antimicrobial activity. Martini et al. [20] reported the antimicrobial activity of flavonoids against Gram-negative bacteria. Tannins are known to be toxic to fungi, bacteria, and yeast. One of the mechanisms by which tannins exhibit their antimicrobial activity is by inhibition of extracellular microbial enzymes [21]. Terpenoids are found in most plants and are known to be active against bacteria. Although their mechanism of action in inhibiting bacteria is not well understood, their action has been related to the disruption of bacterial cell membrane [22]. Taleb-Contini et al. [23] also reported steroids to have significant activity against *Staphylococcus aureus*, *Streptococcus faecalis*, and *Escherichia coli*.

3.5. Bioautography.

Bioautography was used to screen for the presence of antibacterial compounds from *D. lycioides* extracts. Inhibition zones are indicated by the presence of white spot against a purple background. All extracts were unable to inhibit the growth of *E. coli* in all mobile phases (result not shown). The clear zone on TLC eluted in the representative bioautogram (Figure 4) indicates the presence

TABLE 2: R_f values of active compounds with antimicrobial activity eluted in BEA.

Extracts	P. aeruginosa		S. aureus		E. faecalis	
	Number of bands	R_f value	Number of bands	R_f value	Number of bands	R_f value
Ethyl acetate	2	0.10; 0.16	4	0.16; 0.22; 0.27; 0.36	4	0.05; 0.15; 0.17; 0.24; 0.37
Acetone	2	0.12; 0.17	3	0.2; 0.35; 0.45	5	0.05; 0.16; 0.17; 0.24; 0.58
Methanol	—	—	3	0.16; 0.2; 0.27	4	0.05; 0.15; 0.17; 0.24
Hexane	—	—	—	—	4	0.10; 0.39; 0.46; 0.61

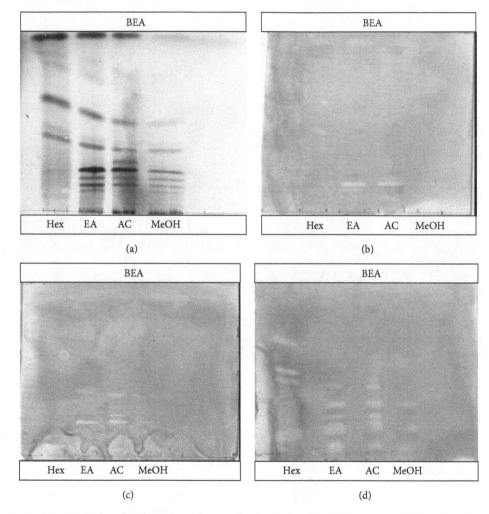

FIGURE 4: Representative bioautography of *D. lycioides* of hexane (hex), ethyl acetate (EA), acetone (AC), and methanol (MeOH) extracts eluted in BEA (a) and sprayed with *P. aeruginosa* (b), *S. aureus* (c), and *E. faecalis* (d).

of compounds within the different extracts with activity against the tested pathogen. Good growths of pathogens were observed with extracts that were eluted in BEA. The R_f value of compounds present in the different extracts against tested pathogens is presented in Table 2. More compounds were contained in the acetone and ethyl acetate extracts active against *S. aureus* and *E. faecalis*.

3.6. *Monitoring of Cytotoxicity in Real-Time Using xCELLigence System.* Acetone extract of *D. lycioides* that displayed the highest number of antibacterial and antioxidant compounds was found to be toxic to BUD-8 cell at concentrations of 500 and 1000 μg/mL. Concentration ranges of 5 to 100 μg/mL were not shown to be toxic at 18 h of exposure, with decrease in cell vailiblity (index) during proplonged exposure

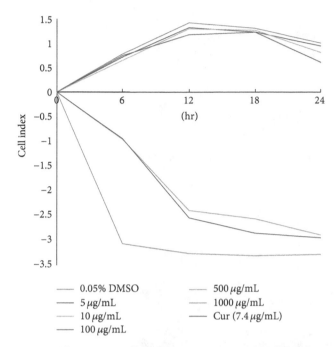

FIGURE 5: The cytotoxic effect of the acetone extract of *D. lycioides* on BUD-8 cells treated with increasing concentrations of crude acetone extract at 6 h interval as evaluated in real-time using xCELLigence system.

time beyond 18 h (Figure 5), with the cells exhibiting a similar trend (decrease in viability) beyond 18 h.

3.7. Effect of Acetone Extract on the Suppression of Migration of HeLa Cells. Since *S. aureus* and *E. coli* are amongst the most common bacteria implicated in vaginitis and associated cellular changes of the cervix; the acetone extract containing the highest number of antibacterial and antioxidant compounds was then tested at noncytotoxic concentrations (0, 150 and 300 μg/mL) for its ability to inhibit the migration of HeLa cells. As shown in Figure 6, the extract was shown to suppress the migration of the cells in a concentration-dependent manner. Cells exposed to the acetone extract were seen to have a reduced ability to migrate and as such prevented the closure of wounds at the various concentrations and exposure times (Figure 6).

3.8. Suppression of the Invasive Ability of HeLa Cells. The anti-invasive efficacy of *D. lycioides* acetone extract was assessed using the Boyden chamber coated with 1 mg/mL matrigel. Curcumin- and extract-treated cells were shown to considerably reduce the passage of cell through the matrigel as compared to untreated cells (Figure 7). Treatment with 300 μg/mL of the extract resulted in greater reduction in invasive ability of the cells than 150 μg/mL, implicative of the anti-invasive activity of the extract to be concentration-dependent with inhibitory activity at the highest concentration tested.

4. Discussion

Diospyros lycioides was selected for this study for screening of antibacterial activity because of its traditional use as

a chewing stick against oral pathogens [5]. In this study, four solvents (hexane, ethyl acetate, acetone, and methanol) were used for extraction of plant material. Methanol, a polar solvent, was the best extracting solvent, signifying that most of the compounds contained in this plant are polar. TLC-fingerprints of *D. lycioides* extracts revealed the presence of various constituents. More compounds were observed in ethyl acetate extract, followed by acetone, while the intermediate polar solvent (CEF) was the best eluent system for the separation of constituents on TLC. Test for the presence of phytochemical constituents in *D. lycioides* revealed the presence of tannins, terpenoids, flavonoids, and steroids and negative for saponins and cardiac glycosides. Free radical scavenging activity of extracts on TLC indicates the presence of antioxidant constituents, most of which were of intermediate polarity. The ferric chloride reducing assay was used to detect the presence of phenolic compounds in the extracts. By comparing the bands that reacted with DPPH and those with ferric chloride and their R_f values, the study concludes with some degree of certainty that phenolic compounds are responsible for the observed antioxidant activities. The quality of antioxidant compounds was high in the methanol extract as compared to the other extracts. This group of compounds is considered to have extensive variety of physiological, antimicrobial, and antioxidant properties [24]. Flavonoids are known to exhibit their antimicrobial activity by penetrating the cell wall of the microorganism and have been reported to be active against Gram-negative bacteria [20].

The antibacterial activities of the extracts were evaluated using bioautography against *S. aureus*, *E. coli*, and *P. aeruginosa*. All the extracts were shown to contain one or more compounds active against tested pathogens except for *E. coli*. This finding was not surprising since previous studies [5] have reported the antimicrobial activity of the methanol extract of this plant against oral pathogens with subsequent isolation of four novel bioactive naphthalene glycosides, diospyroides-A,-B,-C, and -D. The lack of activity observed with this plant against *E. coli* is consistent with previous reports by Fawole et al. [19].

Indeed cancer is a multietiological disease and a manifold of processes maybe involved in cervical carcinogenesis. Tumors have a complex cellular ecology that establishes the malignant potential of the tumor. Since *Staphylococcus aureus* and *Escherichia coli* are amongst the most common bacteria that have been incriminated in vaginitis and associated cellular changes of the cervix [2], and given that macrophages also potentiate the propagation and establishment of metastatic cells and play a role in tumor initiation when inflammation is a causal factor [25, 26], we resolved to test the potential antimetastatic effect of the extract on cervical cancer cells (HeLa).

To archive this, the cytotoxic effects of the acetone extract which contains the highest number of antibacterial constituents and antioxidant activity were tested on BUD-8 cell (human fibroblast cells). Findings revealed the extract to decrease the cell index of normal cells (Bud-8 cells) with an increase in concentration (500 and 1000 μg/mL) following analysis using the real-time-xCELLigence assay.

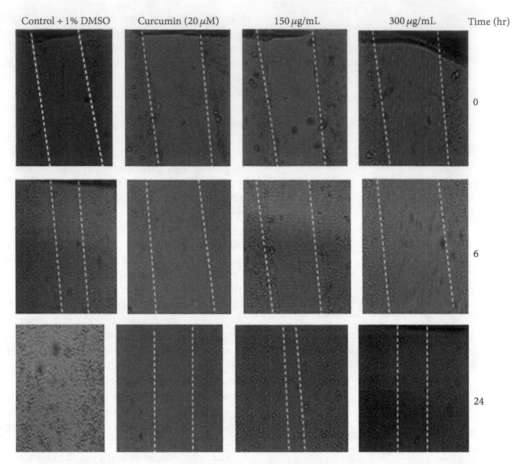

FIGURE 6: Inhibitory effect of the acetone extract of *D. lycioides* on the migration of HeLa cells. Confluent monolayers of cells were scarred, treated with 0, 150, and 300 μg/mL of the extract and 7.4 μg/mL of curcumin (positive control). Wound closure was monitored microscopically at 0, 6, and 24 h and photographed under a phase-contrast microscope at 10x magnification.

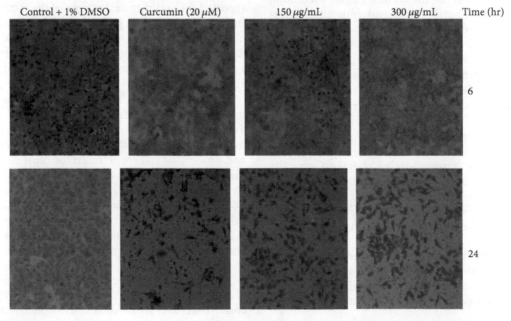

FIGURE 7: Anti-invasive potential of the acetone extract of *D. lycioides* on HeLa cell invasion. HeLa cells were treated with 0, 150, and 300 μg/mL for 6 and 24 h. Curcumin (7.4 μg/mL) was used as the positive control. Cells that penetrated through the matrigel membrane to the lower surface were stained with crystal violet and photographed with a phase-contrast microscope at 10x magnification.

An ideal antimetastatic agent ought to inhibit the metastatic events without affecting normal body cells. The relatively noncytotoxic concentrations of 150 μg/mL and 300 μg/mL of the extract were therefore chosen to access its inhibitory potential in subsequent metastatic-based assays on cervical cancer cells (HeLa cells), since preliminary studies of the extract on these cells in the MTT assay exhibited a >70% viability following 48 h of exposure (results not shown).

Exposure of cells to the acetone extract was shown to suppress the migration and invasive capability of HeLa cells in a time- and concentration-dependent manner. Tumor invasion requires degradation of basement membranes and thus remodelling of the extracellular matrix. Proteins that are mainly involved in degradation of the extracellular matrix are the matrix-metalloproteases (MMP). MMP-9 and MMP-2 are highly expressed in cancer patients. Observed effects suggest the extract to contain substances that can exert their antimetastatic effects by downregulating the activity of MMP-2 and MMP-9. Further study on the effect of the extract on the expression profiles and enzymatic-inhibitory activity of these proteins is necessary.

5. Conclusions

Cervical cancer is a burden in women. The acetone leaf extract of *D. lycioides* was shown to contain a variety of compounds, most of which were phenolics and flavonoids, with antibacterial activity against *S. aureus* and *P. aeruginosa*. Cytotoxicity of the acetone extract was shown to be nontoxic to normal cell at concentrations below 300 μg/mL, with potent antimetastatic effect in the suppression of invasion and migration of HeLa cells, a process that is mediated by the downregulation of MMP-9 and MMP-2. The indication of the presence of compounds in the acetone extracts that can suppress HeLa cell migration and invasion makes it a potential source of drug candidates that can interfere with the metastatic process. Work is ongoing to elucidate the mechanism(s) by which the observed effect(s) is or are asserted.

Abbreviations

TLC: Thin layer chromatography
BEA: Benzene : ethanol : ammonia hydroxide
CEF: Chloroform : ethyl acetate : formic acid
EMW: Ethyl acetate : methanol : water
DPPH: 2,2-Diphenyl-1-picrylhydrazyl
FeCl$_3$:   Ferric chloride
Na$_2$CO$_3$: Sodium bicarbonate
ATCC: American type culture collection
R_f: Retardation factor
MMP: Matrix-metalloproteinases.

Disclosure

This paper contents are solely the responsibility of the authors and do not necessarily represent the official views of the South African Medical Research Council.

Competing Interests

The authors declare that there is no conflict of interests regarding the publication of this paper.

Acknowledgments

Research reported in this publication was supported by the South African Medical Research Council through funding received from the South African National Treasury.

References

[1] C. Grangé, M. Bonal, É. Huyghe, P. Lèguevaque, V. Cances-Lauwers, and S. Motton, "Sexual function and quality of life in locally advanced cervical cancer," *Gynécologie Obstétrique & Fertilité*, vol. 41, no. 2, pp. 116–122, 2013.

[2] H. Al-Hillali, N. A. Hussien, A. Al-Obaidi, and A. A. Jasem, "Association between vaginitis caused by *Staphylococcus aureus*, *Escherichia coli* and *Candida albicans* and Pap smear results," *Qatar Medical Journal*, vol. 8, no. 13, pp. 102–110, 2012.

[3] B. Kocazeybek, "Chronic Chlamydophila pneumoniae infection in lung cancer, a risk factor: a case-control study," *Journal of Medical Microbiology*, vol. 52, no. 8, pp. 721–726, 2003.

[4] A. Hutchings, A. H. Scott, G. Lewis, and A. Cunningham, *Zulu Medicinal Plants: An Inventory*, University of Natal Press, Pietermaritzburg, South Africa, 1996.

[5] L. Cui, G. X. Wei, P. Van der Bijl, and C. D. Wu, "Namibian chewing stick, *Diospyros lycioides*, contains antibacterial compounds against oral pathogens," *Journal of Agricultural and Food Chemistry*, vol. 48, no. 3, pp. 909–914, 2000.

[6] A. Maroyi, "Traditional use of medicinal plants in south-central Zimbabwe: review and perspectives," *Journal of Ethnobiology and Ethnomedicine*, vol. 9, article 31, 2013.

[7] X.-C. Li, P. van der Bijl, and C. D. Wu, "Binaphthalenone glycosides from African chewing sticks, *Diospyros lycioides*," *Journal of Natural Products*, vol. 61, no. 6, pp. 817–820, 1998.

[8] L. M. Van Der Vijver and K. W. Gerritsma, "Naphthoquinones of *Euclea* and *Diospyros* species," *Phytochemistry*, vol. 13, no. 10, pp. 2322–2323, 1974.

[9] M. A. Ferreira, A. C. Costa, and A. Correia, "Identification of isodiospyrine, 7-methyljuglone and 8.8-dihydroxy-4,4-dimethoxy-6,6-dimethyl-2,2-bisnaphtyl1,1-quinone in the bark of roots of Diospyros lycioides Desf. susp. sericea (Bernh. ex Krauss) De Wint)r," *Plant Medicinal Phytotherapy*, vol. 6, no. 1, pp. 32–40, 1972.

[10] A. T. Mbaveng and V. Kuete, "Review of the chemistry and pharmacology of 7-methyljugulone," *African Health Sciences*, vol. 14, no. 1, pp. 201–205, 2014.

[11] S. Sagar, M. Kaur, K. P. Minneman, and V. B. Bajic, "Anti-cancer activities of diospyrin, its derivatives and analogues," *European Journal of Medicinal Chemistry*, vol. 45, no. 9, pp. 3519–3530, 2010.

[12] M. C. Pilane, V. P. Bagla, M. P. Mokgotho et al., "Free radical scavenging activity: antiproliferative and proteomics analyses of the differential expression of apoptotic proteins in MCF-7 cells treated with acetone leaf extract of *Diospyros lycioides* (Ebenaceae)," *Evidence-Based Complementary and Alternative Medicine*, vol. 2015, Article ID 534808, 13 pages, 2015.

[13] T. I. Borokini and O. Omotayo, "Phytochemical and enthnobotanical study of some selected medicinal plants from Nigeria,"

Journal of Medicinal Plants Research, vol. 6, no. 70, pp. 1106–1118, 2012.

[14] M. Kotzé and J. N. Eloff, "Extraction of antibacterial compounds from *Combretum microphyllum* (Combretaceae)," *South African Journal of Botany*, vol. 68, no. 1, pp. 62–67, 2002.

[15] C. Deby and G. Margotteaux, "Relationship between essential fatty acids and tissue antioxidant levels in mice," *C R Seances Society Biology Filiales*, vol. 165, pp. 2675–2681, 1970.

[16] D. Marinova, F. Ribarova, and M. Atanassova, "Total phenolic and total flavonoids in Bulgarian fruits and vegetables," *Journal of the University of Chemical Technology and Metallurgy*, vol. 40, no. 3, pp. 255–260, 2005.

[17] W. J. Begue and R. M. Kline, "The use of tetrazolium salts in bioauthographic procedures," *Journal of Chromatography A*, vol. 64, no. 1, pp. 182–184, 1972.

[18] J. N. Eloff, "Which extractant should be used for the screening and isolation of antimicrobial components from plants?" *Journal of Ethnopharmacology*, vol. 60, no. 1, pp. 1–8, 1998.

[19] O. A. Fawole, J. F. Finnie, and J. Van Staden, "Antimicrobial activity and mutagenic effects of twelve traditional medicinal plants used to treat ailments related to the gastro-intestinal tract in South Africa," *South African Journal of Botany*, vol. 75, no. 2, pp. 356–362, 2009.

[20] N. D. Martini, D. R. P. Katerere, and J. N. Eloff, "Biological activity of the five antibacterial flavonoids from *Combretum erythrophyllum*," *Journal of Enthnopharmacology*, vol. 94, pp. 207–212, 2004.

[21] A. Scalbert, "Antimicrobial properties of tannins," *Phytochemistry*, vol. 30, no. 12, pp. 3875–3883, 1991.

[22] M. M. Cowan, "Plant production as antimicrobial agents," *Clinical Microbiology Review*, vol. 12, no. 4, pp. 564–568, 1999.

[23] S. H. Taleb-Contini, M. J. Salvador, E. Watanabe, I. Y. Ito, and D. C. Rodrigues De Oliveira, "Antimicrobial activity of flavonoids and steroids isolated from two *Chromolaena* species," *Brazilian Journal of Pharmaceutical Sciences*, vol. 39, no. 4, pp. 403–408, 2003.

[24] M. P. Kähkönen, A. I. Hopia, H. J. Vuorela et al., "Antioxidant activity of plant extracts containing phenolic compounds," *Journal of Agricultural and Food Chemistry*, vol. 47, no. 10, pp. 3954–3962, 1999.

[25] J. Condeelis and J. W. Pollard, "Macrophages: obligate partners for tumor cell migration, invasion, and metastasis," *Cell*, vol. 124, no. 2, pp. 263–266, 2006.

[26] J. W. Pollard, "Tumour-educated macrophages promote tumour progression and metastasis," *Nature Reviews Cancer*, vol. 4, no. 1, pp. 71–78, 2004.

Immune Signatures in Patients with Psoriasis Vulgaris of Blood-Heat Syndrome

Xin Li,[1,2] Qing-qing Xiao,[1,2] Fu-lun Li,[1,2] Rong Xu,[1,2] Bin Fan,[1,2] Min-feng Wu,[1,2] Min Zhou,[1,2] Su Li,[1,2] Jie Chen,[1,2] Shi-guang Peng,[3] and Bin Li[1,2]

[1]Department of Dermatology, Yueyang Hospital of Integrated Traditional Chinese and Western Medicine, Shanghai University of Traditional Chinese Medicine, Shanghai 200437, China
[2]Institute of Dermatology, Shanghai Academy of Traditional Chinese Medicine, Shanghai 201203, China
[3]Department of Dermatology, Beijing Chao-Yang Hospital, Capital Medical University, Beijing 100020, China

Correspondence should be addressed to Shi-guang Peng; 18501367719@163.com and Bin Li; 18930568129@163.com

Academic Editor: Juntra Karbwang

Objective. To determine whether immunological serum markers IFN-γ, IL-4, IL-17, IL-23, IL-6, TNF-α, and IL-10 are elevated or decreased in patients compared with healthy controls. *Methods*. A complete search of the literature on this topic within the past 30 years was conducted across seven databases. Seventeen studies including 768 individuals were identified. Differences in serum marker levels between subjects and controls were pooled as MDs using the random-effects model. *Results*. The pooled MDs were higher in patients than in healthy controls for IFN-γ (MD 24.9, 95% CI 12.36–37.43), IL-17 (MD 28.92, 95% CI 17.44–40.40), IL-23 (MD 310.60, 95% CI 4.96–616.24), and TNF-α (MD 19.84, 95% CI 13.80–25.87). Pooled IL-4 (MD −13.5, 95% CI −17.74–−9.26) and IL-10 (MD −10.33, 95% CI −12.03–−8.63) levels were lower in patients. *Conclusion*. The pooled analyses suggest that levels of IFN-γ, IL-17, IL-23, and TNF-α are significantly elevated and that levels of IL-4 and IL-10 are significantly decreased in sera of patients with psoriasis vulgaris of blood-heat syndrome. Measuring progression of blood-heat syndrome of psoriasis vulgaris will require additional high-quality data, with a low risk of bias and adequate sample sizes, before and after antipsoriatic therapy.

1. Introduction

Psoriasis is a chronic immune-mediated skin disease that affects approximately 2–4% of the population in Western countries [1]. Patients with psoriasis may present with the pustular, guttate, arthritic, or erythrodermic variants and may have itching or painful lesions that negatively affect the quality of life. The understanding of the pathogenesis of psoriasis has improved, as has the understanding of the cellular components (mainly keratinocytes and T lymphocytes) involved in psoriasis, and the cytokines produced by the main Th lymphocyte subsets are now known to play a decisive role in pathogenesis [2]. Current evidence suggests that psoriasis is a T-cell-mediated disease driven at least in part by a positive feedback loop from activated T-cells to antigen-presenting cells (APCs) that is mediated by IFN-γ, IL-1, and tumor necrosis factor-α (TNF-α) [3, 4]. It has been shown that the Th1-Th2-Th17 balance is

likely a key functional and genetic determinant of psoriasis [4].

However, current treatments remain unsatisfactory and burdensome, and they often do not meet patients' expectations [5]; thus, therapies collectively called alternative therapies are commonly used. One observational study revealed that 51% of patients with psoriasis opted to use alternative therapies [6]. Traditional Chinese medicine (TCM), one type of alternative therapy, has been used to treat human diseases for more than 2000 years in China. Over the course of history, physicians practicing TCM have accumulated a tremendous amount of knowledge and experience in treating psoriasis. TCM prescribes treatment for psoriasis vulgaris based on syndrome differentiation. According to TCM, the syndromes can be divided into three main categories: blood-heat syndrome, blood-stasis syndrome, and blood-dryness syndrome. Correspondingly, clearing heat and cooling blood, promoting blood circulation to dissipate blood stasis, and adding moisture to reduce blood dryness comprise the treatment principles for the three syndromes of psoriasis vulgaris [7, 8]. The distribution of the three syndromes has been shown to be closely correlated with disease stage: the blood-heat syndrome is the most common at the active stage; the blood-dryness syndrome is the most common at the resting and regressive stages; and the blood-stasis syndrome is the most common at the resting stage [9]. Several investigators have searched for immunological markers of blood-heat syndrome, not only in skin lesions, but also in the circulatory system, using them to measure disease severity or to quantify treatment response. However, the data on serum levels of immunological markers in patients compared with controls are contradictory; some authors have reported elevated levels, whereas others have reported conflicting results. The studies to date have used small sample sizes or have investigated different markers to assess immune status; moreover, measurement of immunological serum markers is often not their primary objective.

We performed a systematic review and meta-analysis to determine whether seven well-known immunological serum markers (IFN-γ, IL-4, IL-17, IL-23, IL-6, TNF-α, and IL-10) are elevated or decreased in patients with psoriasis vulgaris of blood-heat syndrome compared with controls.

2. Materials and Methods

2.1. Eligibility Criteria. Inclusion and exclusion criteria were determined before the search was conducted. We included human studies comparing patients with psoriasis vulgaris of blood-heat syndrome with healthy controls, in which one or more of the following immunological markers was measured in the serum: IFN-γ, IL-4, IL-17, IL-23, IL-6, TNF-α, and IL-10. If several studies reported results from the same study population, the most complete report was included. Case reports and letters were excluded.

2.2. Data Sources and Searches. To identify relevant psoriasis vulgaris of blood-heat syndrome studies that included immunological markers, three reviewers (X. L., Q. Q. X, and F. L. L.) systematically searched MEDLINE, Embase, Cochrane Central Register of Controlled Trials, China National Knowledge Infrastructure database (CNKI), Chinese Scientific Journals Full-Text Database (CQVIP), Wanfang Data Knowledge Service Platform, and Chinese Biomedical Literature Service System (SINOMED). Papers published in English or Chinese and dated from January 1980 to May 2015 were included in this study.

The main descriptors adopted in the search strategy for primary studies were psoriasis, blood-heat syndrome, IFN-γ, IL-4, IL-17, IL-23, IL-6, TNF-α, and IL-10.

The search strategy adopted in the MEDLINE database via PubMed, which was adapted for the other databases analyzed, is presented as follows: psoriasis[tw] AND blood-heat syndrome[tw] AND (interferon-γ[tw] OR IFN-gamma[tw] OR IFN-γ[tw] OR interleukin-4[tw] OR il-4[tw] OR interleukin-17[tw] OR il-17[tw] OR interleukin-23[tw] OR il-23[tw] OR interleukin-6[tw] OR il-6[tw] OR tumor necrosis factor*[tw] OR tnf[tw] OR interleukin-10[tw] OR

il-10[tw]) NOT (animals[mesh] NOT humans[mesh]) NOT (case reports[pt] OR letter[pt]).

2.3. Study Selection. To determine eligibility for inclusion in the review, we screened all titles and abstracts for the following criteria: analyses comparing immunological marker profiles of patients with psoriasis vulgaris of blood-heat syndrome with those of control groups. There were no limitations on the study design, participant's age, gender, or nationality. The selection criteria for inclusion were as follows: (i) human-only studies; (ii) original data; (iii) a healthy control group; and (iv) provision of means and confidence intervals (CIs) for immunological serum markers. We identified 138 articles in the initial search (Figure 1). Through manual review of the citations from these articles, we identified 2 additional articles. After removing 57 duplicate articles and reading 82 individual abstracts, we identified 41 original studies that were eligible for inclusion criteria assessment. After reviewing the full text of these 48 studies, we excluded 24 articles for the following reasons: no healthy control group, duplicate publication of data, missing data from analyses, and no cytokines measured in serum. In the end, we selected 17 studies that met the inclusion criteria for this systematic review [10–26]. A flowchart of the search process is presented in Figure 1.

2.4. Data Extraction and Quality Assessment. Three reviewers independently collected descriptive data for each included study: (i) the first author; (ii) study characteristics (i.e., year, duration, country, and setting); (iii) characteristics of participants (i.e., mean age, male-to-female ratio, numbers of case and control subjects, duration, and mean PASI of cases); and (iv) outcome characteristics (i.e., the mean of immunological serum markers of psoriasis vulgaris blood-heat syndrome along with the standard deviation (SD) and whether results were from primary analysis of the study or were adjusted for comorbidities).

The Newcastle-Ottawa Scale [27] was used to assess study quality. It categorizes studies by three dimensions including selection, comparability, and exposure for case-control studies and selection, comparability, and outcome for cohort studies. Selection included four items, comparability included one item, and exposure included three items.

2.5. Data Synthesis and Analysis. The primary outcome was the identification of differences in mean serum levels of immunological markers between patients with psoriasis vulgaris of blood-heat syndrome and healthy controls for each study (Table 2). The degree of heterogeneity between studies was assessed using the I^2 test. An I^2 value > 50% was considered to indicate substantial heterogeneity. In this case, DerSimonian and Laird random-effects models were considered to compute the global MD. The between-study heterogeneity was not substantial ($I^2 < 50\%$) and the fixed-effect model was suitable. Publication bias was investigated graphically by using funnel plots and was statistically assessed via Egger's regression. The methods and findings of the present review have been reported following the Meta-Analysis of Observational Studies in Epidemiology

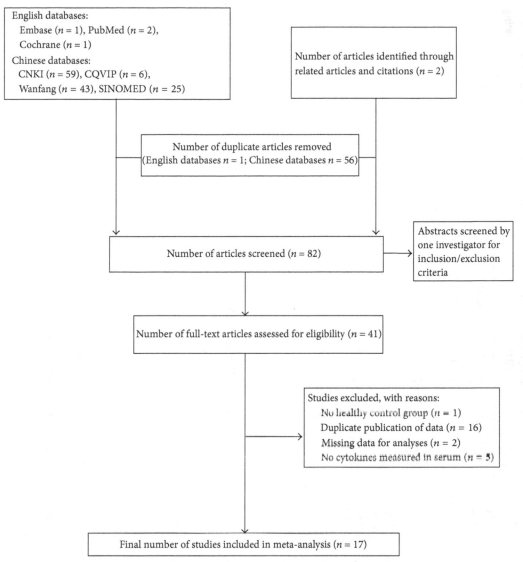

FIGURE 1: Flowchart of literature search and study selection.

group guidelines and checklist [28]. The Cochrane Collaboration Software Review Manager 5.2 was used for meta-analysis (http://ims.cochrane.org/revman). Egger's regression was performed using STATA version 10.0 (STATA Corp., College Station, TX, USA).

3. Results

3.1. Study Selection. Of a total of 139 titles, the full text of 41 potentially relevant studies was reviewed to confirm their eligibility. Among these 41 studies, 24 were excluded, including one with no healthy control group, 23 with duplicate publication of data, two with missing data for analyses, and five with no measurement of cytokines in serum. In total, 17 trials met the inclusion criteria (Figure 1).

3.2. Study Characteristics. The 17 selected studies included data on 768 individuals (443 patients with psoriasis vulgaris of blood-heat syndrome and 325 healthy controls). All of

these seventeen studies were conducted in China; sixteen were published in Chinese and one was published in English. The age and male-to-female ratios of patients with psoriasis vulgaris of blood-heat syndrome and healthy controls were comparable (Table 1). In total, 59% of the studies reported a Psoriasis Area and Severity Index (PASI). Of these, 90% of the patients were from studies reporting a mean PASI > 10, indicating that the majority of the studies included patients with severe disease. The reported Newcastle-Ottawa Scale scores were between 3 and 7, as shown in Table 1. Specifically, fifteen of the studies were deemed as medium-quality (4 to 6 stars), one [20] was deemed as poor-quality (<4 stars), and another [26] was deemed as high-quality (7 or >7 stars).

3.3. Outcomes. Meta-analysis of the results for all markers, including IFN-γ, IL-4, IL-17, IL-23, IL-6, TNF-α, and IL-10, for subjects with psoriasis vulgaris of blood-heat syndrome revealed significant between-study heterogeneity ($I^2 > 75\%$) with random-effects modeling. The MD for studies analyzing

TABLE 1: Characteristics of the included studies and NOS quality assessment.

Author (pub. year)	Study setting	Study period MM/YY–MM/YY	Psoriasis, blood heat syndrome					Healthy control			NOS quality assessment			Overall star rating
			N	Mean age, years, mean (SD)	Males (%)	Mean PASI (SD)	Duration, years, mean (SD)	N	Mean age, years, mean (SD)	Males (%)	Selection	Comparability	Exposure/outcome	
Cao et al. (2014) [10]	China	07/2011–04/2012	16	46.36 (13.04)	63.33	10.35 (5.84)	NR	16	27.31 (1.40)	56.67	++		+++	5
Chen et al. (2014) [11]	China	09/2011–04/2012	15	46.20 (13.97)	53.33	15.8 (8.60)	3.26 (2.98)	16	42.31 (13.61)	53.33	+	++	+++	6
Chen and Yang (2012) [23]	China	01/2010–12/2010	17	31.00 (1.50)	52.94	24.21 (7.03)	7–10	15	30.00 (0.50)	53.33	+	++	+++	6
Fan et al. (2015) [12]	China	11/2010–10/2011	30	37.50 (7.50)	53.33	11.05 (9.10)	0–30	10	40.29 (9.91)	70.00	+	++	+++	6
He et al. (2015) [13]	China	09/2012–09/2013	40	35.92 (12.91)	62.50	18.619 (3.403)	5.53 (5.25)	20	33.30 (10.96)	60.00	+	++	+++	6
Hu and Yang (2015) [24]	China	NR	30	NR	54.44	NR	NR	30	Match	50.00	+	++	+++	6
Li (2010) [14]	China	03/2009–03/2010	30	41.59 (14.73)	70.59	10.99 (11.62)	NR	18	NR	NR	+		+++	4
Li (2011) [15]	China	04/2009–08/2010	24	NR	NR	NR	NR	20	Match	Match		++	+++	5
Lin et al. (2008) [16]	China	10/2005–03/2006	30	33.13 (11.10)	70.00	10.78 (3.51)	10.47 (9.02)	20	Match	Match	+	++	+++	6
Liu (2011) [17]	China	10/2009–10/2010	20	42.45 (13.55)	65.00	12.80 (4.30)	11.98 (10.23)	20	37.05 (14.16)	40.00		++	+++	5
Liu et al. (2012) [18]	China	03/2010–12/2010	20	34.11	60.00	NR	NR	10	30.50	50.00		++	+++	5
Sun and Zhao (2010) [19]	China	10/2008–02/2010	30	33.00 (13.57)	43.33	21.42 (3.06)	6.70 (5.24)	18	31.72 (12.06)	44.44	+	++	+++	6
Wu et al. (2013) [25]	China	NR	30	NR	NR	NR	NR	30	NR	NR	+		+++	4
Zhang (2003) [20]	China	05/2001–01/2003	20	NR	NR	NR	NR	10	NR	NR			+++	3
Zhang et al. (2010) [21]	China	06/2006–05/2009	47	Match	56.00	NR	16.67–34	31	41.50 (9.20)	67.742		++	+++	5
Zhou (2007) [22]	China	06/2006–03/2007	14	Match	Match	NR	NR	31	41.50	64.50		++	+++	5
Zhou and Wang (2011) [26]	China	10/2009–04/2011	30	32.21 (8.33)	70.00	8.92 (2.07)	16.67–32	10	Match	Match	++	++	+++	7

PASI, Psoriasis Area and Severity Index; NR, not reported; NOS, Newcastle-Ottawa Scale; NOS quality assessment: a star system was used to allow a semiquantitative assessment of study quality. A study could be awarded a maximum of one star for each numbered item within the selection and exposure categories. A maximum of two stars could be awarded for comparability. The NOS ranges from zero to nine stars. We consider those that achieve seven or more stars as high-quality studies, those that achieve four to six stars as medium-quality studies, and those that achieve fewer than four stars as poor-quality studies.

TABLE 2: Summary of immunological markers of blood-heat syndrome.

Source	Markers used ELISA measurement methods, mean (SD)						
	IFN-γ (pg/mL)	IL-4 (pg/mL)	IL-17 (pg/mL)	IL-23 (pg/mL)	IL-6 (pg/mL)	TNF-α (pg/mL)	IL-10 (pg/mL)
Cao et al. [10]	Control 47.44 (21.46); psoriasis 91.20 (48.37)	Control 47.41 (14.26); psoriasis 32.73 (7.90)	Control 49.15 (31.18); psoriasis 60.30 (48.08)				
Chen et al. [11]	Control 46.00 (0.67); psoriasis 86.48 (46.44)	Control 48.45 (13.63); psoriasis 32.52 (8.13)					
Chen and Yang [23]			Control 20.70 (13.20); psoriasis 81.40 (15.10)	Control 201.00 (78.00); psoriasis 529.00 (202.00)			
Fan et al. [12]			Control 2.85 (0.64); psoriasis 7.32 (2.01)	Control 814.93 (372.51); psoriasis 1491.80 (464.36)	Control 109.32 (7.22); psoriasis 418.05 (100.83)		
He et al. [13]		Control 30.07 (3.36); psoriasis 11.29 (3.70)				Control 7.40 (1.56); psoriasis 30.58 (7.14)	
Hu and Yang [24]	Control 8.72 (2.04); psoriasis 24.10 (8.13)	Control 30.21 (3.40); psoriasis 19.89 (1.19)				Control 74.30 (24.14); psoriasis 130.26 (21.99)	
Li [14]	Control 69.16 (29.99); psoriasis 98.68 (49.65)					Control 86.65 (41.26); psoriasis 131.24 (41.24)	Control 85.73 (27.96); psoriasis 105.60 (35.27)
Li [15]						Control 6.43 (0.33); psoriasis 15.29 (0.49)	Control 18.25 (1.44); psoriasis 6.51 (0.97)
Lin et al. [16]	Control 8.72 (2.06); psoriasis 24.10 (7.84)						Control 21.27 (4.80); psoriasis 8.59 (4.97)
Liu [17]	Control 10.86 (5.41); psoriasis 14.19 (6.84)	Control 67.65 (17.01); psoriasis 63.69 (20.23)	Control 46.89 (9.13); psoriasis 55.43 (13.76)				Control 24.39 (7.57); psoriasis 16.84 (6.74)

TABLE 2: Continued.

Source	Markers used ELISA measurement methods, mean (SD)						
	IFN-γ (pg/mL)	IL-4 (pg/mL)	IL-17 (pg/mL)	IL-23 (pg/mL)	IL-6 (pg/mL)	TNF-α (pg/mL)	IL-10 (pg/mL)
Liu et al. [18]			Control 6.24 (1.66); psoriasis 23.37 (2.40)	Control 6.95 (0.83); psoriasis 23.12 (1.89)			
Sun and Zho [19]					Control 8.63 (0.88); psoriasis 11.37 (2.80)	Control 21.65 (1.53); psoriasis 39.44 (6.11)	
Wu et al. [25]			Control 46.69 (11.43); psoriasis 114.60 (19.78)				Control 24.39 (2.27); psoriasis 14.14 (1.62)
Zhang [20]						Control 7.37 (0.85); psoriasis 26.67 (17.78)	
Zhang et al. [21]	Control 8.59 (2.59); psoriasis 11.50 (4.48)				Control 78.20 (43.00); psoriasis 239.06 (159.11)	Control 6.5 (3.1); psoriasis 12.8 (7.4)	
Zhou [22]					Control 71.43 (45.90); psoriasis 244.41 (133.25)	Control 5.9 (3.4); psoriasis 11.3 (7.8)	
Zhou and Wang [26]	Control 33.34 (4.50); psoriasis 96.14 (12.29)	Control 25.91 (3.69); psoriasis 12.88 (2.66)				Control 8.09 (1.06); psoriasis 32.64 (6.23)	Control 21.96 (3.16); psoriasis 12.77 (2.70)

ELISA, enzyme-linked immunosorbent assay; SD, standard deviation; IFN, interferon; IL, interleukin; TNF, tumor necrosis factor.

IFN-γ was 24.9 (95% CI 12.36–37.43), indicating a significant difference in serum IFN-γ between the 218 patients with psoriasis vulgaris of blood-heat syndrome and 161 controls (Figure 2(a)). Six studies reported plasma IL-4 levels, in 151 patients and 112 controls. Figure 2(b) shows that a significantly lower level of IL-4 was observed in patients with psoriasis vulgaris of blood-heat syndrome, with a pooled MD of −13.5 (95% CI −17.74–−9.26). Six studies (including 133 patients and 101 controls) showed an elevated MD for IL-17 (28.92, 95% CI 17.44–40.40) (Figure 2(c)). The mean IL-23 across studies was significantly elevated in the 67 patients compared with the 35 controls (MD 310.60; 95% CI 4.96–616.24) (Figure 2(d)). Pooling of IL-6 levels resulted in a small, positive but not statistically significant MD between

121 patients with psoriasis vulgaris of blood-heat syndrome and 90 healthy controls (160.71; 95% CI −10.44–331.86) (Figure 2(e)). In total, nine articles including 265 patients and 188 controls showed a significantly elevated MD for TNF-α between psoriasis and controls (MD 19.84, 95% CI 13.80–25.87) (Figure 2(f)). The combined MD for IL-10 was decreased in 164 patients compared with 118 controls (MD −10.33, 95% CI −12.03–−8.63) (Figure 2(g)).

3.4. Assessment of Publication Bias. The funnel plots for IFN-γ, IL-4, IL-17, IL-23, IL-6, TNF-α, and IL-10 showed evidence of asymmetry (Figure S1 in Supplementary Material available online at http://dx.doi.org/10.1155/2016/9503652; see MOOSE checklist).

Study or subgroup	Blood-heat syndrome			Control			Weight	Mean difference IV, random, 95% CI	Mean difference IV, random, 95% CI
	Mean	SD	Total	Mean	SD	Total			
Cao et al. 2014	91.2	48.37	16	47.44	21.46	16	8.9%	43.76 [17.83, 69.69]	
Chen et al. 2014	86.48	46.44	15	46	0.67	16	9.6%	40.48 [16.98, 63.98]	
Hu 2015	24.1	8.13	30	8.72	2.04	30	14.4%	15.38 [12.38, 18.38]	
Li 2010	98.68	49.65	30	69.16	29.99	18	9.9%	29.52 [6.99, 52.05]	
Lin et al. 2008	24.1	7.84	30	8.72	2.06	20	14.4%	15.38 [12.43, 18.33]	
Liu 2011	14.19	6.84	20	10.86	5.41	20	14.3%	3.33 [−0.49, 7.15]	
Zhang et al. 2010	11.5	4.48	47	8.59	2.59	31	14.4%	2.91 [1.34, 4.48]	
Zhou 2011	96.14	12.29	30	33.34	4.5	10	14.1%	62.80 [57.59, 68.01]	
Total (95% CI)			218			161	100.0%	24.90 [12.36, 37.43]	

Heterogeneity: $\tau^2 = 282.50; \chi^2 = 525.73, df = 7 (P < 0.00001); I^2 = 99\%$
Test for overall effect: $Z = 3.89 (P < 0.0001)$

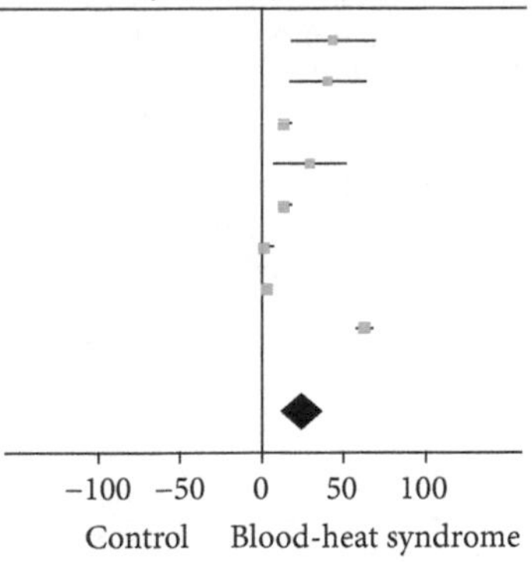

−100 −50 0 50 100
Control   Blood-heat syndrome

(a) IFN-γ

Study or subgroup	Blood-heat syndrome			Control			Weight	Mean difference IV, random, 95% CI	Mean difference IV, random, 95% CI
	Mean	SD	Total	Mean	SD	Total			
Cao et al. 2014	32.73	7.9	16	47.41	14.26	16	12.7%	−14.68 [−22.67, −6.69]	
Chen et al. 2014	32.52	8.13	15	48.45	13.63	16	12.9%	−15.93 [−23.77, −8.09]	
He et al. 2015	11.29	3.7	40	30.07	3.36	20	22.1%	−18.78 [−20.65, −16.91]	
Hu 2015	19.89	1.19	30	30.21	3.4	30	22.6%	−10.32 [−11.61, −9.03]	
Liu 2011	63.69	20.23	20	67.65	17.01	20	8.5%	−3.96 [−15.54, 7.62]	
Zhou 2011	12.88	2.66	30	25.91	3.69	10	21.4%	−13.03 [−15.51, −10.55]	
Total (95% CI)			151			112	100.0%	−13.50 [−17.74, −9.26]	

Heterogeneity: $\tau^2 = 20.34; \chi^2 = 56.48, df = 5 (P < 0.00001); I^2 = 91\%$
Test for overall effect: $Z = 6.24 (P < 0.00001)$

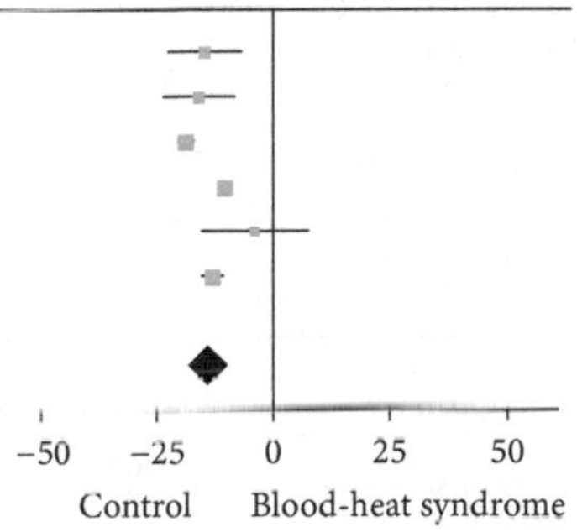

−50 −25 0 25 50
Control   Blood-heat syndrome

(b) IL-4

Study or subgroup	Blood-heat syndrome			Control			Weight	Mean difference IV, random, 95% CI	Mean difference IV, random, 95% CI
	Mean	SD	Total	Mean	SD	Total			
Cao et al. 2014	60.3	48.08	16	49.15	31.18	16	9.0%	11.15 [−16.93, 39.23]	
Chen 2012	81.4	15.1	17	20.7	13.2	15	16.9%	60.70 [50.89, 70.51]	
Fan et al. 2015	7.32	2.01	30	2.85	0.64	10	19.3%	4.47 [3.65, 5.29]	
Liu 2011	55.43	13.76	20	46.89	9.13	20	17.9%	8.54 [1.30, 15.78]	
Liu et al. 2012	23.37	2.4	20	6.24	1.66	10	19.3%	17.13 [15.66, 18.60]	
Wu 2013	114.6	19.78	30	46.69	11.43	30	17.6%	67.91 [59.74, 76.08]	
Total (95% CI)			133			101	100.0%	28.92 [17.44, 40.40]	

Heterogeneity: $\tau^2 = 177.57; \chi^2 = 535.83, df = 5 (P < 0.00001); I^2 = 99\%$
Test for overall effect: $Z = 4.94 (P < 0.00001)$

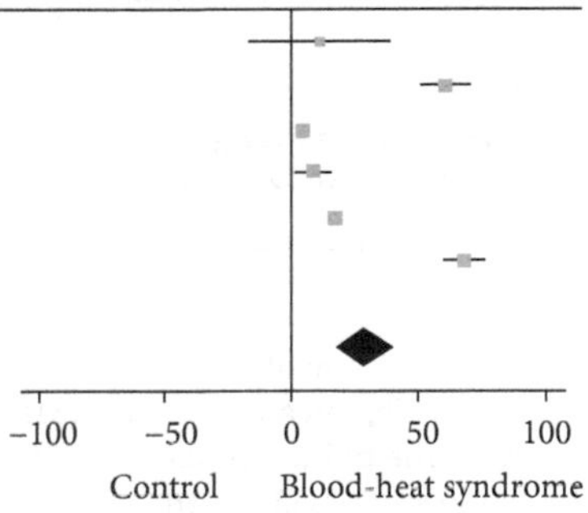

−100 −50 0 50 100
Control   Blood-heat syndrome

(c) IL-17

Study or subgroup	Blood-heat syndrome			Control			Weight	Mean difference IV, random, 95% CI	Mean difference IV, random, 95% CI
	Mean	SD	Total	Mean	SD	Total			
Chen 2012	529	202	17	201	78	15	35.3%	328.00 [224.18, 431.82]	
Fan et al. 2015	1,491.8	464.36	30	814.93	372.51	10	27.9%	676.87 [392.41, 961.33]	
Liu et al. 2012	23.12	1.89	20	6.95	0.83	10	36.8%	16.17 [15.19, 17.15]	
Total (95% CI)			67			35	100.0%	310.60 [4.96, 616.24]	

Heterogeneity: $\tau^2 = 66083.73; \chi^2 = 55.37, df = 2 (P < 0.00001); I^2 = 96\%$
Test for overall effect: $Z = 1.99 (P = 0.05)$

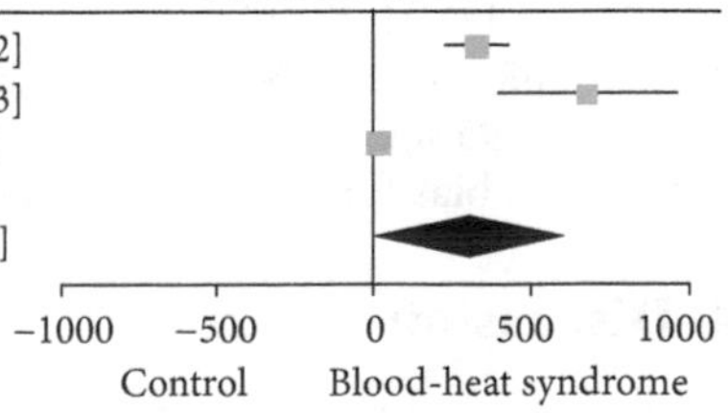

−1000 −500 0 500 1000
Control   Blood-heat syndrome

(d) IL-23

FIGURE 2: Continued.

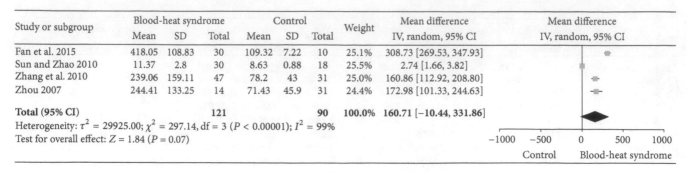

| Study or subgroup | Blood-heat syndrome | | | Control | | | Weight | Mean difference IV, random, 95% CI | Mean difference IV, random, 95% CI |
	Mean	SD	Total	Mean	SD	Total			
Fan et al. 2015	418.05	108.83	30	109.32	7.22	10	25.1%	308.73 [269.53, 347.93]	
Sun and Zhao 2010	11.37	2.8	30	8.63	0.88	18	25.5%	2.74 [1.66, 3.82]	
Zhang et al. 2010	239.06	159.11	47	78.2	43	31	25.0%	160.86 [112.92, 208.80]	
Zhou 2007	244.41	133.25	14	71.43	45.9	31	24.4%	172.98 [101.33, 244.63]	
Total (95% CI)			**121**			**90**	**100.0%**	**160.71 [−10.44, 331.86]**	

Heterogeneity: $\tau^2 = 29925.00; \chi^2 = 297.14, df = 3 (P < 0.00001); I^2 = 99\%$
Test for overall effect: $Z = 1.84 (P = 0.07)$

$-1000 \quad -500 \quad 0 \quad 500 \quad 1000$

Control   Blood-heat syndrome

(e) IL-6

| Study or subgroup | Blood-heat syndrome | | | Control | | | Weight | Mean difference IV, random, 95% CI | Mean difference IV, random, 95% CI |
	Mean	SD	Total	Mean	SD	Total			
He et al. 2015	30.58	7.14	40	7.4	1.56	20	12.8%	23.18 [20.86, 25.50]	
Hu 2015	130.26	21.99	30	74.3	24.14	30	8.8%	55.96 [44.28, 67.64]	
Li 2010	131.24	41.24	30	86.65	41.26	18	4.2%	44.59 [20.48, 68.70]	
Li 2011	15.29	0.49	24	6.43	0.33	20	13.0%	8.86 [8.62, 9.10]	
Sun and Zhao 2010	39.44	6.11	30	21.65	1.53	18	12.8%	17.79 [15.49, 20.09]	
Zhang 2003	26.67	17.78	20	7.37	0.85	10	10.7%	19.30 [11.49, 27.11]	
Zhang et al. 2010	12.8	7.4	47	6.5	3.1	31	12.8%	6.30 [3.92, 8.68]	
Zhou 2007	11.3	7.8	14	5.9	3.4	31	12.2%	5.40 [1.14, 9.66]	
Zhou 2011	32.64	6.23	30	8.09	1.06	10	12.8%	24.55 [22.23, 26.87]	
Total (95% CI)			**265**			**188**	**100.0%**	**19.84 [13.80, 25.87]**	

Heterogeneity: $\tau^2 = 72.90; \chi^2 = 453.39, df = 8 (P < 0.00001); I^2 = 98\%$
Test for overall effect: $Z = 6.44 (P < 0.00001)$

$-50 \quad -25 \quad 0 \quad 25 \quad 50$

Control   Blood-heat syndrome

(f) TNF-α

| Study or subgroup | Blood-heat syndrome | | | Control | | | Weight | Mean difference IV, random, 95% CI | Mean difference IV, random, 95% CI |
	Mean	SD	Total	Mean	SD	Total			
Li 2010	105.6	35.27	30	85.73	27.96	18	0.9%	19.87 [1.81, 37.93]	
Li 2011	6.51	0.97	24	18.25	1.44	20	27.3%	−11.74 [−12.48, −11.00]	
Lin et al. 2008	8.59	4.97	30	21.27	4.8	20	16.4%	−12.68 [−15.43, −9.93]	
Liu 2011	16.84	6.74	20	24.39	7.57	20	9.7%	−7.55 [−11.99, −3.11]	
Wu 2013	14.14	1.62	30	24.39	2.27	30	26.2%	−10.25 [−11.25, −9.25]	
Zhou 2011	12.77	2.7	30	21.96	3.16	10	19.5%	−9.19 [−11.37, −7.01]	
Total (95% CI)			**164**			**118**	**100.0%**	**−10.33 [−12.03, −8.63]**	

Heterogeneity: $\tau^2 = 2.60; \chi^2 = 23.58, df = 5 (P < 0.0003); I^2 = 79\%$
Test for overall effect: $Z = 11.92 (P < 0.00001)$

$-20 \quad -10 \quad 0 \quad 10 \quad 20$

Control   Blood-heat syndrome

(g) IL-10

FIGURE 2: Meta-analysis of serum IFN-γ, IL-4, IL-17, IL-23, IL-6, TNF-α, and IL-10 levels in patients with psoriasis vulgaris of blood-heat syndrome. The mean difference (MD) in IFN-γ, IL-4, IL-17, IL-23, IL-6, TNF-α, and IL-10 levels of patients with psoriasis compared with controls. The point estimate (center of each green square) and statistical size (proportional area of the square) are represented. Horizontal lines indicate 95% confidence intervals. The subtotal and total MDs (diamonds) were calculated using random-effects models.

Egger's test confirmed the presence of publication bias for IFN-γ (9.29, 95% CI 2.30–16.28), IL-4 (−17.74, 95% CI −28.06−−7.42), IL-17 (10.90, 95% CI 2.53–19.28), IL-23 (8.54, 95% CI 1.68–15.42), TNF-α (9.78, 95% CI 5.74–13.83), and IL-10 (−14.61, 95% CI −23.40−−5.81). There appeared to be no publication bias for IL-6 (7.06, 95% CI −1.88–16.01).

4. Discussion

4.1. Summary of Evidence. This review involved a systematic assessment of mainly Chinese-sourced studies reporting immunological serum markers in patients with psoriasis

vulgaris of blood-heat syndrome compared to healthy controls; 17 studies were identified for systematic review and meta-analysis. Although most studies used small sample sizes, analysis of the pooled data showed an elevated MD of serum IFN-γ, IL-17, IL-23, and TNF-α in patients with psoriasis vulgaris of blood-heat syndrome, when compared to the control groups. Pooled IL-4 and IL-10 levels were significantly lower in patients than in controls, but pooled IL-6 levels were not significantly elevated. A simplified model depicting the role of the immunological markers of blood-heat syndrome is presented in Figure 3.

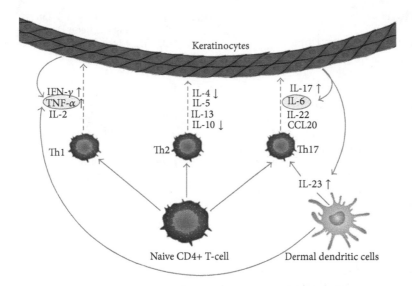

FIGURE 3: A simplified model depicting the role of the immunological markers with psoriasis vulgaris of blood-heat syndrome in this meta-analysis.

4.2. Possible Rationales. According to TCM, patients with psoriasis vulgaris present with one of three syndromes: blood-heat syndrome (53.8%), blood-dryness syndrome (27.4%), or blood-stasis syndrome (18.1%) [9]. At the initiation of the active stage, psoriasis vulgaris usually manifests as blood-heat syndrome; later it may be ameliorated or be converted to blood-dryness/blood-stasis syndrome. The clinical efficacy of TCM, including internal and external applications, in treating psoriasis vulgaris of blood-heat syndrome has been confirmed by a number of previous studies [29–32]. Specifically, the treatment principles of clearing heat and cooling blood are believed to have a positive influence on various pathogenic mechanisms observed in psoriasis because of their anti-inflammatory and antiangiogenic effects, as well as their potential to adjust the Th1/Th2 equilibrium and to change the cytokine balance [15, 26].

Each T-cell subset produces distinct cytokine expression profiles that influence cell fate specification. These different cytokines, released within an inflammatory context, may contribute to psoriasis susceptibility and pathogenesis. Th1 cells develop in the presence of IL-12 and mainly produce IFN-γ, IL-2, and lymphotoxin. Th2 cells differentiate in the presence of IL-4 and produce IL-4, IL-5, and IL-13. In the presence of IL-6 and IL-23, Th17 cells are characterized by their capacity to generate cytokines such as IL-6, IL-17, IL-22, and CCL20 [33, 34]. It has been shown that serum levels of IFN-γ are much higher in patients with psoriasis than in controls and were correlated with the PASI score (psoriasis activity and severity index), whereas levels of Th2 cytokines (IL-4 and IL-10) were reported to be lower [35, 36]. An important cytokine that is generated by Th17 cells, IL-17F, shows significantly higher mRNA expression in lesional skin, and serum levels of the IL-17F protein were substantially increased in a psoriasis(-like) mouse model as well [37–39]. The cytokines IL-6 and TNF-α, which are produced by keratinocytes, play an important role in the activation of innate immunity through activation of dendritic and T-cells [40].

4.3. Limitations of This Review. Our analysis has some limitations. First, we were unable to measure the progression of psoriasis vulgaris of blood-heat syndrome using serum markers in pretherapeutic patients, and only three/four eligible observation studies that reported serum IL-23/IL-6 levels were reviewed. We used two different methods to assess publication bias, and, based on the method used, we found some extent of publication bias. The distorting effects of publication and location bias on systematic reviews and meta-analyses have been well documented [41]. Although we are confident that our search strategy enabled us to locate all relevant studies, a certain degree of uncertainty nevertheless remains. Furthermore, the 17 included studies were mainly observational and consisted of small numbers of patients with psoriasis vulgaris of blood-heat syndrome; more high-quality studies, with a low risk of bias and adequate sample sizes, are required to fully clarify the effects.

5. Conclusion

In summary, patients with psoriasis vulgaris of blood-heat syndrome show significantly elevated levels of IFN-γ, IL-17, IL-23, and TNF-α and decreased levels of IL-4 and IL-10. To investigate the clinical relevance of these findings, a review summarizing the evidence on the effect of clearing heat and cooling blood therapy on markers of immunology would be useful.

Competing Interests

The authors declare that there is no conflict of interests regarding the publication of this paper.

Authors' Contributions

Xin Li and Qing-qing Xiao are equal contributors.

Acknowledgments

This study was supported by a grant from the National Science Foundation (NSFC) of China (81273764 and 81473682 to Bin Li and 81302971 to Xin Li). It was also supported by grants from the Shanghai Science and Technology Committee (nos. 12401903500 and 14401970200 to Bin Li and 14401972703 and 16QA1403800 to Xin Li) and the Shanghai Health Bureau Project (2010Y133, 2011XY004, XYQ2013073, ZY3-CCCX-1-1008, and ZY3-CCCX-3-3033).

References

[1] S. K. Kurd and J. M. Gelfand, "The prevalence of previously diagnosed and undiagnosed psoriasis in US adults: results from NHANES 2003-2004," *Journal of the American Academy of Dermatology*, vol. 60, no. 2, pp. 218–224, 2009.

[2] G. K. Perera, P. Di Meglio, and F. O. Nestle, "Psoriasis," *Annual Review of Pathology: Mechanisms of Disease*, vol. 7, pp. 385–422, 2012.

[3] A. S. Büchau and R. L. Gallo, "Innate immunity and antimicrobial defense systems in psoriasis," *Clinics in Dermatology*, vol. 25, no. 6, pp. 616–624, 2007.

[4] J. T. Elder, A. T. Bruce, J. E. Gudjonsson et al., "Molecular dissection of psoriasis: integrating genetics and biology," *Journal of Investigative Dermatology*, vol. 130, no. 5, pp. 1213–1226, 2010.

[5] J. P. Bartosińska, A. Pietrzak, J. Szepietowski, J. Dreiher, R. Maciejewski, and G. Chodorowska, "Traditional Chinese medicine herbs—are they safe for psoriatic patients?" *Folia Histochemica et Cytobiologica*, vol. 49, no. 2, pp. 201–205, 2011.

[6] A. B. Fleischer Jr., S. R. Feldman, S. R. Rapp, D. M. Reboussin, M. L. Exum, and A. R. Clark, "Alternative therapies commonly used within a population of patients with psoriasis," *Cutis*, vol. 58, no. 3, pp. 216–220, 1996.

[7] J. Koo and S. Arain, "Traditional chinese medicine for the treatment of dermatologic disorders," *Archives of Dermatology*, vol. 134, no. 11, pp. 1388–1393, 1998.

[8] T. W. Tse, "Use of common Chinese herbs in the treatment of psoriasis," *Clinical and Experimental Dermatology*, vol. 28, no. 5, pp. 469–475, 2003.

[9] G.-Z. Zhang, J.-S. Wang, P. Wang et al., "Distribution and development of the TCM syndromes in psoriasis vulgaris," *Journal of Traditional Chinese Medicine*, vol. 29, no. 3, pp. 195–200, 2009.

[10] X. X. Cao, R. Xu, F. L. Li et al., "The expression of Th1/Th2/Th17 in peripheral blood of the patients with blood-heat syndrome of psoriasis," *China Journal of Leprosy and Skin Diseases*, vol. 30, no. 9, pp. 524–526, 2014.

[11] J. Chen, X.-X. Cao, R. Xu et al., "Research on different expressions of peripheral blood Th1/Th2 cells in psoriasis patients of blood heat syndrome and of blood stasis syndrome," *Chinese Journal of Integrated Traditional and Western Medicine*, vol. 34, no. 1, pp. 46–50, 2014.

[12] B. Fan, X. Li, K. Ze et al., "Expression of T-helper 17 cells and signal transducers in patients with psoriasis vulgaris of blood-heat syndrome and blood-stasis syndrome," *Chinese Journal of Integrative Medicine*, vol. 21, no. 1, pp. 10–16, 2015.

[13] S. M. He, H. Y. Zhang, T. F. Liu et al., "Observation the efficacy of Qingre Liangxue Jiedu Decoction in the treatment of psoriasis vulgaris and the influence to TNF-alpha and IL-4 in peripheral blood," *Clinical Journal of Traditional Chinese Medicine*, vol. 27, no. 1, pp. 68–71, 2015.

[14] J. W. Li, *Evaluation of the clinical efficacy and mechanism of of Liangxue Qianyang therapy in patients with blood heat type psoriasis vulgaris [Ph.D. thesis]*, Shanghai University of Traditional Chinese Medicine, 2010.

[15] X. R. Li, *Effect of Qingre Lishi Yin in treatment of psoriasis patients of blood-heat syndrome type and its impact on peripheral Th1/Th2 equilibrium [M.S. thesis]*, Shandong University of Traditional Chinese Medicine, 2011.

[16] Y. Lin, H. Sun, Y. P. Liu, and Y. D. Zou, "Effects of Xiaoyin decoction on the serum levels of interferon-γ and interleukin-10 in patients with psoriasis vulgaris," *Chinese Journal of Dermatovenereology of Integrated Traditional and Western Medicine*, vol. 7, no. 2, pp. 76–79, 2008.

[17] J. Liu, *Effects of the TCM blood-regulating method on cytokine Th1, Th2 & Th17 of common psoriasis patients in different periods [M.S. thesis]*, Shanghai University of Traditional Chinese Medicine, 2011.

[18] T. F. Liu, H. Y. Zhang, X. P. Liu et al., "Ze Qi granule treatment on diffentent TCM syndrome types of PV patients effect on IL-23/Th 17 cell axis," *The Chinese Journal of Dermatovenereology*, vol. 26, no. 5, pp. 442–444, 2012.

[19] H. Sun and F. Q. Zhao, "Clinical effect of Xiaoyin mixture on treating psoriasis vulgaris and detection of correlative serum cytokines," *Chinese Journal of Dermatovenereology of Integrated Traditional and Western Medicine*, vol. 9, no. 6, pp. 358–360, 2010.

[20] C. H. Zhang, *Clinical study on TULing decoction in treating acute psoriasis vulgaris and detection of TNF-α and IL-8 [M.S. thesis]*, Shandong University of Traditional Chinese Medicine, Jinan, China, 2003.

[21] L. Zhang, X. Liu, L. H. Wang, J. X. Zhao, P. Li, and J. S. Wang, "Effect of blood-treating prescriptions on serum IFN-γ, IL-6, and TNF-α of the psoriasis patients with different TCM syndromes," *Journal of Traditional Chinese Medicine*, vol. 51, no. 12, pp. 1083–1085, 1092, 2010.

[22] D. M. Zhou, *Clinical Research of Treatment of Patients with Psoriasis Vulgaris Based on Blood Syndrome Differentiation*, Beijing University of Chinese Medicine, 2007.

[23] J. G. Chen and Z. B. Yang, "Studies on interleukin-17 and interleukin-23 in treatment of patients with psoriasis vulgaris based on blood syndrome differentiation," *Chinese Journal of Dermatology*, vol. 45, no. 2, pp. 140–141, 2012.

[24] X. Y. Hu and W. X. Yang, "The correlation between serum TNF-α, IFN-γ and IL-4 and the syndrome of Traditional Chinese Medicine in psoriasis vulgaris," *Journal of Military Surgeon in in Southwest China*, vol. 17, no. 2, pp. 156–158, 2015.

[25] J. Wu, W. Q. Wang, and A. W. Wu, "Research on the imbalance of Th17/Treg cells in psoriasis patients of blood heat syndrome and blood stasis syndrome," *China Journal of Leprosy and Skin Diseases*, vol. 29, no. 7, pp. 446–448, 2013.

[26] G. J. Zhou and W. Q. Wang, "Evaluation of the clinical efficacy of Xiaoyin decoction in the treatment of the patients with blood-heat syndrome of psoriasis and its influence on Th1/Th2 in peripheral blood," *Fujian Journal of Traditional Chinese Medicine*, vol. 42, no. 6, pp. 1–3, 2011.

[27] A. Stang, "Critical evaluation of the Newcastle-Ottawa scale for the assessment of the quality of nonrandomized studies in meta-analyses," *European Journal of Epidemiology*, vol. 25, no. 9, pp. 603–605, 2010.

[28] D. F. Stroup, J. A. Berlin, S. C. Morton et al., "Meta-analysis of observational studies in epidemiology: a proposal for reporting," *The Journal of the American Medical Association*, vol. 283, no. 15, pp. 2008–2012, 2000.

[29] L.-X. Zhang, Y.-P. Bai, P.-H. Song, L.-P. You, and D.-Q. Yang, "Effect of Chinese herbal medicine combined with acitretin capsule in treating psoriasis of blood-heat syndrome type," *Chinese Journal of Integrative Medicine*, vol. 15, no. 2, pp. 141–144, 2009.

[30] N. Zhou, Y. P. Bai, X. H. Man et al., "Effect of new Pulian Ointment (sic) in treating psoriasis of blood-heat syndrome: a randomized controlled trial," *Chinese Journal of Integrative Medicine*, vol. 15, no. 6, pp. 409–414, 2009.

[31] S. Qiu, S. Tan, J. Zhang, P. Liu, L. Ran, and X. Lei, "Effect of Liangxue Huoxue Tang on serum levels of TNF-α, IFN-γ and IL-6 in psoriasis of blood-heat type," *Journal of Traditional Chinese Medicine*, vol. 25, no. 4, pp. 292–295, 2005.

[32] Y.-J. Dai, Y.-Y. Li, H.-M. Zeng et al., "Effect of Yinxieling decoction on PASI, TNF-α and IL-8 in patients with psoriasis vulgaris," *Asian Pacific Journal of Tropical Medicine*, vol. 7, no. 8, pp. 668–670, 2014.

[33] K. Ghoreschi, A. Laurence, X.-P. Yang, K. Hirahara, and J. J. O'Shea, "T helper 17 cell heterogeneity and pathogenicity in autoimmune disease," *Trends in Immunology*, vol. 32, no. 9, pp. 395–401, 2011.

[34] M. M. D'Elios, G. Del Prete, and A. Amedei, "Targeting IL-23 in human diseases," *Expert Opinion on Therapeutic Targets*, vol. 14, no. 7, pp. 759–774, 2010.

[35] A.-K. Ekman, G. Sigurdardottir, M. Carlström, N. Kartul, M. C. Jenmalm, and C. Enerbäck, "Systemically elevated Th1, Th2 and Th17-associated chemokines in psoriasis vulgaris before and after ultraviolet B treatment," *Acta Dermato-Venereologica*, vol. 93, no. 5, pp. 527–531, 2013.

[36] J. F. Schlaak, M. Buslau, W. Jochum et al., "T cells involved in psoriasis vulgaris belong to the Th1 subset," *Journal of Investigative Dermatology*, vol. 102, no. 2, pp. 145–149, 1994.

[37] M. A. Lowes, T. Kikuchi, J. Fuentes-Duculan et al., "Psoriasis vulgaris lesions contain discrete populations of Th1 and Th17 T cells," *Journal of Investigative Dermatology*, vol. 128, no. 5, pp. 1207–1211, 2008.

[38] H.-L. Ma, S. Liang, J. Li et al., "IL-22 is required for Th17 cell–mediated pathology in a mouse model of psoriasis-like skin inflammation," *The Journal of Clinical Investigation*, vol. 118, no. 2, pp. 597–607, 2008.

[39] N. J. Wilson, K. Boniface, J. R. Chan et al., "Development, cytokine profile and function of human interleukin 17-producing helper T cells," *Nature Immunology*, vol. 8, no. 9, pp. 950–957, 2007.

[40] F. O. Nestle, D. H. Kaplan, and J. Barker, "Mechanisms of disease: Psoriasis," *New England Journal of Medicine*, vol. 361, no. 5, pp. 444–509, 2009.

[41] M. Egger and G. Davey Smith, "Meta-analysis: bias in location and selection of studies," *British Medical Journal*, vol. 316, no. 7124, pp. 61–66, 1998.

Veratri Nigri Rhizoma et Radix (*Veratrum nigrum* L.) and Its Constituent Jervine Prevent Adipogenesis via Activation of the LKB1-AMPKα-ACC Axis *In Vivo* and *In Vitro*

Jinbong Park,[1] Yong-Deok Jeon,[2] Hye-Lin Kim,[3] Dae-Seung Kim,[2] Yo-Han Han,[2] Yunu Jung,[1] Dong-Hyun Youn,[1] JongWook Kang,[1] Daeyeon Yoon,[1] Mi-Young Jeong,[2,3] Jong-Hyun Lee,[4] Seung-Heon Hong,[2] Junhee Lee,[3] and Jae-Young Um[1,3]

[1]*Department of Pharmacology, Graduate School, Kyung Hee University, 26 Kyungheedae-ro, Dongdaemun-gu, Seoul 02447, Republic of Korea*
[2]*Center for Metabolic Function Regulation, Wonkwang University, 460 Iksandae-ro, Iksan, Jeonbuk 54538, Republic of Korea*
[3]*College of Korean Medicine, Kyung Hee University, 26, Kyungheedae-ro, Dongdaemun-gu, Seoul 02447, Republic of Korea*
[4]*College of Pharmacy, Dongduk Women's University, 60 Hwarang-ro 13-gil, Seongbuk-gu, Seoul 02748, Republic of Korea*

Correspondence should be addressed to Junhee Lee; ssljh@daum.net and Jae-Young Um; jyum@khu.ac.kr

Academic Editor: Antonella Fioravanti

This study was performed in order to investigate the antiobese effects of the ethanolic extract of Veratri Nigri Rhizoma et Radix (VN), a herb with limited usage, due to its toxicology. An HPLC analysis identified jervine as a constituent of VN. By an Oil Red O assay and a Real-Time RT-PCR assay, VN showed higher antiadipogenic effects than jervine. In high-fat diet- (HFD-) induced obese C57BL/6J mice, VN administration suppressed body weight gain. The levels of peroxisome proliferator-activated receptor gamma (PPARγ), CCAAT-enhancer-binding protein alpha (C/EBPα), adipocyte fatty-acid-binding protein (aP2), adiponectin, resistin, and LIPIN1 were suppressed by VN, while SIRT1 was upregulated. Furthermore, VN activated phosphorylation of the liver kinase B1- (LKB1-) AMP-activated protein kinase alpha- (AMPKα-) acetyl CoA carboxylase (ACC) axis. Further investigation of cotreatment of VN with the AMPK agonist AICAR or AMPK inhibitor Compound C showed that VN can activate the phosphorylation of AMPKα in compensation to the inhibition of Compound C. In conclusion, VN shows antiobesity effects in HFD-induced obese C57BL/6J mice. In 3T3-L1 adipocytes, VN has antiadipogenic features, which is due to activating the LKB1-AMPKα-ACC axis. These results suggest that VN has a potential benefit in preventing obesity.

1. Introduction

Obesity has become a public health dilemma recently, especially in developed countries. According to the report of the World Health Organization, over 1.4 billion of 20-year-old or older individuals worldwide are overweight [1]. Obesity is closely related to chronic diseases such as hyperlipidemia, hypertension, and type 2 diabetes mellitus [2]. Adipogenesis is a process by which undifferentiated preadipocytes are converted into fully differentiated adipocytes, such as fat cells [3]. The mouse preadipocyte cell line 3T3-L1 is one of the best characterized models for studying the conversion process of preadipocytes into adipocytes. Adipogenesis is known as a closely related process to the etiologies of obesity involving several genes and proteins at different stages [4].

During the adipogenesis of 3T3-L1 cells, among the several adipogenic transcription factors, peroxisome proliferator-activated receptor gamma (PPARγ) and CCAAT-enhancer-binding protein alpha (C/EBPα) are known to act as the key regulators [5]. PPARγ acts as a regulator of development of adipocytes and is known as the only factor that can induce the adipocyte-like phenotype in nonadipogenic cell types [6]. C/EBPα, a member of the leucine zipper transcription factor family, plays an important role in the terminal differentiation in adipocytes [7]. These two factors are not expressed in preadipocytes but are activated during adipocyte differentiation [8]. Adipocyte fatty-acid-binding protein (aP2) acts as cytoplasmic lipid chaperones and plays a role in several lipid signals [9], while resistin, a newly identified adipokine, is secreted by adipocytes and has antagonistic effects on insulin actions [10]. A novel protein, LIPIN1, is primarily expressed in adipose tissues, liver, and skeletal muscles [11]. SIRT1 has been found to suppress adipocyte differentiation and to prevent TG accumulation in white adipose tissue through repression of PPARγ [12]. Similarly, AMP-activated protein kinase (AMPK) activation inhibits adipocyte differentiation and lipogenesis [13, 14].

The fuel-sensing enzyme AMPK is a heterotrimeric protein kinase consisting of three subunits: α, β, and γ [15]. The increased AMP/ATP ratio affects the γ subunit to induce phosphorylation of a threonine residue within the activation domain of the α subunit, by the upstream kinase, liver kinase B1 (LKB1) [16]. AMPK can be activated by inhibition of ATP, that is, hypoxia, ischemia, oxidative stress, and glucose deprivation [15] but, importantly, can be activated by adipokines leptin and adiponectin, the important regulators of energy metabolism [17]. Activation of AMPK results in the repression of ATP-consuming anabolic processes and activation of ATP-producing catabolic processes [17, 18]. AMPK mediates these effects through the phosphorylation of metabolic enzymes, such as acetyl CoA carboxylase (ACC), the rate-limiting enzyme for fatty acid oxidation [19].

Veratrum nigrum L., commonly known as black false hellebore, is a coarse, poisonous perennial herb native to Asia and Europe [20]. The stems and roots of this plant are used under the name of Veratri Nigri Rhizoma et Radix. Due to its ability to cause nausea and vomiting, it is applied to dyspnea in epilepsy or stroke patients in Traditional Korean Medicine. Previous studies report that *Veratrum nigrum* L. is a potential agonist of β2-adrenoceptor [21] and is also able to prevent hepatic ischemia injury in rats [22]. However, the effect of the ethanolic extract of Veratri Nigri Rhizoma et Radix (VN) or its constituent, jervine (($3\beta,23\beta$)-17,23-epoxy-3-hydroxyveratraman-11-one; Figure 1), on obesity has not been reported to date. Thus, this study was performed to investigate the effects of VN and jervine on obesity *in vivo* and *in vitro*.

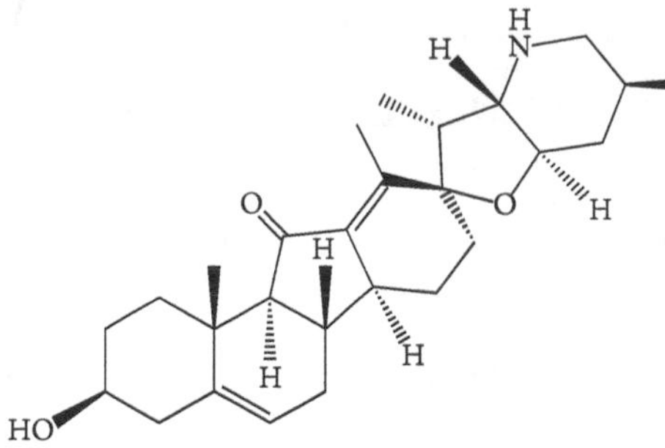

2. Materials and Methods

2.1. Sample Collection. The stems and roots of *Veratrum nigrum* L. (Veratri Nigri Rhizoma et Radix), known as "black false hellebore," were obtained from Omniherb (Daejeon, Republic of Korea). A voucher specimen of the plant has been deposited in our laboratory. The Veratri Nigri Rhizoma et Radix was already processed into dried and chopped pieces before purchase. 100 g of Veratri Nigri Rhizoma et Radixslices was extracted for 2 h 20 min using a heating mantle with 1000 mL of 70% aqueous ethanol. The extract was filtered through a 0.22 μm syringe filter, evaporated, and then stored at −20°C until usage.

2.2. Reagents. Dulbecco's modified Eagle's medium (DMEM), penicillin-streptomycin-glutamine, bovine serum

FIGURE 1: Structure of jervine.

(BS), and fetal bovine serum (FBS) were purchased from Gibco BRL (Grand Island, NY, USA). Insulin, 3-isobutylmethylxanthine (IBMX), dexamethasone (DEX), Oil Red O powder, and 5-amino-4-imidazolecarboxamide riboside (AICAR) were from Sigma Chemical Co. (St. Louis, MO, USA). 6-[4-(2-Piperidin-1-ylethoxy)phenyl]-3-pyridin-4-ylpyrazolo[1,5-a]pyrimidine (Compound C) was obtained from Calbiochem (La Jolla, CA, USA). The antibodies for C/EBPα and glyceraldehyde-3-phosphate dehydrogenase (GAPDH) were purchased from Santa Cruz Biotechnology (Santa Cruz, CA, USA), and PPARγ, phospho-LKB1, phospho-ACC, phospho-AMPKα, and AMPKα were obtained from Cell Signaling technology (Beverly, MA, USA). Jervine (PubChem CID: 10098) was purchased from Sigma Chemical Co. (St. Louis, MO, USA).

2.3. HPLC Analysis. The chromatographic system consisted of Jasco HPLC-LC-2000 Plus (Tokyo, Japan) equipped with a Jasco MD-2018 Plus Photodiode Array Detector, using the Mightysil RP-18(L) GP column (5 μm, 4.6 × 150 mm, Kanto Chemical Co. Inc., Japan). The column temperature was set to 40°C. The mobile phase consisted of acetonitrile as solvent A and acetic acid in water (0.05%) as solvent B using gradients elution. The initial mobile phase composition was 10% of solvent A, and the following gradient system was used: 10–20% (0–10 min), 20% (10–15 min), 20–35% (15–25 min), 35% (25–30 min), 35–40% (30–35 min), 40% (35–45 min), 40–10% (45–50 min), and 10% of solvent A (50–60 min). The total running time was 60 min, and the flow rate was 1.0 mL/min. Data acquisition was performed in the range of 190–650 nm. The retention times of these compounds were obtained as follows: jervine, 26.3 min.

2.4. Animal Experiments. The animal obesity model experiment was conducted based on previous reports [20, 23–25]. Male C57BL/6J mice, weighing 17-18 g at the age of 4 weeks, were purchased from the Dae-Han Experimental Animal Center (Eumsung, Republic of Korea). The animal experiment was proceeded in conditions in accordance with the regulations issued by the Institutional Review Board of Kyung Hee University (confirmation number: KHUASP (SE)-13-012). The mice were maintained for 1 week prior to the experiments in a 12-hour light/dark cycle at humidity of 70% and constant temperature of 23 ± 2°C. The animals were then divided into four groups ($n = 5$–7 per group): a normal control group fed normal chow diet (CJ Feed Co. Ltd., Seoul, Republic of Korea), a high-fat diet (HFD) group fed 60% fat HFD (Rodent diet D12492, Research diet, New Brunswick, NJ, USA) for 14 weeks, a VN group and slinti group which were fed HFD for 4 weeks in order to induce obesity and then fed for 10 additive weeks with HFD plus VN or HFD plus slinti (Myungmoon Pharm. Co. LTD., Seoul, Republic of Korea), respectively. Slinti, which consisted of Theae Folium Powder 250 mg and Orthosiphon Powder 150 mg, was used as a positive control according to the antiobese effects reported on our previous studies [20, 24]. The components of the diets are described in S1 Table (in Supplementary Material available online at http://dx.doi.org/10.1155/2016/8674397). The body weight and food intake amount were recorded every other day. At the end of the period of total 14 weeks, the animals were fasted overnight. The next day, they were anesthetized under CO_2 asphyxiation and plasma was separated at 4,000 g for 30 min immediately after blood collection via cardiac puncture. The total cholesterol, low-density lipoprotein (LDL) and high-density lipoprotein (HDL) cholesterol, alanine transaminase (ALT), and creatinine were assessed by Seoul Medical Science Institute (Seoul, Republic of Korea). Animals were killed by cervical dislocation. Subcutaneous white adipose tissues (sWATs) were weighed.

2.5. Cell Culture and Differentiation.

3T3-L1 mouse embryo fibroblasts were obtained from the American Type Culture Collection (ATCC, Rockville, MD, USA). Cells were grown in DMEM plus 10% BS containing penicillin-streptomycin-glutamine solution (100 UI/mL) in a 10 cm dish. After reaching passage 10, the cells were then moved to 6-well plates for final differentiation in DMEM plus 10% FBS containing antibiotics described above. Until 100% confluence (Day 0), the cells were maintained in a cell incubator at 37°C, 5% CO_2, and 95% humidity. Two days after confluence (Day 2), the cells were stimulated to differentiation with differentiation media (DM) composed of DMEM plus 10% FBS and differentiation inducers (MDI: 1 μM DEX, 500 μM IBMX, and 1 μg/mL insulin). After 2 days, the DM was removed and replaced with DMEM plus 10% FBS containing 1 μg/mL insulin (Day 4). After another additional 2 days, the media were replaced with DMEM plus 10% FBS containing 1 μg/mL insulin again (Day 6). The cells were cultured for 2 more days, at which time more than 90% of cells were mature adipocytes with accumulated fat droplets, and then harvested for further experiments (Day 8). The VN or jervine was treated at Day 4, dissolved in the culture media. AICAR or Compound C was administered 30 min before the VN or jervine treatment dissolved in the culture media.

2.6. MTS Assay.

The 3T3-L1 preadipocytes were seeded (2×10^4 cell/well) and incubated in DMEM plus 10% FBS for 24 h. Then the cells were incubated in the same media containing an ethanol extract of VN for an additional 48 h. Cell viability was monitored using the cell proliferation MTS kit by the Promega Corporation (Madison, WI, USA) as recommended by the manufacturer. Prior to measuring the viability, the media were removed and replaced with 200 μL of fresh DMEM plus 10% FBS medium and 10 μL of 3-(4,5-dimethylthiazol-2-yl)-5-(3-carboxymethoxyphenyl)-2-(4-sulfophenyl)-2H-tetrazolium (MTS) solution. The cells were then incubated in the incubator for 4 h. The absorbance was measured at 490 nm in a VersaMax microplate reader (Molecular Devices, Sunnyvale, CA, USA) to determine the formazan concentration, which is proportional to the number of live cells.

2.7. Oil Red O Staining.

Intracellular lipid accumulation was measured using Oil Red O. The Oil Red O working solution was prepared as described by Ramírez-Zacarías et al. [26]. Briefly, Oil Red O stock solution was prepared Oil Red O (Sigma-Aldrich, St. Louis, MO, USA) dissolved in isopropanol at the concentration of 3.5 mg/mL, and the Oil Red O working solution was prepared 60% Oil Red O stock solution mixed with 40% distilled water. 3T3-L1 adipocytes were harvested 6 days after the initiation of differentiation. Cells were washed twice with phosphate buffered saline (PBS, pH 7.4) and then fixed with 10% neutral formalin for 2 hours at room temperature. After washing with 60% isopropanol, the cells were stained with Oil Red O working solution for 30 min and then were washed 4 times with water in order to remove the unbound dye. The stained cells were observed by an Olympus IX71 Research Inverted Phase microscope (Olympus Co., Tokyo, Japan). Following the microscopic observation, 100% isopropanol was added as an extraction solution to extract the staining dye of cells. The absorbance of the extracted dye was measured spectrophotometrically at 500 nm in a VersaMax microplate reader (Molecular Devices, Sunnyvale, CA, USA).

2.8. RNA Isolation and Real-Time RT-PCR.

Total cellular RNA was isolated from 3T3-L1 adipocytes using QIAzol lysis reagent (Qiagen Sciences, Maryland, USA). Total RNA was used as a template for first-strand cDNA synthesis performed using a Power cDNA Synthesis Kit (iNtRON Biotechnology, Seoul, Korea) according to the manufacturer's instructions. The Real-Time RT-PCR mixture, with a final volume of 20 μL, consisted of Fast SYBR Green PCR Master Mix (Applied Biosystems, Foster City, CA, USA), 1 μM of a forward primer, 1 μM of a reverse primer, and 0.1 μg of a cDNA sample. The thermal cycling conditions were as follows: holding stage, 10 s at 95°C and 40 cycles of 15 s at 95°C and 1 min at 60°C, and then melt curve stage, 15 s at 95°C, 1 min at 60°C, and 15 s at 95°C. PCR products were measured with a StepOnePlus Real-Time RT-PCR System (Applied Biosystems, Foster City, CA, USA), and the relative gene expression was calculated based on the comparative CT method using a StepOne Software v2.1 (Applied Biosystems, Foster City, CA, USA). The mRNA expression of GAPDH was used as an endogenous control. The target cDNA was amplified using the sense and antisense primers described in S2 Table.

2.9. Western Blot Analysis.

After experimental treatment, cells were washed twice with ice-cold PBS and lysed with RIPA lysis buffer, which consisted of 50 mM Tris-HCl

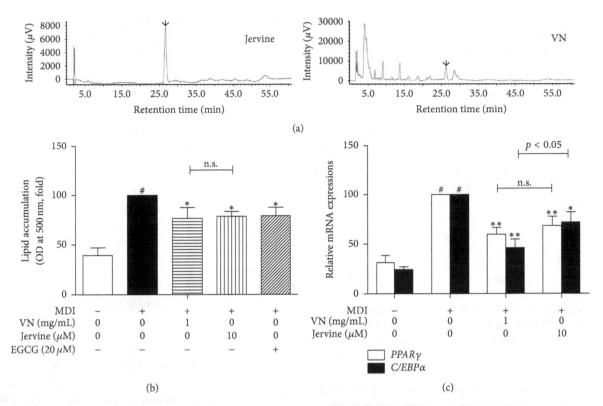

FIGURE 2: HPLC analysis of VN and effects of VN and its compound jervine on 3T3-L1 adipocytes. (a) HPLC-PDA measurement of VN demonstrated various chromatographic peaks. By comparing chromatographic peaks with reference chromatographic peaks, jervine was identified. (b) The effects of VN and jervine on lipid accumulation during 3T3-L1 adipogenesis were compared by an Oil Red O staining assay. (c) The effects of VN and jervine on adipogenic genes, PPARγ and C/EBPα, expressions were compared using a Real-Time RT-PCR assay. Data are expressed as mean ± SD of three or more experiments. $^{#}p < 0.05$ versus MDI-uninduced preadipocytes, $^{*}p < 0.05$, and $^{**}p < 0.01$ versus MDI-induced adipocytes.

(pH 7.5), 0.1% sodium dodecyl sulphate (SDS), 0.1% Triton X-100, 1% Nonidet P-40, 0.5% sodium deoxycholate, 150 mM NaCl, and 1 mM phenylmethylsulfonyl fluoride. Insoluble materials were removed by centrifugation at 13,000 rpm for 20 min at 4°C. The total concentration of extracted proteins was determined using the method of Bradford [27]. The proteins in the supernatants were separated by 8% SDS-polyacrylamide gel electrophoresis and transferred onto polyvinylidene difluoride (PVDF) membranes. After blocking with 10 mM Tris, 150 mM NaCl, and 0.05% Tween-20 (TBST) (pH 7.6) containing 5% skim milk for 1 h at room temperature, the membranes were washed with TBST and then incubated with the appropriate primary antibodies against PPARγ, C/EBPα, phospho-AMPKα, AMPKα, phospho-ACC, phospho-LKB1, or GAPDH at 4°C overnight. After washing with TBST, the blots were subsequently incubated with horseradish peroxidase- (HRP-) conjugated AffiniPure Goat anti-rabbit IgG (Jackson ImmunoResearch Lab., West Grove, PA, USA) or HRP-conjugated AffiniPure Goat anti-mouse IgG (Jackson ImmunoResearch Lab., West Grove, PA, USA) in 5% skim milk-TBST at room temperature for 1 h. Protein signals were developed by using the ECL Western Blotting Detection Reagent (Amersham Bioscience, Piscataway, NJ, USA). All experiments were repeated at least three times. PVDF membranes were purchased from

Millipore (EMD Millipore Co., Billerica, MA, USA), and the protein assay reagents were obtained from Bio-Rad (Bio-Rad Laboratories, Hercules, CA, USA).

2.10. Statistical Analysis. Data were expressed as the mean ± standard deviation (SD). Significant differences between groups were determined using Student's *t*-test and one-way ANOVA followed by *post hoc* Tukey's multiple comparisons tests. All statistical analyses were performed using SPSS statistical analysis software version 11.5 (SPSS Inc., Chicago, IL, USA). A probability value of $p < 0.05$ was considered as statistical significance.

3. Results

3.1. HPLC Analysis of VN. For qualitative analysis of VN to confirm jervine, we performed an HPLC analysis. HPLC-PDA measurement of the ethanolic extraction of VN demonstrated various chromatographic peaks. Comparing the analyzed chromatographic peaks with reference chromatographic peaks, jervine was identified (Figure 2(a)).

3.2. Comparisons of Antiadipogenic Effects of VN and Its Compound Jervine. As the HPLC analysis identified jervine as a compound of VN, investigation to compare the two substances was proceeded. Ahead of any further *in vitro* experiments, a cell viability test was performed. As a result, VN did not show any cytotoxicity at the concentration of 0.01–1 mg/mL (Supplementary Figure 1(a)). Due to this result, further assays were performed at concentrations of 0.01, 0.1, and 1 mg/mL. The MTS assay also showed that jervine had no cytotoxicity at the concentration up to 10 μM (Supplementary Figure 1(b)). In order to compare the effects of VN and jervine on lipid accumulation, an Oil Red O assay was performed. The assay result showed that 1 mg/mL of VN had a slightly higher inhibition rate (23.46%) on lipid accumulation than 10 μM of jervine (21.31%), but there were no significant differences between the two (Figure 2(b)). A Real-Time RT-PCR assay was performed to investigate the effects on adipogenic genes *PPARγ* and *C/EBPα*. As in Figure 2(c), VN had higher inhibition rate on both genes and, especially on *C/EBPα* expression, it showed a significantly higher inhibition rate (53.69%) compared to jervine (28.17%). These results suggest that VN and jervine both have antiobese features, while VN might have higher effects than its compound jervine. Therefore, further experiments were performed in order to investigate the effects of VN, not jervine.

3.3. VN Has Beneficial Effects on HFD-Induced Obese C57BL/6J Mice.

To investigate the antiobesity effects of VN *in vivo*, an animal experiment was performed as described in the materials and methods section. As shown in Figure 3(a), VN treatment significantly suppressed body weight gain (12.37 ± 1.04 g) when compared to the HFD group (27.49 ± 1.01 g), which was even greater than the positive control, slinti group (20.59 ± 1.25 g). Furthermore, the weight of the sWATs between the VN group and HFD group showed significant difference (Figure 3(b)). The blood serum analysis revealed the beneficial effects of VN on total cholesterol, triglyceride, and LDL-cholesterol levels (Figures 3(c), 3(d), and 3(e)). In particular, the serum LDL-cholesterol level of the VN group was highly downregulated compared to that of the HFD group. In addition, in spite of the concern on toxic features of VN, the VN group did not show any toxicity in the liver and kidney as proved by the serum ALT and creatinine levels (Supplementary Figure 2).

3.4. VN Inhibits Lipid Accumulation in 3T3-L1 Adipocytes.

Next, to investigate the effects of VN on adipocyte differentiation, the lipid accumulation was measured using the Oil Red O staining method. As in Figures 4(a) and 4(b), VN significantly suppressed lipid accumulation at the dose of 0.1 and 1 mg/mL, suggesting its antiadipogenic effect. Epigallocatechin-3-gallate (EGCG), a green tea compound previously reported to show antiobese features [28], was used as a positive control.

3.5. VN Modulates Adipogenic Gene Expressions in 3T3-L1 Adipocytes.

Among the several related factors in adipogenesis, PPARγ and C/EBPα especially are well known as the two major regulators in managing adipogenesis [29]. Figure 5(a) shows that VN treatment suppressed *PPARγ* and *C/EBPα* gene expression at 0.1 and 1 mg/mL. Further investigations on protein levels were performed in order to confirm the antiadipogenic effects of VN. As shown in Figure 5(b), VN treatment successfully downregulated the protein levels of PPARγ and C/EBPα.

We also examined the effects of VN on adipogenic genes *aP2*, *resistin*, and *adiponectin*. The downstream target genes of *PPARγ* and *C/EBPα*, such as *aP2* and *adiponectin*, are involved in maintaining the adipocyte phenotype [30], and *resistin* has been reported as a link between obesity and diabetes [10]. These three adipokines were also downregulated by VN treatment, at a dose-dependent manner (Figure 5(c)).

LIPIN1 is an adipokine which has an important role in the regulation of cellular lipid and energy metabolism [31]. As in Figure 5(d), *LIPIN1* was suppressed by VN at a dose-dependent manner.

These results suggest the beneficial effects of VN on obesity, as it suppresses adipogenic factors expressed during the differentiation of 3T3-L1 adipocytes, at both the mRNA and protein levels.

3.6. VN Activates Phosphorylation of the LKB1-AMPKα-ACC Axis in 3T3-L1 Adipocytes.

Next, we investigated whether VN can influence the SIRT1-AMPK axis. SIRT1, one of the seven mammalian orthologs (SIRT1–SIRT7), is a conserved NAD$^+$-dependent protein deacetylase [32], which is known to suppress adipogenesis [12]. *SIRT1* was upregulated by the VN treatment, but only at the highest concentration of 1 mg/mL (Figure 6(a)). As SIRT1 is a closely related factor to AMPKα in obesity, we assessed the effects of VN on AMPKα and its upstream and downstream targets, LKB1 and ACC.

As our hypothesis, VN treatment could induce the phosphorylation of AMPKα (Figure 6(b)). AMPKα is a key player in energy homeostasis, and its activation results in inhibition of adipocyte differentiation [13] and lipogenesis via increased ACC phosphorylation [14]. AMPKα phosphorylation was successfully activated in the VN treated cells. However, interestingly, VN treatment failed to activate phosphorylation of both the AMPK upstream kinase LKB1 and the AMPK downstream target ACC (Figure 6(b)). The Western blot results suggested that VN treatment activates phosphorylation of AMPK directly, without affecting the phosphorylation levels of LKB1 or ACC.

AICAR is an AMPK agonist and, in contrast, Compound C acts as an inhibitor of AMPK. Sullivan and colleagues reported that AICAR was able to activate AMPK in a time- and dose-dependent manner and therefore inhibit lipogenesis [14]. On the other hand, Compound C, also known in the name dorsomorphin, is reported to be the only available agent that is used as a cell-permeable AMPK inhibitor [33]. As in Figure 6(c), AICAR treatment upregulated AMPKα phosphorylation while Compound C was able to suppress the phosphorylation of AMPKα. VN treatment could not boost up the effect of AICAR but, on the other hand, it was able to show compensation to the AMPKα inhibition of Compound C and highly upregulated the phosphorylation of AMPKα. These results confirm the antiadipogenic effects of VN, supposably by its ability to activate AMPKα phosphorylation.

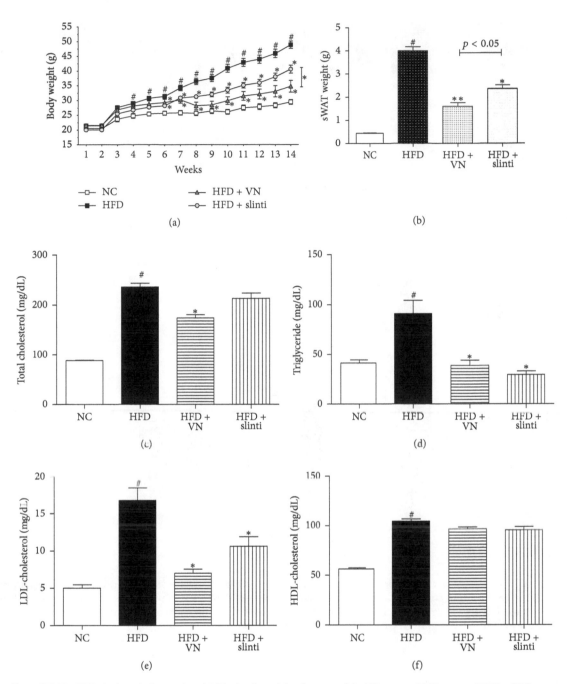

FIGURE 3: Effect of VN in HFD-induced obese mice. (a) The body weight changes of the NC group, HFD group, HFD + VN group, and HFD + slinti group were measured every week. (b) The subcutaneous adipose tissue weights were measured after the termination of the experiment. The serum levels of (c) total cholesterol, (d) triglyceride, (e) LDL-cholesterol, and (f) HDL-cholesterol were measured. Data are expressed as mean ± SD (n = 5–7). $^{#}p < 0.05$ versus NC group, $^{*}p < 0.05$, and $^{**}p < 0.01$ versus HFD-induced obese group.

4. Discussion

In this study, we have evaluated the effects of VN and its constituent jervine on obesity using the *in vivo* HFD-induced obese mouse model and the *in vitro* 3T3-L1 adipocyte model, for the first time.

Obesity is a chronic metabolic disorder caused by an imbalanced energy intake-expenditure status [34]. The prevalence of obesity is growing; in the year 2008, the worldwide obesity has nearly doubled since 1980 [1]. Current medications for the treatment of obesity include mixed noradrenergic-serotonergic agents (sibutramine) [35] and absorption-reducing agents (orlistat) [36]. However, these two drugs show adverse effects at high frequencies. For example, sibutramine is reported to cause cardiac arrhythmias, constipation, and headache with only minimum weight

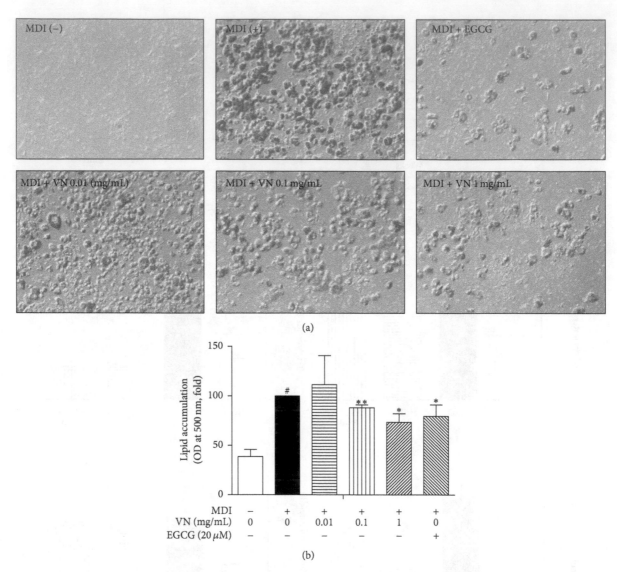

(a)

(b)

FIGURE 4: Effect of VN on lipid accumulation during 3T3-L1 adipocyte differentiation. (a) The lipid droplets were observed at the magnification of 100x. (b) The lipid content was quantified by resolving the Oil Red O stain in isopropanol and measuring absorbance at 500 nm. EGCG was used as a positive control. Data are expressed as mean ± SD of three or more experiments. $^{\#}p < 0.05$ versus MDI-uninduced preadipocytes, $^{*}p < 0.05$, and $^{**}p < 0.01$ versus MDI-induced adipocytes.

loss [35], and orlistat can show steatorrhea and lipid-soluble-vitamin-deficiency [36]. Due to the limits of currently available drugs, the necessity for new drugs for the treatment of obesity is rapidly growing, and the interest in natural products especially is increasing.

Veratrum nigrum L. is a medicinal plant used in Traditional Chinese and Korean Medicine native to Asia and Europe. In the plant, mainly the stem and root of *Veratrum nigrum* L., Veratri Nigri Rhizoma et Radix, are administered internally as an emetic medicine in cases of strokes or epilepsies or also topically treated in order to kill parasites or to stop pruritus [37]. But because of its toxicology, Veratri Nigri Rhizoma et Radix is not widely used, as it is difficult to prepare a safe yet effective dose [38]. Therefore, only few reports on Veratri Nigri Rhizoma et Radix are currently

published. Among those studies, none has reported the effects of VN on obesity or adipogenesis.

Jervine ($C_{27}H_{39}O_3N$), a steroidal alkaloid derived from the *Veratrum* genus [39], which is reported to have antitumor effects [40, 41], was detected as an active compound of VN by the HPLC analysis. Jervine and VN both successfully suppressed lipid accumulation and expressions of adipogenic genes *PPARγ* and *C/EBPα* in 3T3-L1 adipocytes. However, the antiadipogenic effects of VN were higher than jervine, and thus further investigations were performed in order to assess the effects of VN.

As the basic *in vitro* experiments preceded suggested positive effects on obesity, an *in vivo* experiment was carried on using C57BL/6J mice. As expected, VN had beneficial effects on obesity in the animal model, too. The weight

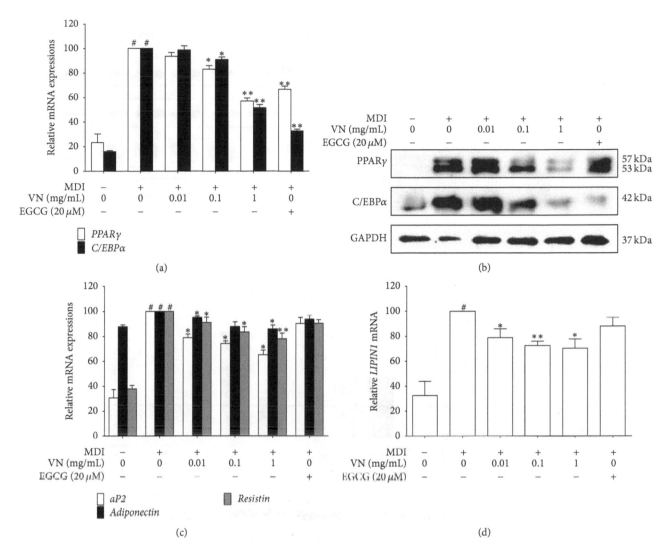

FIGURE 5: Effect of VN on adipogenesis-related factors in 3T3-L1 adipocytes. The mRNA expression levels of (a) *PPARγ* and *C/EBPα*, (c) *aP2*, *adiponectin*, and *resistin*, and (d) *LIPIN1* were measured by the Real-Time RT-PCR assays. (b) The expressions PPARγ and C/EBPα were measured using a Western blot assay. GAPDH was used as an endogenous control. EGCG was used as a positive control. Data are expressed as mean ± SD of three or more experiments. $^{#}p < 0.05$ versus MDI-uninduced preadipocytes, $^{*}p < 0.05$, and $^{**}p < 0.01$ versus MDI-induced adipocytes.

gains and sWAT weights were significantly suppressed in the VN administered group. Serum analyses also confirmed the beneficial effects of VN on obesity. On the other hand, ALT and creatinine, the barometers measuring liver and kidney toxicity, respectively, were not negatively affected but showed lower levels than the HFD group. These results are conflict to the formerly known toxicity of *Veratrum nigrum* [38, 42]. The *in vivo* results do not only prove the beneficial effects of VN in obesity, but the toxicity-safe dosage of VN also shows potential application to human treatment as well, leading to expansion of the limited oral use of VN.

Based on the positive *in vivo* results on obesity, we then performed more experiments back at the cell level, in order to find out which responsible mechanism was giving the beneficial effects. First, an Oil Red O staining assay showed suppressed lipid accumulation by VN treatment.

In addition, the mRNA levels of adipogenic genes including *PPARγ*, *C/EBPα*, *aP2*, *adiponectin*, *resistin*, and *LIPIN1* were downregulated. The suppression of the genes suggested the inhibiting effect on adipogenesis by VN treatment. PPARγ and C/EBPα are well known as important regulators of adipogenesis [5–7], while adipose-derived adipokines, aP2, adiponectin, and resistin possess their roles in adipocytes in lipid signaling [9], glucose regulation [43], and insulin resistance [10], respectively. On the other hand, *LIPIN1* is a candidate gene for lipodystrophy [11]. In addition to these genes, the level of *SIRT1*, the NAD^{+}-dependent protein deacetylase [12], which is able to suppress adipogenesis, was significantly upregulated by VN at the highest dose of 1 mg/mL. The elevated *SIRT1* expression suggested the effects of VN on the SIRT1-AMPKα axis, which is a key factor in the etiology of obesity.

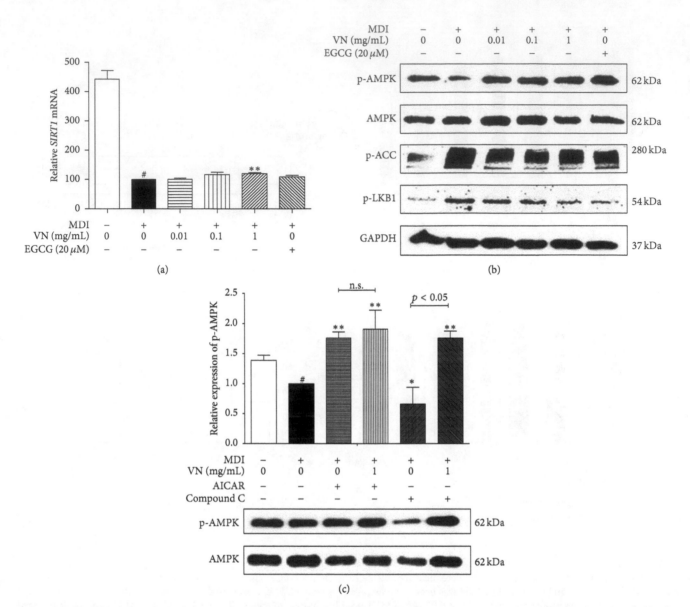

FIGURE 6: Effect of VN on AMPKα pathway-related factors in 3T3-L1 adipocytes. (a) The mRNA expression level of SIRT1 was measured by the Real-Time RT-PCR assay. (b) The expressions of p-AMPKα, p-ACCα, and p-LKB1 were measured using a Western blot assay. (c) The effects of VN on the AMPKα modulation when administered with AMPK activator AICAR or AMPK inhibitor Compound C were evaluated by a Western blot assay. AMPKα was used as an endogenous control for p-AMPKα measurement. GAPDH was used as an endogenous control. EGCG was used as a positive control. Data are expressed as mean ± SD. of three or more experiments. $^{\#}p < 0.05$ versus MDI-uninduced preadipocytes, $^{*}p < 0.05$, and $^{**}p < 0.01$ versus MDI-induced adipocytes.

Previous studies have reported the detailed role of SIRT1-AMPKα axis in obesity. According to Ruderman et al., AMPKα is suggested to play a central role in metabolic syndromes [44]. Other numerous studies also link the phosphorylation of AMPK to obesity in 3T3-L1 models [3, 8, 24, 45, 46]. Several genetic rodent models with a metabolic syndrome phenotype, such as *ob/ob* mice or *fa/fa* rats, show decreased AMPK activity [47], and when the decreased AMPK activity is restored by AICAR, they showed improved glucose homeostasis [48, 49]. Sirtuins, a group of histone/protein deacetylases, are regulated by the NAD$^+$/NADH ratio. SIRT1 is the most well-known member

of this family, which is reported to respond to changes in energy expenditure [47], which is similar to AMPK. Other studies revealed that SIRT1 can activate AMPK by deacetylating LKB1, the upstream kinase of AMPK [50, 51], and vice versa AMPK can activate SIRT1 by increasing the NAD$^+$/NADH ratio [52]. Therefore, these previous reports suggest the important role of SIRT1-AMPKα axis, or circle, in obesity.

The Real-Time RT-PCR result showing the upregulation of the antiadipogenic gene *SIRT1* by VN treatment suggested the possible effects of VN on the SIRT1-AMPKα circle. As we expected, a Western blot analysis confirmed the effect of VN on AMPKα phosphorylation, subsequently to the previous results. VN treatment also suppressed the expression of PPARγ and C/EBPα at the protein levels. Unlike AMPKα, however, the phosphorylation of ACC and LKB1, the upstream and downstream enzymes of AMPKα, respectively, were not upregulated as we expected. These results were conflict to our former researches, in which the protein expressions of p-ACC or p-LKB1 were successfully elevated by treatments showing antiobese features [8, 24]. LKB1, also known as serine/threonine kinase 11, is a protein kinase encoded from the LKB1 gene [53]. Originally known as a tumor suppressor, LKB1 is also related to obesity due to its role as an upstream factor of the energy homeostasis regulator, AMPK [54]. The downstream target of AMPK, ACC, is dephosphorylated by AMPK inhibition [55], and activation of AMPK leads to inhibition of cholesterol synthesis by direct phosphorylation of ACC [56]. However, recent studies report that p-LKB1 [57] or p-ACC [58] is not essential in the cascade of AMPK phosphorylation.

In contrast to the p-ACC and p-LKB1 expressions, the effect of VN on AMPKα activation was surely confirmed, as we coadministered the AMPK activator AICAR and the AMPK inhibitor Compound C with VN. AICAR and Compound C were able to activate or attenuate the phosphorylation of AMPKα. In addition, the treatment of VN was able to restore the inhibited AMPKα phosphorylation by Compound C, nearly up to the AMPK level by AICAR activation. These cotreatment results suggest the effect of VN on the LKB1-AMPKα-ACC axis, by solely affecting the AMPK activation only.

Our results on sole phosphorylation of AMPK in the LKB1-AMPK-ACC pathway suggest that the antiadipogenic features of VN resulted from direct activation of AMPK by VN and proceed through SIRT1 activation, which leads to inhibition of PPARγ and C/EBPα. However, the detailed mechanism for how VN regulates adipogenesis regarding sole activation of AMPK within the LKB1-AMPK-ACC axis requires further investigation.

5. Conclusions

In summary, our results demonstrated that VN contains jervine, and they both can attenuate lipid accumulation during 3T3-L1 adipogenesis. VN showed beneficial effects on obesity in a HFD-induced obese C57BL/6J mouse model. In 3T3-L1 adipocytes, VN was able to attenuate adipogenic factors and upregulate SIRT1 and AMPKα phosphorylation, suggesting its ability to activate the SIRT1-AMPKα circle. These results led to further investigations involving the LKB1-AMPKα-ACC axis. VN treatment was able to compensate for the action of the AMPK inhibitor, Compound C. These results suggest the potential of VN as an AMPKα axis-modulating antiobese agent.

Competing Interests

The authors declare that they have no competing interests.

Acknowledgments

This work was supported by the National Research Foundation of Korea (NRF) grant funded by the Korea government (NRF-2011-0012113).

References

[1] WHO, "WHO Media Centre Fact Sheets: Obesity and Overweight," 2015, http://www.who.int/mediacentre/factsheets/fs311/en/.

[2] P. G. Kopelman, "Obesity as a medical problem," Nature, vol. 404, no. 6778, pp. 635–643, 2000.

[3] H.-L. Kim, J.-E. Sim, H.-M. Choi et al., "The AMPK pathway mediates an anti-adipogenic effect of fruits of Hovenia dulcis Thunb," Food and Function, vol. 5, no. 11, pp. 2961–2968, 2014.

[4] J. M. Ntambi and Y.-C. Kim, "Adipocyte differentiation and gene expression," The Journal of Nutrition, vol. 130, no. 12, pp. 3122S–3126S, 2000.

[5] Z. Wu, E. D. Rosen, R. Brun et al., "Cross-regulation of C/EBPα and PPARγ controls the transcriptional pathway of adipogenesis and insulin sensitivity," Molecular Cell, vol. 3, no. 2, pp. 151–158, 1999.

[6] P. Tontonoz and B. M. Spiegelman, "Fat and beyond: the diverse biology of PPARγ," Annual Review of Biochemistry, vol. 77, pp. 289–312, 2008.

[7] R. P. Brun, J. B. Kim, E. Hu, S. Altiok, and B. M. Spiegelman, "Adipocyte differentiation: a transcriptional regulatory cascade," Current Opinion in Cell Biology, vol. 8, no. 6, pp. 826–832, 1996.

[8] M.-Y. Jeong, H.-L. Kim, J. Park et al., "Rubi fructus (Rubus coreanus) inhibits differentiation to adipocytes in 3T3-L1 cells," Evidence-Based Complementary and Alternative Medicine, vol. 2013, Article ID 475386, 10 pages, 2013.

[9] G. Tuncman, E. Erbay, X. Hom et al., "A genetic variant at the fatty acid-binding protein aP2 locus reduces the risk for hypertriglyceridemia, type 2 diabetes, and cardiovascular disease," Proceedings of the National Academy of Sciences of the United States of America, vol. 103, no. 18, pp. 6970–6975, 2006.

[10] C. M. Steppan, S. T. Bailey, S. Bhat et al., "The hormone resistin links obesity to diabetes," Nature, vol. 409, no. 6818, pp. 307–312, 2001.

[11] M. Péterfy, J. Phan, P. Xu, and K. Reue, "Lipodystrophy in the fld mouse results from mutation of a new gene encoding a nuclear protein, lipin," Nature Genetics, vol. 27, no. 1, pp. 121–124, 2001.

[12] F. Picard, M. Kurtev, N. Chung et al., "Sirt1 promotes fat mobilization in white adipocytes by repressing PPAR-γ," Nature, vol. 429, no. 6993, pp. 771–776, 2004.

[13] S. A. Habinowski and L. A. Witters, "The effects of AICAR on adipocyte differentiation of 3T3-L1 cells," Biochemical and Biophysical Research Communications, vol. 286, no. 5, pp. 852–856, 2001.

[14] J. E. Sullivan, K. J. Brocklehurst, A. E. Marley, F. Carey, D. Carling, and R. K. Beri, "Inhibition of lipolysis and lipogenesis in isolated rat adipocytes with AICAR, a cell-permeable activator of AMP-activated protein kinase," FEBS Letters, vol. 353, no. 1, pp. 33–36, 1994.

[15] Y. C. Long and J. R. Zierath, "AMP-activated protein kinase signaling in metabolic regulation," The Journal of Clinical Investigation, vol. 116, no. 7, pp. 1776–1783, 2006.

[16] R. J. Shaw, M. Kosmatka, N. Bardeesy et al., "The tumor suppressor LKB1 kinase directly activates AMP-activated kinase and regulates apoptosis in response to energy stress," *Proceedings of the National Academy of Sciences of the United States of America*, vol. 101, no. 10, pp. 3329–3335, 2004.

[17] M. C. Towler and D. G. Hardie, "AMP-activated protein kinase in metabolic control and insulin signaling," *Circulation Research*, vol. 100, no. 3, pp. 328–341, 2007.

[18] G. R. Steinberg, S. L. Macaulay, M. A. Febbraio, and B. E. Kemp, "AMP-activated protein kinase—the fat controller of the energy railroad," *Canadian Journal of Physiology and Pharmacology*, vol. 84, no. 7, pp. 655–665, 2006.

[19] W. W. Winder, H. A. Wilson, D. G. Hardie et al., "Phosphorylation of rat muscle acetyl-CoA carboxylase by AMP-activated protein kinase and protein kinase A," *Journal of Applied Physiology*, vol. 82, no. 1, pp. 219–225, 1997.

[20] J. Park, Y.-D. Jeon, H.-L. Kim et al., "Interaction of Veratrum nigrum with Panax ginseng against obesity: a sang-ban relationship," *Evidence-Based Complementary and Alternative Medicine*, vol. 2013, Article ID 732126, 13 pages, 2013.

[21] H. Wang, S.-Y. Li, C.-K. Zhao, and X. Zeng, "A system for screening agonists targeting $\beta2$- adrenoceptor from Chinese medicinal herbs," *Journal of Zhejiang University: Science B*, vol. 10, no. 4, pp. 243–250, 2009.

[22] Z.-Z. Wang, W.-J. Zhao, X.-S. Zhang et al., "Protection of Veratrum nigrum L. var. ussuriense Nakai alkaloids against ischemia-reperfusion injury of the rat liver," *World Journal of Gastroenterology*, vol. 13, no. 4, pp. 564–571, 2007.

[23] K.-S. Kim, H. J. Yang, E.-K. Choi et al., "The effects of complex herbal medicine composed of Cornus fructus, Dioscoreae rhizoma, Aurantii fructus, and Mori folium in obese type-2 diabetes mice model," *Oriental Pharmacy and Experimental Medicine*, vol. 13, no. 1, pp. 69–75, 2013.

[24] H.-L. Kim, Y.-D. Jeon, J. Park et al., "Corni fructus containing formulation attenuates weight gain in mice with diet-induced obesity and regulates adipogenesis through AMPK," *Evidence-Based Complementary and Alternative Medicine*, vol. 2013, Article ID 423741, 11 pages, 2013.

[25] M.-Y. Jeong, H.-L. Kim, J. Park et al., "Rubi Fructus (*Rubus coreanus*) activates the expression of thermogenic genes in vivo and in vitro," *International Journal of Obesity*, vol. 39, no. 3, pp. 456–464, 2015.

[26] J. L. Ramírez-Zacarías, F. Castro-Muñozledo, and W. Kuri-Harcuch, "Quantitation of adipose conversion and triglycerides by staining intracytoplasmic lipids with oil red O," *Histochemistry*, vol. 97, no. 6, pp. 493–497, 1992.

[27] M. M. Bradford, "A rapid and sensitive method for the quantitation of microgram quantities of protein utilizing the principle of protein-dye binding," *Analytical Biochemistry*, vol. 72, no. 1-2, pp. 248–254, 1976.

[28] N.-H. Kim, S.-K. Choi, S.-J. Kim et al., "Green tea seed oil reduces weight gain in C57BL/6J mice and influences adipocyte differentiation by suppressing peroxisome proliferator-activated receptor-γ," *Pflugers Archiv*, vol. 457, no. 2, pp. 293–302, 2008.

[29] Z. Wu, Y. Xie, N. L. R. Bucher, and S. R. Farmer, "Conditional ectopic expression of C/EBPβ in NIH-3T3 cells induces PPARγ and stimulates adipogenesis," *Genes and Development*, vol. 9, no. 19, pp. 2350–2363, 1995.

[30] Y. Xing, F. Yan, Y. Liu, Y. Liu, and Y. Zhao, "Matrine inhibits 3T3-L1 preadipocyte differentiation associated with suppression of ERK1/2 phosphorylation," *Biochemical and Biophysical Research Communications*, vol. 396, no. 3, pp. 691–695, 2010.

[31] A. Yao-Borengasser, N. Rasouli, V. Varma et al., "Lipin expression is attenuated in adipose tissue of insulin-resistant human subjects and increases with peroxisome proliferator-activated receptor γ activation," *Diabetes*, vol. 55, no. 10, pp. 2811–2818, 2006.

[32] M. Fulco and V. Sartorelli, "Comparing and contrasting the roles of AMPK and SIRT1 in metabolic tissues," *Cell Cycle*, vol. 7, no. 23, pp. 3669–3679, 2008.

[33] X. Liu, R. R. Chhipa, I. Nakano, and B. Dasgupta, "The AMPK inhibitor compound C is a potent AMPK-independent antiglioma agent," *Molecular Cancer Therapeutics*, vol. 13, no. 3, pp. 596–605, 2014.

[34] B. M. Spiegelman and J. S. Flier, "Obesity and the regulation of energy balance," *Cell*, vol. 104, no. 4, pp. 531–543, 2001.

[35] C. A. Luque and J. A. Rey, "Sibutramine: a serotonin-norepinephrine reuptake-inhibitor for the treatment of obesity," *Annals of Pharmacotherapy*, vol. 33, no. 9, pp. 968–978, 1999.

[36] A. M. Heck, J. A. Yanovski, and K. A. Calis, "Orlistat, a new lipase inhibitor for the management of obesity," *Pharmacotherapy*, vol. 20, no. 3, pp. 270–279, 2000.

[37] J. Heo, *Dongeuibogam(1613)*, Dongeuibogam Publishing Company, Seoul, Republic of Korea, 1st edition, 2006.

[38] D. Bensky, S. Clavey, and E. Stöger, *Chinese Herbal Medicine: Materia Medica*, Eastland Press, Seattle, Wash, USA, 3rd edition, 2004.

[39] W. A. Jacobs and Y. Sato, "The veratrine alkaloids; the structure of jervine," *The Journal of Biological Chemistry*, vol. 175, no. 1, pp. 57–65, 1948.

[40] J. Tang, H.-L. Li, Y.-H. Shen et al., "Antitumor activity of extracts and compounds from the rhizomes of Veratrum dahuricum," *Phytotherapy Research*, vol. 22, no. 8, pp. 1093–1096, 2008.

[41] J. Tang, H.-L. Li, Y.-H. Shen et al., "Antitumor and antiplatelet activity of alkaloids from Veratrum dahuricum," *Phytotherapy Research*, vol. 24, no. 6, pp. 821–826, 2010.

[42] K. C. Huang, *The Pharmacology of Chinese Herbs, Second Edition*, Taylor & Francis, New York, NY, USA, 2nd edition, 1998.

[43] J. J. Díez and P. Iglesias, "The role of the novel adipocyte-derived protein adiponectin in human disease: an update," *Mini-Reviews in Medicinal Chemistry*, vol. 10, no. 9, pp. 856–869, 2010.

[44] N. B. Ruderman, D. Carling, M. Prentki, and J. M. Cacicedo, "AMPK, insulin resistance, and the metabolic syndrome," *The Journal of Clinical Investigation*, vol. 123, no. 7, pp. 2764–2772, 2013.

[45] B. Huang, H. D. Yuan, D. Y. Kim, H. Y. Quan, and S. H. Chung, "Cinnamaldehyde prevents adipocyte differentiation and adipogenesis via regulation of peroxisome proliferator-activated receptor-γ (PPARγ) and AMP-activated protein kinase (AMPK) pathways," *Journal of Agricultural and Food Chemistry*, vol. 59, no. 8, pp. 3666–3673, 2011.

[46] H. Kim and S.-Y. Choung, "Anti-obesity effects of *Boussingaultia gracilis* miers var. pseudobaselloides bailey via activation of AMP-activated protein kinase in 3T3-L1 cells," *Journal of Medicinal Food*, vol. 15, no. 9, pp. 811–817, 2012.

[47] N. B. Ruderman, X. J. Xu, L. Nelson et al., "AMPK and SIRT1: a long-standing partnership?" *American Journal of Physiology, Endocrinology and Metabolism*, vol. 298, no. 4, pp. E751–E760, 2010.

[48] E. S. Buhl, N. Jessen, R. Pold et al., "Long-term AICAR administration reduces metabolic disturbances and lowers blood pressure in rats displaying features of the insulin resistance syndrome," *Diabetes*, vol. 51, no. 7, pp. 2199–2206, 2002.

[49] X. M. Song, M. Fiedler, D. Galuska et al., "5-Aminoimidazole-4-carboxamide ribonucleoside treatment improves glucose homeostasis in insulin-resistant diabetic (ob/ob) mice," *Diabetologia*, vol. 45, no. 1, pp. 56–65, 2002.

[50] X. Hou, S. Xu, K. A. Maitland-Toolan et al., "SIRT1 regulates hepatocyte lipid metabolism through activating AMP-activated protein kinase," *The Journal of Biological Chemistry*, vol. 283, no. 29, pp. 20015–20026, 2008.

[51] N. L. Price, A. P. Gomes, A. J. Y. Ling et al., "SIRT1 is required for AMPK activation and the beneficial effects of resveratrol on mitochondrial function," *Cell Metabolism*, vol. 15, no. 5, pp. 675–690, 2012.

[52] C. Cantó, Z. Gerhart-Hines, J. N. Feige et al., "AMPK regulates energy expenditure by modulating NAD^+ metabolism and SIRT1 activity," *Nature*, vol. 458, no. 7241, pp. 1056–1060, 2009.

[53] A. Hemminki, D. Markie, I. Tomlinson et al., "A serine/threonine kinase gene defective in Peutz-Jeghers syndrome," *Nature*, vol. 391, no. 6663, pp. 184–187, 1998.

[54] G. J. Gowans, S. A. Hawley, F. A. Ross, and D. G. Hardie, "AMP is a true physiological regulator of AMP-activated protein kinase by both allosteric activation and enhancing net phosphorylation," *Cell Metabolism*, vol. 18, no. 4, pp. 556–566, 2013.

[55] L. A. Witters, T. D. Watts, D. L. Daniels, and J. L. Evans, "Insulin stimulates the dephosphorylation and activation of acetyl-CoA carboxylase," *Proceedings of the National Academy of Sciences of the United States of America*, vol. 85, no. 15, pp. 5473–5477, 1988.

[56] D. Carling, V. A. Zammit, and D. G. Hardie, "A common bicyclic protein kinase cascade inactivates the regulatory enzymes of fatty acid and cholesterol biosynthesis," *FEBS Letters*, vol. 223, no. 2, pp. 217–222, 1987.

[57] L. Luo, S. Jiang, D. Huang, N. Lu, and Z. Luo, "MLK3 phophorylates AMPK independently of LKB1," *PLoS ONE*, vol. 10, no. 4, Article ID e0123927, 2015.

[58] B. N. M. Zordoky, J. Nagendran, T. Pulinilkunnil et al., "AMPK-dependent inhibitory phosphorylation of ACC is not essential for maintaining myocardial fatty acid oxidation," *Circulation Research*, vol. 115, no. 5, pp. 518–524, 2014.

Systems Pharmacology Uncovers the Multiple Mechanisms of Xijiao Dihuang Decoction for the Treatment of Viral Hemorrhagic Fever

Jianling Liu,[1,2] Tianli Pei,[1,2] Jiexin Mu,[1,2] Chunli Zheng,[2] Xuetong Chen,[2] Chao Huang,[2] Yingxue Fu,[2] Zongsuo Liang,[3] and Yonghua Wang[2]

[1]College of Life Science, Northwest University, Xi'an, Shaanxi 710069, China
[2]Center of Bioinformatics, College of Life Science, Northwest A&F University, Yangling, Shaanxi 712100, China
[3]College of Life Science, Zhejiang Sci-Tech University, Hangzhou, Zhejiang 310000, China

Correspondence should be addressed to Yonghua Wang; yh_wang@nwsuaf.edu.cn

Academic Editor: Hyunsu Bae

Background. Viral hemorrhagic fevers (VHF) are a group of systemic diseases characterized by fever and bleeding, which have posed a formidable potential threat to public health with high morbidity and mortality. Traditional Chinese Medicine (TCM) formulas have been acknowledged with striking effects in treatment of hemorrhagic fever syndromes in China's history. Nevertheless, their accurate mechanisms of action are still confusing. *Objective.* To systematically dissect the mechanisms of action of Chinese medicinal formula Xijiao Dihuang (XJDH) decoction as an effective treatment for VHF. *Methods.* In this study, a systems pharmacology method integrating absorption, distribution, metabolism, and excretion (ADME) screening, drug targeting, network, and pathway analysis was developed. *Results.* 23 active compounds of XJDH were obtained and 118 VHF-related targets were identified to have interactions with them. Moreover, systematic analysis of drug-target network and the integrated VHF pathway indicate that XJDH probably acts through multiple mechanisms to benefit VHF patients, which can be classified as boosting immune system, restraining inflammatory responses, repairing the vascular system, and blocking virus spread. *Conclusions.* The integrated systems pharmacology method provides precise probe to illuminate the molecular mechanisms of XJDH for VHF, which will also facilitate the application of traditional medicine in modern medicine.

1. Introduction

Viral hemorrhagic fevers (VHF) are a group of systemic diseases caused by certain viruses, such as Ebola, Lassa, Dengue, and Crimean-Congo hemorrhagic fever viruses. Patients with VHF show the common cardinal symptoms, including fever, hemorrhages, and shock [1]. Data obtained over the past years indicate that these diseases are characterized by intense inflammatory responses with generalized signs of increased vascular permeability, severely impaired immune functions, diffuse vascular dysregulation, and coagulation abnormalities [2, 3]. VHF are generally prevalent in developing countries, which have posed a serious public health threat with high mortality, morbidity, and infectivity in recent years [4].

Currently, many large pharmaceutical companies are pursuing an effective antiviral therapy for VHF. Although the broad-spectra antiviral drug ribavirin is approved for treatment of several types of VHF, there remains a need for a safe and more effective medication to replace the antiviral drug [5].

Traditional Chinese Medicine (TCM) formulas consisting of complex mixtures of multiple plants play an outstanding role in the treatment of various acute infectious diseases because of the pharmacological and pharmacokinetic synergistic effects of the abundant bioactive ingredients [6]. A series of TCM prescriptions for hemorrhagic fever syndromes have been described in history [7, 8]. For example, XJDH is a famous TCM formula for treating hemorrhagic fever syndromes [9]. XJDH originally comes from "Prescriptions Worth A Thousand Gold" which is written by the "Medicinal King" Sun Simiao in the Tang Dynasty (around 700 AD) [10, 11]. The components of the formula include *Rhino horn* (substituted by *Buffalo Horn* now, Shui Niujiao in Chinese), *Rehmannia dried* rhizome (Sheng Dihuang in Chinese), *Paeonia lactiflora* Pall. (Shao Yao in Chinese), and *Paeonia suffruticosa* Andr. (Mu Danpi in Chinese). Actually, XJDH has been normally used for cooling the blood for hemostasis, stopping bleeding accompanied with fever, removing toxic substances, and treating the cases of high fever and sweating, spontaneous bleeding, hemoptysis, and nosebleeds [12, 13]. Although the therapeutic efficiency of XJDH in the treatment of VHF is attractive, several fundamental questions are still unclear. What are the potential active ingredients of XJDH? What are the underlying molecular mechanisms of action of the formula in the treatment of VHF? What are the precise targets of these medicines? Since the multiple components-multiple targets interaction model of TCM formulas, traditional experimental research methods show up the shortcomings of long-term investment.

Fortunately, as an emerging discipline, systems pharmacology provides a new way to solve the complex pharmacological problems [14]. Systems pharmacology integrates pharmacokinetic data (ADME/T characteristics of a drug) screening together with targets prediction, networks, and pathways analyses to explore the drug actions from molecular and cellular levels to tissue and organism levels. It also provides an analysis platform for decoding molecular mechanisms of TCM formulas. In our previous work, a series of systems pharmacology methods have been exploited to uncover the underlying mechanisms of action of TCM formulas for cardiovascular diseases, depression, and cancer [15–17].

The purpose of the present study is to investigate the underlying molecular mechanisms of XJDH in treating VHF based on systems pharmacology method. Firstly, four pharmacokinetic models, including oral bioavailability (OB), drug-likeness (DL), Caco-2 permeability, and drug half-life (HL), were employed to filter out the potential active ingredients with favorable ADME profiles from XJDH. Then, based on an integrated target prediction method which combined the biological and mathematical models, the corresponding targets of these active ingredients were identified. Finally, the network pharmacology and VHF-related signaling pathways analysis was carried out to systematically disclose the underlying interactions between drugs, target proteins, and pathways. The detailed flowchart of the systems pharmacology method is shown in Figure 1.

2. Materials and Methods

2.1. Active Compounds Database.

All chemicals of these four medicines in XJDH were manually collected from a wide-scale text mining and our in-house developed database: the Traditional Chinese Medicine Systems Pharmacology Database (TCMSP, http://lsp.nwsuaf.edu.cn/tcmsp.php) [18]. In order to obtain the potential active compounds from these medicines, we applied a method incorporating OB, DL, Caco-2 permeability, and drug HL evaluation in this work.

2.1.1. OB Prediction. OB is defined as "the ratio of how many active components absorbed into the circulatory system to play a role at the site of action." OB is one of the vital pharmacokinetic profiles in active compounds screening processes. In this work, the OB screening was calculated by a robust in-house system, OBioavail1.1 [19], and components with OB ≥ 30% were selected as the candidate molecules for further study. The following two basic sections describe the design principles of the threshold: (1) information from the studied medicines is obtained as much as possible using the least number of compounds and (2) the established model can be elucidated within reason by the reported pharmacological data [6].

2.1.2. DL Prediction. DL generally means "molecule which holds functional groups and/or has physical properties consistent with the majority of known drugs" [20]. In this study, we performed a self-constructed model pre-DL (predicts drug-likeness) based on the molecular descriptors and Tanimoto coefficient [21]. The DL index of the compounds was calculated by Tanimoto coefficient defined as

$$T(A, B) = \frac{A \cdot B}{\|A\|^2 + \|B\|^2 - A \cdot B}, \qquad (1)$$

where A is the molecular descriptors of herbal compounds, B represents the average molecular properties of all compounds in DrugBank database (http://www.drugbank.ca/) [22]. The DL ≥ 0.18 (average value for DrugBank) was defined as the criterion to select those drug-like compounds which are chemically suitable for drugs.

2.1.3. Caco-2 Permeability Prediction. The majority of orally administered drugs absorption occurs in the small intestine where the surface absorptivity greatly improves with the presence of villi and microvilli [23]. Previously, researchers have developed a quantity of *in silico* drug absorption models using *in vitro* Caco-2 permeability in drug discovery and development processes [24]. In this study, based on 100 drug molecules with satisfactory statistical results, a robust *in silico* Caco-2 permeability prediction model pre-Caco-2 (predicts Caco-2 permeability) was employed to predict the compound's intestinal absorption [25]. Finally, on the account of the fact that compounds with Caco-2 value less than 0 are not permeable, in the study, the threshold of Caco-2 permeability was set to 0.

2.1.4. Drug HL Prediction. An *in silico* pre-HL (predicts half-life) has been developed in our previous work to calculate the drug HL by using the C-partial least square (C-PLS) algorithm which is supported by 169 drugs with known half-life values [26–28]. HL evaluates the time needed for compounds in the body to fall by half, and components with long HL were selected as the candidate molecules.

In order to obtain the potential active ingredients, the screening principle was defined as follows: OB ≥ 30%; Caco-2 ≥ 0; DL ≥ 0.18; or long HL.

2.2. Drug Targeting.

Apart from screening out the active compounds, the therapeutic targets exploration is also a vital

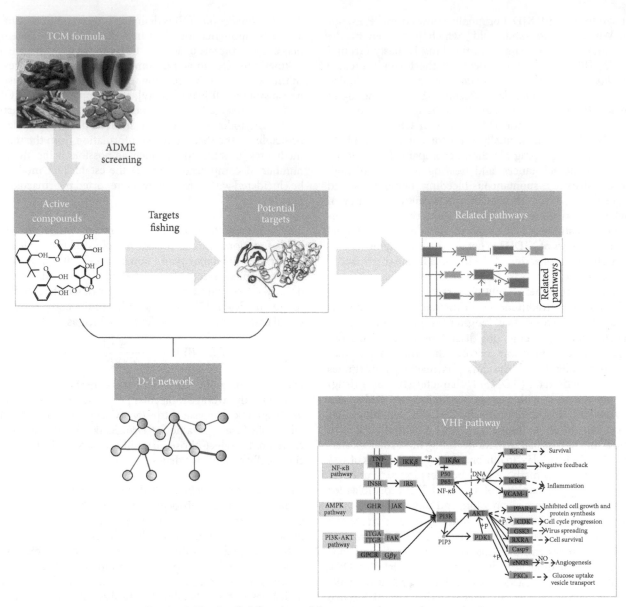

FIGURE 1: The detailed flowchart of the systems pharmacology method.

stage. Firstly, the potential targets exploration was fulfilled based on the systematic drug targeting tool (SysDT) as described in our previous work. Based on two mathematical tools, Random Forest (RF) and Support Vector Machine (SVM), the method can comprehensively ascertain the compound-target interaction profiles [29]. These two models exert great property of predicting the drug-target mutual effects with a concordance of 82.83%, a sensitivity of 81.33%, and a specificity of 93.62%. In this work, the compound-target interactions with SVM score ≥ 0.8 and the RF score ≥ 0.7 were selected for further research. Secondly, a recently developed computational model named weighted ensemble similarity (WES) was also introduced to detect drug direct targets [30]. For internal validation, this model performed remarkably well in predicting the binding (average sensitivity 72%, SEN) and the nonbinding (average specificity 82%, SPE)

patterns, with the average areas under the receiver operating curves (ROC, AUC) of 85.2% and an average concordance of 77.5%. Thirdly, the obtained protein targets were mapped to the database UniProt (http://www.uniprot.org/) for normalization [31]. Finally, in order to identify and analyze the specific biological properties of the potential targets, the Gene Ontology (GO) biological processes were introduced to dissect target genes in a hierarchically structured way based on biological terms [32]. The GlueGO, a Cytoscape plug-in, was utilized to interpret the biology processes of large lists of genes.

2.3. Network Construction and Analysis. In order to explore the multiple mechanisms of action of XJDH for VHF, currently we analyzed the relationship between candidate compounds and potential targets by constructing the drug-target network (D-T network), in which all active compounds are connected to their targets. The network was generated by Cytoscape 2.8.1 [33]. In the network, compounds and targets are represented by nodes, while the interactions between them are represented by edges. In addition, a vital topological parameter, namely, degree was analyzed by the plugin NetworkAnalyzer of Cytoscape [34]. The degree of a node is defined as the number of edges connected to the node.

2.4. Pathway Construction and Analysis. At the pathway level, in order to probe into the action mechanisms of the formula for VHF, an incorporated "VHF pathway" was established based on the current knowledge of VHF pathology. Firstly, the obtained human target proteins were collected to be input into the Kyoto Encyclopedia of Genes and Genomes (KEGG, http://www.kegg.jp/) database to acquire the information of pathways. Then, based on the obtained information of basic pathways, we assembled an incorporated "VHF pathway" by picking out closely linked pathways related with VHF pathology.

3. Results

3.1. Active Compounds Screening. We employed four ADME parameters to screen out the potential active components of XJDH. As a result, from the 136 compounds of XJDH (as shown in supporting information, Table S1, in Supplementary Material available online at http://dx.doi.org/10.1155/2016/9025036), a total of 20 active compounds pass through the criteria of OB $\geq$ 30%, Caco-2 $\geq$ 0, DL $\geq$ 0.18, or long HL. Besides, in order to obtain a more accurate result, some certain rejected compounds, which have relatively poor pharmacokinetic properties, but are the most abundant and active ingredients of certain herbs, were also selected as the active components for further research. For example, although catalpol (MOL108) has poor OB, Caco-2, and HL properties, it has been reported to be rich in the roots of *Rehmannia dried* rhizome. And rehmaglutin D (MOL116) and paeoniflorin (MOL046) with poor OB (14.43%) take a large proportion in *Paeonia lactiflora* Pall. Thus, the three compounds were also retained for further analysis. Finally, a total of 23 active ingredients were obtained in this study (as shown in Table 1).

For all these 23 ingredients, many of them have been reported to demonstrate significant biologic activity including anti-inflammatory, antivirus, antipyretic, and immune-regulatory activities and protection effect of vascular endothelial cell. For instance, methyl gallate (MOL006, OB = 30.91%, Caco-2 = 0.26, and long HL), obtained from *Paeonia lactiflora* Pall., shows antivirus activity by interacting with virus proteins and altering the adsorption and penetration of the virion [35]. Salicylic acid (MOL045, OB = 32.13%, Caco-2 = 0.63, and long HL) and paeoniflorin (MOL046) with poor OB from *Paeonia lactiflora* Pall. exhibit antipyretic, anti-inflammatory, and immune-regulatory activities [36, 37]. In addition, kaempferol (MOL060, OB = 69.61%, Caco-2 = 0.15, DL = 0.24, and long HL), paeonol (MOL072, OB = 30.98%, Caco-2 = 0.91, long HL), and eugenol (MOL070, OB = 44.47%, Caco-2 = 1.36, and long HL), the main active compounds of the radix of *Paeonia suffruticosa* Andr.,

have been reported to have potential therapeutic effect for inflammation and vascular injury disorders [38–40]. Besides, it is worth noting that β-sitosterol (MOL018, OB = 36.9%, DL = 0.75) is a common ingredient of *Rehmannia dried* rhizome, *Paeonia lactiflora* Pall., and *Paeonia suffruticosa* Andr., indicating that these active compounds may show synergetic pharmacological effects on VHF.

3.2. Drug Targeting and Functional Analysis. Traditional information retrieval approaches of therapeutic targets of drugs are expatiatory and complicated [41]. To overcome this barrier, we introduced our previous developed target prediction model [29, 30] to dissect interactions between drugs and proteins. As a result, 23 candidate compounds are linked with 118 candidate targets (as shown in Table 2). The results show that many components simultaneously can act on more than one target and many targets can connect to all of the four medicines, demonstrating the promiscuous actions and analogous pharmacological effects of the bioactive molecules. For instance, kaempferol (MOL060) not only serves as the restrainer of Prostaglandin G/H synthase 2 [42] but also acts as the inhibitor of tumor necrosis factor [43]. And β-sitosterol (MOL018), which is shared by *Rehmannia dried* rhizome, *Paeonia lactiflora* Pall., and *Paeonia suffruticosa* Andr., acts as the activator of estrogen receptor [44] and transcription factor AP-1 [45]. Meanwhile, the results show that different drugs in XJDH can immediately impact on the common targets such as DNA ligase 1 (LIG1), indicating the synergism or cumulative effects of the drug molecules.

In general, vascular system, particularly the endothelium, plays a key role in VHF development [3]. A strong inflammatory response characterized by high circulating concentrations of cytokines and chemokines occurs early during the VHF infectious process [46]. And the patients' immune functions might also be severely impaired; innate defenses are further hindered by the loss of natural killer cells [47]. The relevant biological processes of above targets were revealed by GlueGO (as shown in supporting information, Table S2). Figure 2 provides primary biological processes of these targets by cluster analysis. It is interesting to note that these targets are involved in a variety of biological processes including regulation of macrophage derived from cell differentiation, regulation of vasoconstriction and vasodilation, nitric oxide biosynthetic process, and vascular process in circulatory system. These biological processes largely fall into three groups: controlling inflammation response, modulating the immune system, and accommodation of vascular system. For example, peroxisome proliferator-activated receptor gamma (PPARγ), tumor necrosis factor receptor superfamily member 1A (TNFRSF1A), beta-2 adrenergic receptor (ADRB2), and so forth are involved in the regulation of acute inflammatory response. Nitric oxide synthase, inducible (NOS2), dipeptidyl peptidase 4 (DPP4), and so forth are associated with regulation of immune effector process, while nitric oxide synthase, endothelial (NOS3), NOS2, Krüppel-like factor 5 (KLF5), and so forth are directly connected to blood vessel remodeling and blood vessel morphogenesis. These suggest that XJDH might exert the therapeutic effect on VHF mainly through anti-inflammation, enhancing immunity and vascular repair therapy.

TABLE 1: 23 potential compounds of XJDH and their network parameters.

MOL_ID	Compounds	Structure	OB	Caco-2	DL	HL	Degree	Medicines
MOL001	Cholesterol		37.87	1.31	0.68	Long	16	*Buffalo Horn*
MOL004	2,2-Dimethylcyclohexanol		82.54	1.22	0.02	Long	12	*Paeonia lactiflora* Pall.
MOL005	Dibutylphenol		38.90	1.73	0.06	Long	15	*Paeonia lactiflora* Pall.
MOL006	Methyl gallate		30.91	0.26	0.05	Long	17	*Paeonia lactiflora* Pall.
MOL014	(−)-Alpha-cedrene		55.56	1.81	0.10	Long	16	*Paeonia lactiflora* Pall.

TABLE 1: Continued.

MOL_ID	Compounds	Structure	OB	Caco-2	DL	HL	Degree	Medicines
MOL018	β-Sitosterol		36.91	1.34	0.75	Short	21	*Paeonia lactiflora Pall, Paeonia suffruticosa Andr, Rehmannia dried rhizome*
MOL025	Dipropyl Phthalate		66.30	0.78	0.10	Long	8	*Paeonia lactiflora Pall.*
MOL031	Mairin		55.38	0.73	0.78	Short	14	*Paeonia lactiflora Pall.*
MOL041	Acetyl oxide		45.13	0.65	0	Long	12	*Paeonia lactiflora Pall.*
MOL045	Salicylic acid		32.13	0.63	0.027	Long	19	*Paeonia lactiflora Pall.*
MOL046	Paeoniflorin		14.43	−1.38	0.79	Short	5	*Paeonia lactiflora Pall.*

TABLE 1: Continued.

MOL_ID	Compounds	Structure	OB	Caco-2	DL	HL	Degree	Medicines
MOL053	Apocynin		31.71	0.74	0.04	Long	22	*Paeonia suffruticosa* Andr.
MOL060	Kaempferol		69.61	0.15	0.24	Long	41	*Paeonia suffruticosa* Andr.
MOL066	Methyl salicylate		42.55	1.05	0.03	Long	17	*Paeonia suffruticosa* Andr.
MOL070	Eugenol		44.47	1.36	0.04	Long	34	*Paeonia suffruticosa* Andr.
MOL072	Paeonol		30.98	0.91	0.04	Long	27	*Paeonia suffruticosa* Andr.
MOL073	5-[[5-(4-Methoxyphenyl)-2-furyl]methylene]barbituric acid		43.44	0.09	0.30	Long	10	*Paeonia suffruticosa* Andr.

TABLE 1: Continued.

MOL_ID	Compounds	Structure	OB	Caco-2	DL	HL	Degree	Medicines
MOL075	1-(2,3-Dihydroxy-4-methoxyphenyl)ethanone		32.96	0.81	0.05	Long	25	*Paeonia suffruticosa* Andr.
MOL077	Vanillic acid		35.47	0.43	0.04	Long	13	*Paeonia suffruticosa* Andr.
MOL078	(1R)-(+)-Nopinone		57.86	1.23	0.05	Long	7	*Paeonia suffruticosa* Andr.
MOL096	Stigmasterol		43.83	1.44	0.76	Short	18	*Rehmannia dried rhizome*
MOL108	Catalpol		14.78	−2.10	0.44	Short	6	*Rehmannia dried rhizome*
MOL116	Rehmaglutin D		62.9	−0.31	0.1	Long	7	*Rehmannia dried rhizome*

TABLE 2: The VHF-related targets information.

UniProt ID	Name	Gene name	Species
O14920	Inhibitor of nuclear factor kappa-B kinase subunit beta	IKBKB	*Homo sapiens*
P19320	Vascular cell adhesion protein 1	VCAM1	*Homo sapiens*
P31749	RAC-alpha serine/threonine-protein kinase	AKT1	*Homo sapiens*
P19838	Nuclear factor NF-kappa-B p105 subunit	NFKB1	*Homo sapiens*
P25963	NF-kappa-B inhibitor alpha	NFKBIA	*Homo sapiens*
A1L156	LTB4R2 protein	LTB4R2	*Homo sapiens*
F1D8P7	Liver X nuclear receptor beta	NR1H2	*Homo sapiens*
O00748	Cocaine esterase	CES2	*Homo sapiens*
O14757	Serine/threonine-protein kinase Chk1	CHEK1	*Homo sapiens*
O15528	25-Hydroxyvitamin D-1 alpha hydroxylase, mitochondrial	CYP27B1	*Homo sapiens*
O43570	Carbonic anhydrase 12	CA12	*Homo sapiens*
O60218	Aldo-keto reductase family 1 member B10	AKR1B10	*Homo sapiens*
O95622	Adenylate cyclase type 5	ADCY5	*Homo sapiens*
P00325	Alcohol dehydrogenase 1B	ADH1B	*Homo sapiens*
P00734	Prothrombin	F2	*Homo sapiens*
P00797	Renin	REN	*Homo sapiens*
P00915	Carbonic anhydrase 1	CA1	*Homo sapiens*
P00918	Carbonic anhydrase 2	CA2	*Homo sapiens*
P03372	Estrogen receptor	ESR1	*Homo sapiens*
P04150	Glucocorticoid receptor	NR3C1	*Homo sapiens*
P04798	Cytochrome P450 1A1	CYP1A1	*Homo sapiens*
P05067	Amyloid beta A4 protein	APP	*Homo sapiens*
P05091	Aldehyde dehydrogenase, mitochondrial	ALDH2	*Homo sapiens*
P05093	Steroid 17-alpha-hydroxylase/17,20 lyase	CYP17A1	*Homo sapiens*
P05177	Cytochrome P450 1A2	CYP1A2	*Homo sapiens*
P06276	Cholinesterase	BCHE	*Homo sapiens*
P06746	DNA polymerase beta	POLB	*Homo sapiens*
P07550	Beta-2 adrenergic receptor	ADRB2	*Homo sapiens*
P07686	Beta-hexosaminidase subunit beta	HEXB	*Homo sapiens*
P07900	Heat shock protein HSP 90-alpha	HSP90AA1	*Homo sapiens*
P08172	Muscarinic acetylcholine receptor M2	CHRM2	*Homo sapiens*
P08183	Multidrug resistance protein 1	ABCB1	*Homo sapiens*
P08235	Mineralocorticoid receptor	NR3C2	*Homo sapiens*
P08588	Beta-1 adrenergic receptor	ADRB1	*Homo sapiens*
P08913	Alpha-2A adrenergic receptor	ADRA2A	*Homo sapiens*
P09917	Arachidonate 5-lipoxygenase	ALOX5	*Homo sapiens*
P10253	Lysosomal alpha-glucosidase	GAA	*Homo sapiens*
P10275	Androgen receptor	AR	*Homo sapiens*
P10636	Microtubule-associated protein tau	MAPT	*Homo sapiens*
P11229	Muscarinic acetylcholine receptor M1	CHRM1	*Homo sapiens*
P11309	Serine/threonine-protein kinase pim-1	PIM1	*Homo sapiens*
P11413	Glucose-6-phosphate 1-dehydrogenase	G6PD	*Homo sapiens*
P11413	Glucose-6-phosphate 1-dehydrogenase	G6PD	*Homo sapiens*
P11473	Vitamin D3 receptor	VDR	*Homo sapiens*
P11509	Cytochrome P450 2A6	CYP2A6	*Homo sapiens*
P11712	Cytochrome P450 2C9	CYP2C9	*Homo sapiens*
P12931	Proto-oncogene tyrosine-protein kinase Src	SRC	*Homo sapiens*
P14222	Perforin-1	PRF1	*Homo sapiens*
P14867	Gamma-aminobutyric-acid receptor subunit alpha-1	GABRA1	*Homo sapiens*
P15121	Aldose reductase	AKR1B1	*Homo sapiens*
P16152	Carbonyl reductase [NADPH] 1	CBR1	*Homo sapiens*

TABLE 2: Continued.

UniProt ID	Name	Gene name	Species
P16278	Beta-galactosidase	GLB1	*Homo sapiens*
P16662	UDP-glucuronosyltransferase 2B7	UGT2B7	*Homo sapiens*
P17538	Chymotrypsinogen B	CTRB1	*Homo sapiens*
P18031	Tyrosine-protein phosphatase nonreceptor type 1	PTPN1	*Homo sapiens*
P18089	Alpha-2B adrenergic receptor	ADRA2B	*Homo sapiens*
P18825	Alpha-2C adrenergic receptor	ADRA2C	*Homo sapiens*
P18858	DNA ligase 1	LIG1	*Homo sapiens*
P19438	Tumor necrosis factor receptor superfamily member 1A	TNFRSF1A	*Homo sapiens*
P19801	Amiloride-sensitive amine oxidase [copper-containing]	AOC1	*Homo sapiens*
P20248	Cyclin-A2	CCNA2	*Homo sapiens*
P20309	Muscarinic acetylcholine receptor M3	CHRM3	*Homo sapiens*
P21397	Amine oxidase [flavin-containing] A	MAOA	*Homo sapiens*
P21728	D(1A) dopamine receptor	DRD1	*Homo sapiens*
P22303	Acetylcholinesterase	ACHE	*Homo sapiens*
P23219	Prostaglandin G/H synthase 1	PTGS1	*Homo sapiens*
P23368	NAD-dependent malic enzyme, mitochondrial	ME2	*Homo sapiens*
P23945	Follicle-stimulating hormone receptor	FSHR	*Homo sapiens*
P23975	Sodium-dependent noradrenaline transporter	SLC6A2	*Homo sapiens*
P24941	Cell division protein kinase 2	CDK2	*Homo sapiens*
P25100	Alpha-1D adrenergic receptor	ADRA1D	*Homo sapiens*
P27338	Amine oxidase [flavin-containing] B	MAOB	*Homo sapiens*
P27487	Dipeptidyl peptidase 4	DPP4	*Homo sapiens*
P28223	5-Hydroxytryptamine 2A receptor	HTR2A	*Homo sapiens*
P29474	Nitric oxide synthase, endothelial	NOS3	*Homo sapiens*
P29475	Nitric oxide synthase, brain	NOS1	*Homo sapiens*
P31350	Ribonucleoside diphosphate reductase subunit M2	RRM2	*Homo sapiens*
P33527	Multidrug resistance-associated protein 1	ABCC1	*Homo sapiens*
P35228	Nitric oxide synthase, inducible	NOS2	*Homo sapiens*
P35348	Alpha-1A adrenergic receptor	ADRA1A	*Homo sapiens*
P35354	Prostaglandin G/H synthase 2	PTGS2	*Homo sapiens*
P35869	Aryl hydrocarbon receptor	AHR	*Homo sapiens*
P36888	Receptor-type tyrosine-protein kinase FLT3	FLT3	*Homo sapiens*
P37231	Peroxisome proliferator-activated receptor gamma	PPARG	*Homo sapiens*
P43681	Neuronal acetylcholine receptor subunit alpha-4	CHRNA4	*Homo sapiens*
P47989	Xanthine dehydrogenase/oxidase [includes xanthine dehydrogenase]	XDH	*Homo sapiens*
P48736	Phosphatidylinositol-4,5-bisphosphate 3-kinase catalytic subunit gamma isoform	PIK3CG	*Homo sapiens*
P49841	Glycogen synthase kinase-3 beta	GSK3B	*Homo sapiens*
P51684	C-C chemokine receptor type 6	CCR6	*Homo sapiens*
P51843	Nuclear receptor subfamily 0 group B member 1	NR0B1	*Homo sapiens*
P53634	Dipeptidyl peptidase 1	CTSC	*Homo sapiens*
P60174	Triose-phosphate isomerase	TPI1	*Homo sapiens*
P80365	Corticosteroid 11-beta-dehydrogenase isozyme 2	HSD11B2	*Homo sapiens*
P80404	4-Aminobutyrate aminotransferase, mitochondrial	ABAT	*Homo sapiens*
P84022	Mothers against decapentaplegic homolog 3	SMAD3	*Homo sapiens*
Q00534	Cyclin-dependent kinase 6	CDK6	*Homo sapiens*
Q04760	Lactoylglutathione lyase	GLO1	*Homo sapiens*
Q07075	Glutamyl aminopeptidase	ENPEP	*Homo sapiens*
Q07973	1,25-Dihydroxyvitamin D(3) 24-hydroxylase, mitochondrial	CYP24A1	*Homo sapiens*
Q12791	Calcium-activated potassium channel subunit alpha-1	KCNMA1	*Homo sapiens*
Q12882	Dihydropyrimidine dehydrogenase [NADP(+)]	DPYD	*Homo sapiens*
Q13822	Ectonucleotide pyrophosphatase/phosphodiesterase family member 2	ENPP2	*Homo sapiens*

TABLE 2: Continued.

UniProt ID	Name	Gene name	Species
Q13887	Krüppel-like factor 5	KLF5	*Homo sapiens*
Q14524	Sodium channel protein type 5 subunit alpha	SCN5A	*Homo sapiens*
Q14973	Sodium/bile acid cotransporter	SLC10A1	*Homo sapiens*
Q16539	Mitogen-activated protein kinase 14	MAPK14	*Homo sapiens*
Q16602	Calcitonin gene-related peptide type 1 receptor	CALCRL	*Homo sapiens*
Q16678	Cytochrome P450 1B1	CYP1B1	*Homo sapiens*
Q16853	Membrane primary amine oxidase	AOC3	*Homo sapiens*
Q92731	Estrogen receptor beta	ESR2	*Homo sapiens*
Q96IY4	Carboxypeptidase B2	CPB2	*Homo sapiens*
Q9H5J4	Elongation of very long chain fatty acids protein 6	ELOVL6	*Homo sapiens*
Q9HBH1	Peptide deformylase, mitochondrial	PDF	*Homo sapiens*
Q9NPH5	NADPH oxidase 4	NOX4	*Homo sapiens*
Q9NYA1	Sphingosine kinase 1	SPHK1	*Homo sapiens*
Q9UBM7	7-Dehydrocholesterol reductase	DHCR7	*Homo sapiens*
Q9UNQ0	ATP-binding cassette subfamily G member 2	ABCG2	*Homo sapiens*
Q9Y263	Phospholipase A-2-activating protein	PLAA	*Homo sapiens*
Q9Y2I1	Nischarin	NISCH	*Homo sapiens*

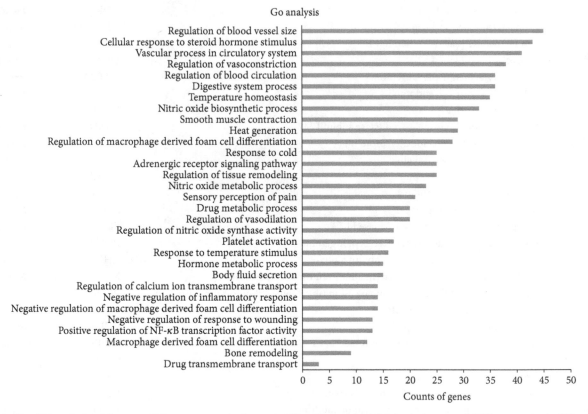

FIGURE 2: ClueGO analysis of the potential targets. y-axis shows significantly enriched "biological process" (BP) categories in GO relative to the target genes, and x-axis shows the counts of targets.

3.3. *Drug-Target Network Construction and Analysis.* As shown in Figure 3, D-T network is constructed including 141 nodes (23 active compounds and 118 potential targets) and 382 edges. The degrees of the candidate compounds are shown in Table 1; this provides us with an intuitionistic concept to distinguish those highly connected vital compounds or targets from the others in the network. The results of network analysis show that 18 out of 23 candidate compounds are linked with more than ten targets, among which kaempferol (MOL060) displays the highest number of target

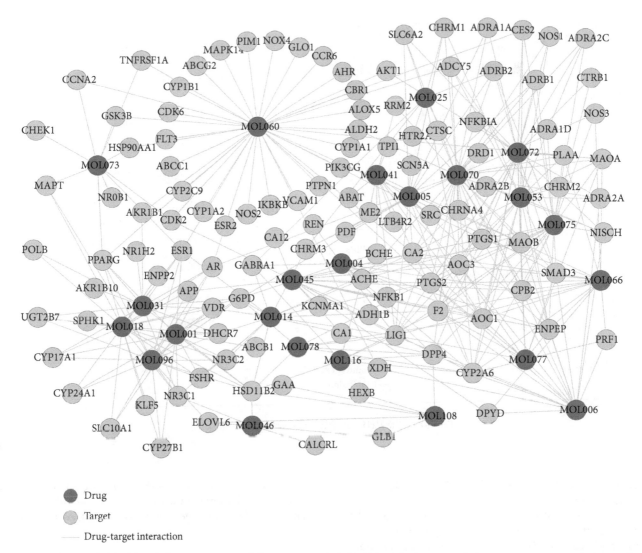

FIGURE 3: D-T network. The blue circles represent candidate compounds in XJDH, while the green circles represent target proteins, and each edge represents the interaction between them.

interactions (degree = 41), followed by eugenol (MOL070, degree = 34) and paeonol (MOL072, degree = 27). This confirms the multitarget properties of herbal compounds. We speculate that the top three ingredients might be the crucial elements in the treatment of VHF. For instance, kaempferol (MOL060) is predicted to interact with 41 targets like calcitonin gene-related peptide type 1 receptor (MAPK14), PPARγ, and phosphatidylinositol-4,5-bisphosphate 3-kinase catalytic subunit gamma isoform (PIK3CG). MAPK14 takes part in the vascular endothelial growth factor (VEGF) synthesis through the mediation of angiotensin II [48]. VEGF can induce angiogenesis and improve the increased vascular permeability, so as to prevent bleeding in patients with VHF [49]. Besides, kaempferol is also found to significantly upregulate the transcriptional activity of PPARγ, which acts as an inhibitor of inflammatory gene expression and vandalizes proinflammatory transcription factor signaling pathways in vascular cells [50]. Additionally, previous finding suggests

that PIK3CG interacting with kaempferol can participate in inflammation processes and influence the innate immune system [51]. Thus, these key active ingredients of XJDH work mainly by modulating inflammatory factor, innate immune system, and VEGF.

Meanwhile, the results also show that one target can be hit by multiple compounds from different medicines, indicating synergism or summation effects of the formula. According to the D-T network analysis, 64 out of the 118 targets have at least two links with the components of different herbs. XJDH exerts its therapeutic effect for VHF by binding and regulating particular protein targets. For instance, prostaglandin G/H synthase 2 (PTGS2) is simultaneously targeted by 10 active compounds including eugenol (MOL070, from *Paeonia suffruticosa* Andr.), paeonol (MOL072, from *Paeonia suffruticosa* Andr.), and salicylic acid (MOL045, from *Paeonia lactiflora* Pall.). PTGS2 is possibly an effective marker of platelet dysfunction; a reduced PTGS2 expression in the VHF

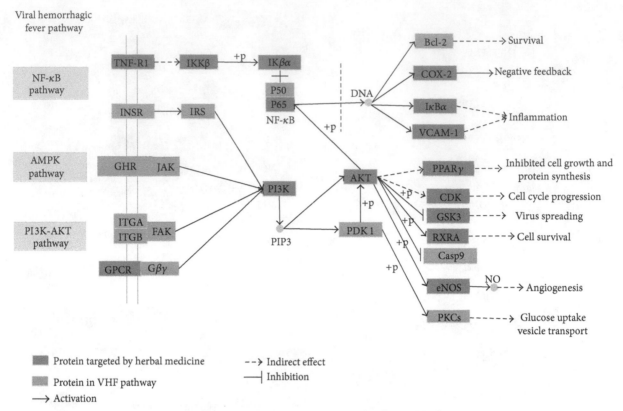

FIGURE 4: The VHF pathway and therapeutic modules.

primate model cells could directly result in platelet dysfunction [52]. Fortunately, in agreement with our study, previous findings suggest that eugenol and paeonol can control the expression of PTGS2 through the suppression of NF-κB in macrophage [53–55], so as to recover the function of thrombocyte. Study shows that severe disseminated intravascular coagulation is the mechanisms of bleeding in all VHF [3]. Prothrombin (F2), the precursor substances of clotting enzyme, plays a crucial role in optimizing the procoagulant activity through controlling the anticoagulant function of meizothrombin [56]. Thus, these 10 ingredients such as methyl gallate (MOL006, from *Paeonia lactiflora* Pall.), salicylic acid (MOL045, from *Paeonia lactiflora* Pall.), and apocynin (MOL053, *Paeonia suffruticosa* Andr.) interacting with F2 may be the key factors in the treatment of bleeding in patients with VHF. By analyzing the above D-T network, we can conclude that XJDH produces the healing efficacy for VHF probably by three different ways, intervening in the process of inflammation, boosting immune reaction, and repairing vascular system.

3.4. Pathway Analysis. To explore the integral regulation of XJDH for the treatment of VHF, we assembled an integrated "VHF pathway" (Figure 4) on the basis of the current knowledge of VHF pathogenesis. By means of inputting the obtained human target proteins into KEGG pathway database, result shows that 110 of the 118 targets can be mapped to the KEGG pathways, including NF-κB signaling pathway,

AMPK pathway, and PI3K-AKT signaling pathway. Now, three detailed therapeutic modules are provided (inflammation module, angiogenesis module, and virus spreading module).

3.4.1. Inflammation Module. As shown in Figure 4, 7 key proteins targeted by XJDH are mapped onto a key inflammation process, namely, NF-κB signaling pathway, indicating the anti-inflammatory action may play a vital role in the treatment of VHF. Patients with VHF have a strong inflammatory response with high inflammatory cytokines and chemokines levels such as IL-1β, TNF, and IL-6 in the early phase of VHF [46]. The expression of inflammatory cytokines (TNF-α, IL-1β, IL-6, and IL-8) is mediated by NF-κB [57], and NF-κB is one of the most important regulators of proinflammatory gene expression. The result demonstrates that paeoniflorin (MOL046) from *Paeonia lactiflora* Pall. and *Paeonia suffruticosa* Andr. can regulate transcription factor NF-κB activity. Meanwhile, other researchers have verified that paeoniflorin can restrain the activation of the NF-κB pathway via inhibiting IκB kinase [58]. In addition, vascular adhesion molecule 1 (VCAM-1), a cell adhesion molecule, also plays an important role in the pathogenesis of inflammatory and immune processes [59]. Our work indicates that kaempferol (MOL060) and β-sitosterol (MOL018) can regulate the expression of inflammatory cytokines by targeting vascular adhesion molecule 1 (VCAM-1). Consequently, the foregoing analysis shows that XJDH has the effect of ameliorating the symptoms of inflammation disorders of patients with VHF.

3.4.2. Virus Spreading Module.

In Figure 4, the phosphoinositide-3 kinase (PI3K) pathway is a significant cell signaling pathway that regulates diverse cellular activities including cell proliferation, differentiation, apoptosis, and vesicular trafficking. Notably, our research shows that, in line with previous studies, kaempferol (MOL060) is predicted to modulate PI3Ks activity, and AKT is also a target for kaempferol (MOL060) and paeonol (MOL072) [60–62]. Besides, PI3Ks, a family of lipid kinases, can prevent hemorrhagic fever virus entry into host cells by regulating cellular activities of vesicular trafficking [63]. AKT is a major downstream effector of the PI3K pathway, and this target protein can control the expression of many molecules directly or indirectly. Moreover, evidence also suggests that activity of PI3K/Akt pathway is required for hemorrhagic fever virus intruding into the host cells [63]. Therefore, depressors of PI3K and AKT dramatically reduced the risk of hemorrhagic fever virus infection at an early step during the replication cycle. These above analyses show that XJDH could make effective control of hemorrhagic fever virus entry into cells, thus blocking virus spread by interfering with the PI3K-AKT signaling pathway.

3.4.3. Angiogenesis Module.

VHF is a severe multisystem syndrome characterized by diffuse vascular damage. The vascular system, particularly the vascular endothelium, seems to be directly and indirectly targeted by hemorrhagic fever viruses [3]. In the VHF pathway shown in Figure 4, PI3K pathway and AMPK pathway are involved in regulating the angiogenesis progress. We find out that apocynin (MOL053), kaempferol (MOL060), methyl salicylate (MOL066), and eugenol (MOL070) can affect the activity of endothelial NO synthase (eNOS) and then bring about NO production changes in endothelial cell. Moreover, at present, a large number of researches indicate that the synthesis of bioactive endothelium-derived NO is required for the progress of angiogenesis [64–66]. Therefore, the evidence presented enables us to reasonably conclude that the XJDH takes part in regulation of angiogenesis progress through PI3K signaling pathway and AMPK pathway.

4. Discussion

Actually, XJDH has been normally used for cooling the blood for hemostasis, stopping bleeding accompanied with fever, removing toxic substances, and treating the cases of high fever and sweating, spontaneous bleeding, hemoptysis, and nosebleeds [13, 67]. Although XJDH has been used historically for treating hemorrhagic fever syndromes, the specific bioactive molecules responsible for VHF and their precise mechanisms of action are still unclear. Thus, in this work, a systems pharmacology method combining the screening active components, drug targeting, network, and pathway analysis was carried out, so as to uncover the active ingredients, targets, and pathways of XJDH and systematically decipher its therapeutic mechanism of actions.

Our results show that 23 active ingredients were obtained from XJDH, and 118 potential targets were predicted. These manifest that the characteristics of XJDH are multicomponent botanical therapeutics and multitargets synergetic therapeutic effects. The GO analysis of targets and integrated D-T network analysis demonstrate the synergistic effects of XJDH for the treatment of VHF mainly through boosting of immune system, inhibiting inflammatory response, and repairing vascular system. Meanwhile, the integrated "VHF pathway" analysis in our work shows that XJDH might simultaneously regulate multitargets/pathways coupled with a range of therapeutic modules, for example, anti-inflammation, antivirus, and angiogenesis.

Now most researchers believe that VHF can be attributed to the simultaneous occurrence of multiple pathogenic mechanisms. They are mainly as follows: hemorrhagic fever virus infection stimulates macrophages to release cytokines, chemokines, and other mediators, causing fever, malaise, alterations in vascular function, and a shift in the coagulation system toward a procoagulant state, and immune functions might also be severely impaired [2]. Besides, hemorrhagic fever virus can target the vascular system directly and indirectly and cause endothelial activation and dysfunction [3]. In this study, we show here for the first time using GO enrichment analysis, network analysis, and integrated pathway analysis that XJDH significantly enriches target genes involved in reducing the inflammation response, enhancing immunity, combating the spreading virus, and preventing vascular dysfunction. And more experiments are needed to verify the validity of the results in further research works.

5. Conclusions

The result of this study provides bioactive ingredients, vital targets, and pathways of XJDH. We have come to the conclusion that the action mechanisms of XJDH for VHF mainly include restoring the immune system and enhancing immune response, ameliorating the symptoms of inflammation disorders, improving their vascular endothelial dysfunction, and combating the spreading virus. The systems pharmacology method established in our work provides preliminary clues that the multilayer networks of drug-target paradigm may be valuable for the modernization of TCM formulas at molecular level and then push forward their acceptance into mainstream medicine.

Competing Interests

The authors declare that there are no competing interests with respect to this study.

Authors' Contributions

Jianling Liu and Tianli Pei contributed equally to this work.

Acknowledgments

This work was supported by Grants from Northwest A&F University, National Natural Science Foundation of China

(31170796 and 81373892), and Science and Technology Department of Shaanxi Province, Natural Science Fund Projects (2014JM3063). It was also supported in part by China Academy of Chinese Medical Sciences (ZZ0608).

References

[1] P. B. Jahrling, A. M. Marty, and T. W. Geisbert, "Viral hemorrhagic fevers," in *Medical Aspects of Biological Warfare*, pp. 271–310, Office of the Surgeon General, United States Army, and Borden Institute, Walter Reed Army Medical Center, Washington, DC, USA, 2007.

[2] M. Bray, "Pathogenesis of viral hemorrhagic fever," *Current Opinion in Immunology*, vol. 17, no. 4, pp. 399–403, 2005.

[3] H.-J. Schnittler and H. Feldmann, "Viral hemorrhagic fever-a vascular disease?" *Thrombosis and Haemostasis*, vol. 89, no. 6, pp. 967–972, 2003.

[4] L. Borio, T. Inglesby, C. J. Peters et al., "Hemorrhagic fever viruses as biological weapons: medical and public health management," *JAMA*, vol. 287, no. 18, pp. 2391–2405, 2002.

[5] M. Bray, "Highly pathogenic RNA viral infections: challenges for antiviral research," *Antiviral Research*, vol. 78, no. 1, pp. 1–8, 2008.

[6] X. Wang, X. Xu, Y. Li et al., "Systems pharmacology uncovers Janus functions of botanical drugs: activation of host defense system and inhibition of influenza virus replication," *Integrative Biology*, vol. 5, no. 2, pp. 351–371, 2013.

[7] Y.-P. Zhu and H. J. Woerdenbag, "Traditional Chinese herbal medicine," *Pharmacy World and Science*, vol. 17, no. 4, pp. 103–112, 1995.

[8] Z.-A. Yina, Y.-Y. He, L. Long et al., "Prevention and treatment idea of Chinese medicine on ebola hemorrhagic fever," *Journal of Acupuncture and Herbs*, vol. 2, no. 2014, pp. 55–62, 2014.

[9] S. Dharmananda, "Treatment of leukemia using integrated Chinese and western medicine," *International Journal of Oriental Medicine*, vol. 22, pp. 169–183, 1997.

[10] J. Cai and Y. Zhen, "Medicine in ancient China," in *Medicine Across Cultures*, pp. 49–73, Springer, Berlin, Germany, 2003.

[11] S. Dharmananda, *Sun Simiao*, vol. 1, Deutsche Übersetzung in ZTCM, 2004.

[12] S. Jing and Z. Xiaojiang, "Professor Zhang Shiqing's experience on treating pediatric allergic purpura with Xijiao Dihuang decoction," *Journal of Gansu College of Traditional Chinese Medicine*, vol. 3, article 3, 2005.

[13] B.-R. Zheng, J.-P. Shen, H.-F. Zhuang, S.-Y. Lin, Y.-P. Shen, and Y.-H. Zhou, "Treatment of severe aplastic anemia by immunosuppressor anti-lymphocyte globulin/anti-thymus globulin as the chief medicine in combination with Chinese drugs," *Chinese Journal of Integrative Medicine*, vol. 15, no. 2, pp. 145–148, 2009.

[14] S. I. Berger and R. Iyengar, "Network analyses in systems pharmacology," *Bioinformatics*, vol. 25, no. 19, pp. 2466–2472, 2009.

[15] C. Huang, C. Zheng, Y. Li, Y. Wang, A. Lu, and L. Yang, "Systems pharmacology in drug discovery and therapeutic insight for herbal medicines," *Briefings in Bioinformatics*, vol. 15, no. 5, Article ID bbt035, pp. 710–733, 2013.

[16] X. Li, X. Xu, J. Wang et al., "A system-level investigation into the mechanisms of Chinese traditional medicine: compound danshen formula for cardiovascular disease treatment," *PLoS ONE*, vol. 7, no. 9, Article ID e43918, 2012.

[17] W. Tao, X. Xu, X. Wang et al., "Network pharmacology-based prediction of the active ingredients and potential targets of Chinese herbal Radix Curcumae formula for application to cardiovascular disease," *Journal of Ethnopharmacology*, vol. 145, no. 1, pp. 1–10, 2013.

[18] J. Ru, P. Li, J. Wang et al., "TCMSP: a database of systems pharmacology for drug discovery from herbal medicines," *Journal of Cheminformatics*, vol. 6, no. 1, article 13, 2014.

[19] X. Xu, W. Zhang, C. Huang et al., "A novel chemometric method for the prediction of human oral bioavailability," *International Journal of Molecular Sciences*, vol. 13, no. 6, pp. 6964–6982, 2012.

[20] W. P. Walters and M. A. Murcko, "Prediction of 'drug-likeness'," *Advanced Drug Delivery Reviews*, vol. 54, no. 3, pp. 255–271, 2002.

[21] H. Liu, J. Wang, W. Zhou, Y. Wang, and L. Yang, "Systems approaches and polypharmacology for drug discovery from herbal medicines: an example using licorice," *Journal of Ethnopharmacology*, vol. 146, no. 3, pp. 773–793, 2013.

[22] D. S. Wishart, C. Knox, A. C. Guo et al., "DrugBank: a comprehensive resource for in silico drug discovery and exploration," *Nucleic Acids Research*, vol. 34, supplement 1, pp. D668–D672, 2006.

[23] K. S. Pang, "Modeling of intestinal drug absorption: roles of transporters and metabolic enzymes (for the gillette review series)," *Drug Metabolism and Disposition*, vol. 31, no. 12, pp. 1507–1519, 2003.

[24] A. Kam, K. M. Li, V. Razmovski-Naumovski et al., "The protective effects of natural products on blood-brain barrier breakdown," *Current Medicinal Chemistry*, vol. 19, no. 12, pp. 1830–1845, 2012.

[25] L. Li, Y. Li, Y. Wang, S. Zhang, and L. Yang, "Prediction of human intestinal absorption based on molecular indices," *Journal of Molecular Science*, vol. 23, pp. 286–291, 2007.

[26] A.-L. Boulesteix, "PLS dimension reduction for classification with microarray data," *Statistical Applications in Genetics and Molecular Biology*, vol. 3, no. 1, 2004.

[27] D. Chung and S. Keles, "Sparse partial least squares classification for high dimensional data," *Statistical Applications in Genetics and Molecular Biology*, vol. 9, no. 1, 2010.

[28] C. Knox, V. Law, T. Jewison et al., "DrugBank 3.0: a comprehensive resource for 'omics' research on drugs," *Nucleic Acids Research*, vol. 39, supplement 1, pp. D1035–D1041, 2011.

[29] H. Yu, J. Chen, X. Xu et al., "A systematic prediction of multiple drug-target interactions from chemical, genomic, and pharmacological data," *PLoS ONE*, vol. 7, no. 5, Article ID e37608, 2012.

[30] C. Zheng, Z. Guo, C. Huang et al., "Large-scale direct targeting for drug repositioning and discovery," *Scientific Reports*, vol. 5, 2015.

[31] C. H. Wu, R. Apweiler, A. Bairoch et al., "The Universal Protein Resource (UniProt): an expanding universe of protein information," *Nucleic Acids Research*, vol. 34, supplement 1, pp. D187–D191, 2006.

[32] G. Bindea, B. Mlecnik, H. Hackl et al., "ClueGO: a Cytoscape plug-in to decipher functionally grouped gene ontology and pathway annotation networks," *Bioinformatics*, vol. 25, no. 8, pp. 1091–1093, 2009.

[33] M. E. Smoot, K. Ono, J. Ruscheinski, P.-L. Wang, and T. Ideker, "Cytoscape 2.8: new features for data integration and network visualization," *Bioinformatics*, vol. 27, no. 3, Article ID btq675, pp. 431–432, 2011.

[34] P. Shannon, A. Markiel, O. Ozier et al., "Cytoscape: a software environment for integrated models of biomolecular interaction networks," *Genome Research*, vol. 13, no. 11, pp. 2498–2504, 2003.

[35] C. J. M. Kane, J. H. Menna, C.-C. Sung, and Y.-C. Yeh, "Methyl gallate, methyl-3,4,5-trihydroxybenzoate, is a potent and highly specific inhibitor of herpes simplex virus in vitro. II. Antiviral activity of methyl gallate and its derivatives," *Bioscience Reports*, vol. 8, no. 1, pp. 95–102, 1988.

[36] T. Grosser, E. Smyth, and G. FitzGerald, "Antiinflammatory, antipyretic and analgesic agents," in *Goodman and Gilman's the Pharmacological Basis of Therapeutics*, L. Bruton, B. A. Chabner, and B. C. Knollmann, Eds., p. 985, McGraw-Hill Education, 2011.

[37] X.-X. Xu, X.-M. Qi, W. Zhang et al., "Effects of total glucosides of paeony on immune regulatory toll-like receptors TLR2 and 4 in the kidney from diabetic rats," *Phytomedicine*, vol. 21, no. 6, pp. 815–823, 2014.

[38] L. L. Pan and M. Dai, "Paeonol from *Paeonia suffruticosa* prevents TNF-α-induced monocytic cell adhesion to rat aortic endothelial cells by suppression of VCAM-1 expression," *Phytomedicine*, vol. 16, no. 11, pp. 1027–1032, 2009.

[39] P. Prakash and N. Gupta, "Therapeutic uses of *Ocimum sanctum* Linn (Tulsi) with a note on eugenol and its pharmacological actions: a short review," *Indian Journal of Physiology and Pharmacology*, vol. 49, no. 2, pp. 125–131, 2005.

[40] K. Markowitz, M. Moynihan, M. Liu, and S. Kim, "Biologic properties of eugenol and zinc oxide-eugenol: a clinically oriented review," *Oral Surgery, Oral Medicine, Oral Pathology*, vol. 73, no. 6, pp. 729–737, 1992.

[41] B. Lomenick, R. W. Olsen, and J. Huang, "Identification of direct protein targets of small molecules," *ACS Chemical Biology*, vol. 6, no. 1, pp. 34–46, 2010.

[42] K. M. Lee, K. W. Lee, S. K. Jung et al., "Kaempferol inhibits UVB-induced COX-2 expression by suppressing Src kinase activity," *Biochemical Pharmacology*, vol. 80, no. 12, pp. 2042–2049, 2010.

[43] J. L. Pang, D. A. Ricupero, S. Huang et al., "Differential activity of kaempferol and quercetin in attenuating tumor necrosis factor receptor family signaling in bone cells," *Biochemical Pharmacology*, vol. 71, no. 6, pp. 818–826, 2006.

[44] C. Shi, F. Wu, X. Zhu, and J. Xu, "Incorporation of β-sitosterol into the membrane increases resistance to oxidative stress and lipid peroxidation via estrogen receptor-mediated PI3K/GSK3β signaling," *Biochimica et Biophysica Acta (BBA)—General Subjects*, vol. 1830, no. 3, pp. 2538–2544, 2013.

[45] S. Loizou, I. Lekakis, G. P. Chrousos, and P. Moutsatsou, "β-Sitosterol exhibits anti-inflammatory activity in human aortic endothelial cells," *Molecular Nutrition and Food Research*, vol. 54, no. 4, pp. 551–558, 2010.

[46] E. M. Leroy, S. Baize, V. E. Volchkov et al., "Human asymptomatic Ebola infection and strong inflammatory response," *The Lancet*, vol. 355, no. 9222, pp. 2210–2215, 2000.

[47] D. S. Reed, L. E. Hensley, J. B. Geisbert, P. B. Jahrling, and T. W. Geisbert, "Depletion of peripheral blood T lymphocytes and NK cells during the course of Ebola hemorrhagic fever in cynomolgus macaques," *Viral Immunology*, vol. 17, no. 3, pp. 390–400, 2004.

[48] Y. S. Kang, Y. G. Park, B. K. Kim et al., "Angiotensin II stimulates the synthesis of vascular endothelial growth factor through the p38 mitogen activated protein kinase pathway in cultured mouse podocytes," *Journal of Molecular Endocrinology*, vol. 36, no. 2, pp. 377–388, 2006.

[49] A. Srikiatkhachorn, C. Ajariyakhajorn, T. P. Endy et al., "Virus-induced decline in soluble vascular endothelial growth receptor 2 is associated with plasma leakage in dengue hemorrhagic fever," *Journal of Virology*, vol. 81, no. 4, pp. 1592–1600, 2007.

[50] L. A. Moraes, L. Piqueras, and D. Bishop-Bailey, "Peroxisome proliferator-activated receptors and inflammation," *Pharmacology & Therapeutics*, vol. 110, no. 3, pp. 371–385, 2006.

[51] K. Wojciechowska-Durczynska, K. Krawczyk-Rusiecka, A. Cyniak-Magierska, A. Zygmunt, S. Sporny, and A. Lewinski, "The role of phosphoinositide 3-kinase subunits in chronic thyroiditis," *Thyroid Research*, vol. 5, no. 1, article 22, 4 pages, 2012.

[52] S. Fisher-Hoch, J. B. McCormick, D. Sasso, and R. B. Craven, "Hematologic dysfunction in Lassa fever," *Journal of Medical Virology*, vol. 26, no. 2, pp. 127–135, 1988.

[53] M.-S. Kim and S.-H. Kim, "Inhibitory effect of astragalin on expression of lipopolysaccharideinduced inflammatory mediators through NF-κB in macrophages," *Archives of Pharmacal Research*, vol. 34, no. 12, pp. 2101–2107, 2011.

[54] A. N. Daniel, S. M. Sartoretto, G. Schmidt, S. M. Caparroz-Assef, C. A. Bersani-Amado, and R. K. N. Cuman, "Anti-inflammatory and antinociceptive activities of eugenol essential oil in experimental animal models," *Revista Brasileira de Farmacognosia*, vol. 19, no. 1, pp. 212–217, 2009.

[55] T.-C. Chou, "Anti-inflammatory and analgesic effects of paeonol in carrageenan-evoked thermal hyperalgesia," *British Journal of Pharmacology*, vol. 139, no. 6, pp. 1146–1152, 2003.

[56] J. P. Wood, J. R. Silveira, N. M. Maille, L. M. Haynes, and P. B. Tracy, "Prothrombin activation on the activated platelet surface optimizes expression of procoagulant activity," *Blood*, vol. 117, no. 5, pp. 1710–1718, 2011.

[57] P. P. Tak and G. S. Firestein, "NF-κB: a key role in inflammatory diseases," *The Journal of Clinical Investigation*, vol. 107, no. 1, pp. 7–11, 2001.

[58] W.-L. Jiang, X.-G. Chen, H.-B. Zhu, Y.-B. Gao, J.-W. Tian, and F.-H. Fu, "Paeoniflorininhibits systemic inflammation and improves survival in experimental sepsis," *Basic & Clinical Pharmacology and Toxicology*, vol. 105, no. 1, pp. 64–71, 2009.

[59] M. I. Cybulsky, J. W. U. Fries, A. J. Williams et al., "Gene structure, chromosomal location, and basis for alternative mRNA splicing of the human VCAM1 gene," *Proceedings of the National Academy of Sciences of the United States of America*, vol. 88, no. 17, pp. 7859–7863, 1991.

[60] G. Marfe, M. Tafani, M. Indelicato et al., "Kaempferol induces apoptosis in two different cell lines via Akt inactivation, bax and SIRT3 activation, and mitochondrial dysfunction," *Journal of Cellular Biochemistry*, vol. 106, no. 4, pp. 643–650, 2009.

[61] W.-T. Kuo, Y.-C. Tsai, H.-C. Wu et al., "Radiosensitization of non-small cell lung cancer by kaempferol," *Oncology Reports*, vol. 34, no. 5, pp. 2351–2356, 2015.

[62] H. S. Lee, H. J. Cho, G. T. Kwon, and J. H. Park, "Kaempferol downregulates insulin-like growth factor-I receptor and ErbB3 signaling in HT-29 human colon cancer cells," *Journal of Cancer Prevention*, vol. 19, no. 3, pp. 161–169, 2014.

[63] M. F. Saeed, A. A. Kolokoltsov, A. N. Freiberg, M. R. Holbrook, and R. A. Davey, "Phosphoinositide-3 kinase-akt pathway controls cellular entry of ebola virus," *PLoS Pathogens*, vol. 4, no. 8, Article ID e1000141, 2008.

[64] J. P. Cooke, "NO and angiogenesis," *Atherosclerosis Supplements*, vol. 4, no. 4, pp. 53–60, 2003.

[65] D. Fulton, J.-P. Gratton, T. J. McCabe et al., "Regulation of endo-thelium-derived nitric oxide production by the protein kinase Akt," *Nature*, vol. 399, no. 6736, pp. 597–601, 1999.

[66] S. Babaei, K. Teichert-Kuliszewska, Q. Zhang, N. Jones, D. J. Dumont, and D. J. Stewart, "Angiogenic actions of angiopoietin-1 require endothelium-derived nitric oxide," *The American Journal of Pathology*, vol. 162, no. 6, pp. 1927–1936, 2003.

[67] S. Jing and Z. Xiaojiang, "Professor Zhang Shiqing's experience on treating pediatric allergic purpura with Xijiao Dihuang decoction," *Journal of Gansu College of Traditional Chinese Medicine*, vol. 3, article 003, 2005.

Electroacupuncture Attenuates Cerebral Ischemia and Reperfusion Injury in Middle Cerebral Artery Occlusion of Rat via Modulation of Apoptosis, Inflammation, Oxidative Stress, and Excitotoxicity

Mei-hong Shen,[1] Chun-bing Zhang,[2,3] Jia-hui Zhang,[2] and Peng-fei Li[3]

[1]*The Second Clinical College, Nanjing University of Chinese Medicine, Nanjing, Jiangsu 210046, China*
[2]*College of Basic Medicine, Nanjing University of Chinese Medicine, Nanjing, Jiangsu 210046, China*
[3]*Department of Clinical Laboratory, Jiangsu Province Hospital of Traditional Chinese Medicine,*
  Affiliated Hospital of Nanjing University of Chinese Medicine, Nanjing, Jiangsu 210029, China

Correspondence should be addressed to Mei-hong Shen; 13815894855@163.com

Academic Editor: Francesca Mancianti

Electroacupuncture (EA) has several properties such as antioxidant, antiapoptosis, and anti-inflammatory properties. The current study was to investigate the effects of EA on the prevention and treatment of cerebral ischemia-reperfusion (I/R) injury and to elucidate possible molecular mechanisms. Sprague-Dawley rats were subjected to middle cerebral artery occlusion (MCAO) for 2 h followed by reperfusion for 24 h. EA stimulation was applied to both *Baihui* and *Dazhui* acupoints for 30 min in each rat per day for 5 successive days before MCAO (pretreatment) or when the reperfusion was initiated (treatment). Neurologic deficit scores, infarction volumes, brain water content, and neuronal apoptosis were evaluated. The expressions of related inflammatory cytokines, apoptotic molecules, antioxidant systems, and excitotoxic receptors in the brain were also investigated. Results showed that both EA pretreatment and treatment significantly reduced infarct volumes, decreased brain water content, and alleviated neuronal injury in MCAO rats. Notably, EA exerts neuroprotection against I/R injury through improving neurological function, attenuating the inflammation cytokines, upregulating antioxidant systems, and reducing the excitotoxicity. This study provides a better understanding of the molecular mechanism underlying the traditional use of EA.

1. Introduction

Stroke, a serious threat to human's health, is a major cause of death and disability in the world. Moreover, stroke has been a leading cause of death in China [1]. It is well known that stroke can be classified into ischemic stroke (IS) and hemorrhagic stroke (HS). Approximately, 87% of the stroke cases are ischemic in origin [2]. Although the exact molecular mechanisms of cerebral ischemia and reperfusion (I/R) injury are not fully known, several evidences indicate that excitotoxicity, oxidative stress, apoptosis, and inflammatory events that occur during cerebral ischemia are critical for the pathogenesis of tissue injury in IS [3–6]. So far, the thrombolytic agent tissue plasminogen activator (tPA) is the

only FDA approved therapy for acute IS [7]. However, tPA has potential shortcomings including the risk of hemorrhagic transformation and narrow time window [8]. Therefore, new strategies that protect against ischemia are urgently needed.

Electroacupuncture (EA) was derived from traditional Chinese medicine and has been widely applied for treatment of many diseases as an alternative therapy method [9–11]. Increasing experimental evidences demonstrate that EA possesses many beneficial properties, such as neuroprotective, anti-inflammatory, and antiapoptotic effects in various animal models [12, 13]. EA has recently been shown to effectively exert neuroprotective effects on stroke patients [14] and in animal middle cerebral artery occlusion (MCAO) models [15]. Moreover, this neuroprotection is closely related to anti-inflammatory and antiapoptotic pathways [16–18]. Our previous studies demonstrated that EA at *Baihui* (GV20) and *Dazhui* (GV14) in MCAO rats protected cerebral cortical cells from injury by clearing away excessive oxygen free radicals [19]. However, the precise mechanism of EA's neuroprotective efficacy is still not well defined.

Therefore, the present study was conducted to investigate whether EA pretreatment or treatment at the *Baihui* (GV20) and *Dazhui* (GV14) acupoints improves cerebral I/R injury in rat. Furthermore, we elucidated the underlying mechanism which was related to the functional recovery.

2. Materials and Methods

2.1. Animals and Groups. Eight-month-old specific-pathogen-free adult male Sprague-Dawley rats, weighing 280 to 320 g, were provided by SLRC Laboratory Animals (Shanghai, China) (certification no. SCXK (Hu) 2007-0005) and housed under diurnal lighting conditions (12 h light/dark cycle). The study conformed to the Guide for the Care and Use of Laboratory Animals published by the US National Institutes of Health (NIH publication no. 85-23, revised 1996), and the experimental procedures were consistent with the ethical requirements established by the Ethics Committee for Animal Experimentation of Nanjing University of Chinese Medicine. Rats were divided randomly into four groups: Sham-operation group (Sham), middle cerebral artery occlusion model-no treatment group (MCAO), EA pretreatment-MCAO group (EA pretreatment), and MCAO-EA treatment group (EA treatment).

2.2. Middle Cerebral Artery Occlusion Model. Rats were allowed free access to food and water but were fasted 12 h before surgery. The MCAO model was performed as described previously, with minor modifications [20]. During the procedure, room temperature was maintained at 27°C. Briefly, rats were anesthetized by intraperitoneal injection of 10% chloral hydrate (Abbott, Illinois, USA); the right common carotid artery, internal carotid artery, and external carotid artery were exposed through a ventral midline neck incision. The internal carotid artery was then isolated and coagulated, and the proximal common carotid artery was ligated. A 4-0 monofilament nylon suture (Beijing Sunbio Biotech Co. Ltd., Beijing, China) with a rounded tip was inserted into the internal carotid artery from the common carotid artery through the external carotid artery stump and gently advanced 18 to 20 mm to occlude the middle cerebral artery. Body temperature was maintained between 37 and 37.5°C by means of heating pad. After 2 h of MCAO, the suture was removed to restore blood flow (reperfusion). Sham-operation rats underwent identical surgery except that the suture was not inserted. During the experiments, Laser-Doppler Flowmetry (LDF) (MoorDRT4; Biopac Systems, Inc., Goleta, CA, USA) was used to monitor cerebral blood flow (CBF) before and after MCAO. Rats were anesthetized with 2% diethyl ether. The flexible 0.5 mm fiber optic probe was perpendicularly placed at 1 mm above the skull surface of the MCA territory (4 mm lateral and 2 mm posterior from bregma). This blood flow rate was maintained for at least 1 h,

with the exception of the 0 h time-point. The MCAO model was considered successful only when the drop in cerebral blood flow was ≥70% of baseline during occlusion.

2.3. EA Stimulation. EA was applied to the acupuncture points *Baihui* (GV20) and *Dazhui* (GV14) with a pair of bipolar stimulation electrodes after placing the rats under intraperitoneal injection of 10% chloral hydrate (Abbott, Illinois, USA). Stainless acupuncture needles of 0.3 mm in diameter (HuaTuo, Suzhou Medical Appliance Factory) were applied to both *Baihui* (GV20) and *Dazhui* (GV14) acupoints in each rat (10 mm EA penetration depth, sparse-dense wave with a frequency of 2/15 Hz and a current intensity of 1~3 mA) using an electrical needle stimulator (WQ1002K, Electro-Acupuncture Equipment Company, China). For the EA pretreatment group, the animals underwent acupuncture once per day for a duration of 30 min for 5 consecutive days and then received MCAO. For the EA treatment group, after 2 h of MCAO, rats received EA stimulation for 30 min. Moreover, the stimulation parameters were the same as EA pretreatment.

2.4. Neurological Function Assessment. At 24 h after reperfusion, a neurological assessment of the rats in different groups was performed by a blind investigator using the 18-point scoring system reported by Garcia et al. [21]. The system consisted of the following six tests: (1) spontaneous activity, (2) symmetry in the movement of four limbs, (3) forepaw outstretching, (4) climbing, (5) body proprioception, and (6) response to vibrissae touch. The score given to each rat at the completion of the evaluation was the summation of all six individual test scores. Minimum neurologic score was 3 and maximum score was 18.

2.5. Quantification of Brain Water Content. The brain edema was determined by evaluating the brain water content according to the wet-dry method [22]. In brief, rats were decapitated under deep anesthesia with 10% chloral hydrate at 24 h of reperfusion and their brains were immediately acquired. A neutral filter paper was used to absorb and remove blood stains from the brain. The ipsilateral and contralateral hemispheres were dissected and the wet weight of the tissue was determined by an electronic scale (wet weight). Subsequently, the tissues were dried overnight at 105°C in a desiccating oven and the dry weight was obtained. Then, the brain water content was calculated using the following formula: brain water content (g) = (wet weight − dry weight).

2.6. Measurement of Infarct Volume. After neurological evaluation, rats were decapitated and the brains were rapidly removed and mildly frozen to keep the morphology intact during slicing. Infarct volume was measured as described previously [23]. In brief, the brain was rapidly dissected and sectioned into five coronal blocks in brain matrix with an approximate thickness of 2 mm and stained with 2% (w/v) 2,3,5-triphenyltetrazolium chloride (TTC) (Sigma, USA) for 30 min at 37°C followed by overnight immersion in 4% (w/v) paraformaldehyde. The infarct tissue area remained unstained (white), whereas normal tissue was stained red.

The infarct areas on each slice were demarcated and analyzed by Image J software (National Institutes of Health, Bethesda, MD, USA). The infarct volumes were calculated via the method according to the following formula: ((total contralateral hemispheric volume) – (total ipsilateral hemispheric stained volume))/(total contralateral hemispheric volume) × 100%.

2.7. Histopathological Examination. Hematoxylin and eosin (HE) staining was performed to show the morphological features of injured neurons in the cerebral cortex. At 24 h after MCAO, rats were sacrificed and brains were fixed by transcardial perfusion with saline, followed by perfusion and immersion in 4% paraformaldehyde. Brains were then dehydrated in a graded series of alcohols and embedded in paraffin. A series of 5 μm thick sections were cut from the block. Finally, the sections were stained with HE reagents for pathological histological examination. The slices were observed and photographed with an Olympus BX50 microscope (Tokyo, Japan).

2.8. Transmission Electron Microscopy (TEM). Fresh brain tissue was taken from the ischemic cortex, cut into 1 mm^3 size cubes and fixed in 1% freshly made paraformaldehyde with 2.5% glutaraldehyde for 24 h. Samples were fixed in 1% osmium tetroxide for 2 h and dehydrated in graded ethanol and embedded in araldite. Sections were cut at 50 nm and stained with uranyl acetate and lead citrate. Finally, the ultrastructures of the pyramidal cells, astrocyte, and the blood brain barrier (BBB) were observed with Tecnai 12 transmission electron microscope (Philips, Netherlands).

2.9. Quantitative Real-Time PCR. At 24 h after MCAO, rats were sacrificed and the ischemic cortex was dissected. Total RNA was extracted using TRIzol reagent (Invitrogen, Carlsbad, CA) according to the manufacturer's protocol. cDNA synthesis was performed using random hexamer primers and the TaqMan reverse transcription kit (Applied Biosystems, Foster City, CA, USA). Samples were subjected to real-time PCR analysis on a 7500 Sequence Detection System (Applied Biosystems) in accordance with the manufacturer's instructions. The primers and probes for rat glutamylcysteine synthetase high subunit (*GCSh*), glutamylcysteine synthetase light subunit (*GCSl*), nuclear factor erythroid 2-related factor 2 (*Nrf2*), tumor necrosis factor-α (*TNF-α*), interleukin-1β (*IL-1β*), interleukin-6 (*IL-6*), and *GAPDH* were designed using Primer Express 3.0 software (Applied Biosystems) based on respective GeneBank accession number. All the primers used were listed in Table 1. *GAPDH* was used as an internal control. The absolute quantities of each mRNA were calculated according to respective standard curve. Each sample was assayed in triplicate.

2.10. Measurement of Glutathione and Glutathione Peroxidase. The blood samples were centrifuged at 3,000 g/min at 4°C for 15 min, and serum was extracted and stored at −80°C until analyzed. The glutathione (GSH) and glutathione peroxidase (GSH-Px) activities in the serum were measured using commercial kits (Jiancheng Bioengineering Institute, Nanjing, Jiangsu, China). The activities of GSH and GSH-Px were expressed as g/L and units, respectively.

2.11. Enzyme-Linked Immunosorbent Assay (ELISA). Blood samples were collected at 24 h after MCAO. Whole blood was centrifuged (13000 ×g for 15 min) and supernatants were collected to determine the level of TNF-α, IL-1β, and IL-6 in serum by available quantitative sandwich ELISA kits (R&D, USA). All use of ELISA kits was in strict accordance with the manufacturer's protocols. The concentrations of the samples were calculated according to the standard curve. The serum TNF-α, IL-1β, and IL-6 levels were all expressed as ng/L.

2.12. Immunohistochemistry Analysis. The immunohistochemistry staining was performed to evaluate the Bax, Bcl-2, Nrf2, and N-methyl-d-aspartate (NMDA) receptors 2A (NR2A) and 2B (NR2B) expression in brain. The hippocampal tissues were separated and fixed in 4% paraformaldehyde overnight at room temperature. The 5 μm thick sections were deparaffinized and treated with 3% H$_2$O$_2$ methanol solution to eliminate endogenous peroxidase activity followed by blocking with 5% goat serum in tris-buffered saline. Then, the sections were incubated with anti-rat Bax (1:150), Bcl-2 (1:200), Nrf2 (1:100), NR2A (1:150), and NR2B (1:150) rabbit antibodies (Abcam, Cambridge, UK) in 0.01 mol/L PBS overnight at 4°C. After a PBS wash, the sections were incubated with horseradish peroxidase-conjugated goat antibodies against rabbit as the second antibody at 37°C for 30 min. After the sections were stained with diaminobenzidine kit (Zhongshan Goldenbridge Biotechnology, Beijing, China), images were acquired using a light microscope (Leica DM4000, Germany) at 400x magnification. The morphometric examination was performed in a blinded manner by two independent investigators. For each section, five visual fields were chosen at random for statistical analysis. Results were expressed as the mean number of the positive cells.

2.13. Statistical Analysis. All data are expressed as mean ± standard error of the mean (SEM). Statistical significance was assessed using one-way analysis of variance (ANOVA) followed by Tukey's multiple comparison tests for multiple comparisons. Values of $P < 0.05$ were considered statistically significant. All statistical analyses were performed using GraphPad Prism v5.0 (GraphPad Software, La Jolla, CA, USA).

3. Results

3.1. Effects of EA on the Neurological Deficits and Brain Water Content after I/R. To investigate whether EA can influence neurological function in MCAO model rats, neurological testing was performed. After 2 h of ischemia followed by 24 h of reperfusion, rats subjected to MCAO showed significant motor behavioral deficits. Neurological function scores were significantly decreased in the MCAO group ($P < 0.01$, Figure 1(a)). Rats in both EA pretreatment and EA treatment group showed significant improvements in

TABLE 1: All the primers information used in quantitative real-time PCR.

Gene		Primer sequence
GCSh	Forward primer	5'-TATCTGCCCAATTGTTATGGCTTT-3'
	Reverse primer	5'-TCCTCCCGTGTTCTATCATCTACA-3'
	Probe	5'-CATCGCCATTTTACCGAGGCTACGTG-3'
GCSl	Forward primer	5'-GGGCACAGGTAAAACCCAATAG-3'
	Reverse primer	5'-TTGGGTCATTGTGAGTCAGTAGCT-3'
	Probe	5'-TTAATCTTGCCTCCTGCTGTGTGATGCC-3'
Nrf2	Forward primer	5'-CCATTCCCGAGTTACAGTGTCTT-3'
	Reverse primer	5'-GATCGATGAGTAAAAATGGTAATTGC-3'
	Probe	5'-CAGCCCAGAGGCCACACTGACAGA-3'
IL-1β	Forward primer	5'-TGTGATGAAAGACGGCACAC-3'
	Reverse primer	5'-CTTCTTCTTTGGGTATTGTTTGG-3'
	Probe	5'-AGCTGGAG-3'
TNF-α	Forward primer	5'-TGAACTTCGGGGGTGATCG-3'
	Reverse primer	5'-GGGCTTGTCACTCGAGTTTT-3'
	Probe	5'-AGGAGGAG-3'
IL-6	Forward primer	5'-CCCTTCAGGAACAGCTATGAA-3'
	Reverse primer	5'-ACAACATCAGTCCCAAGAAGG-3'
	Probe	5'-CCAGCCAG-3'
GAPDH	Forward primer	5'-CCTCAAGATTGTCAGCAATGCA-3'
	Reverse primer	5'-TGGCAGTGATGGCATGGA-3'
	Probe	5'-CACCACCAACTGCTTAGCCCCCCT-3'

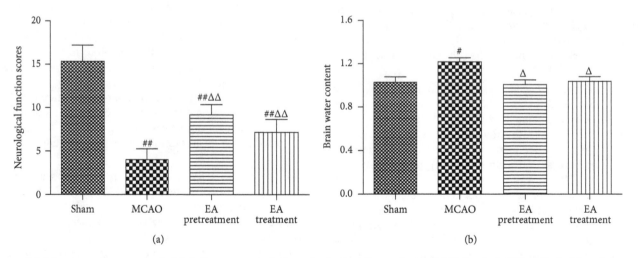

FIGURE 1: EA improves the neurological function scores and attenuates brain water content in MCAO rats. (a) Neurological function scores at 24 h after reperfusion ($n = 6$ animals per group). Rats receiving EA pretreatment and EA treatment showed significant improvement in neurological function compared with the MCAO model groups. (b) Both EA pretreatment and EA treatment significantly reduced brain water weight compared with the MCAO group ($n = 6$ animals per group). Data are represented as mean ± SEM. $^{#}P < 0.05$ and $^{##}P < 0.01$ versus Sham; $^{\Delta}P < 0.05$ and $^{\Delta\Delta}P < 0.01$ versus MCAO. EA, electroacupuncture; MCAO, middle cerebral artery occlusion.

neurological function scores compared with MCAO group ($P < 0.01$, Figure 1(a)). Furthermore, brain water content was determined to assess brain edema in both ipsilateral and contralateral hemispheres of all the groups. Brain water content was remarkably increased in the ipsilateral hemisphere in the MCAO group ($P < 0.05$, Figure 1(b)). In contrast, EA pretreatment or EA treatment after MCAO significantly

decreased brain water content in comparison with the MCAO group ($P < 0.05$, Figure 1(b)).

3.2. Effects of EA on Infarct Volumes in Ischemic Brains.
Infarct volume, as a measure of stroke severity, was also determined in the different groups. Extensive infarction was detected by TTC staining in the cerebral cortex in rats

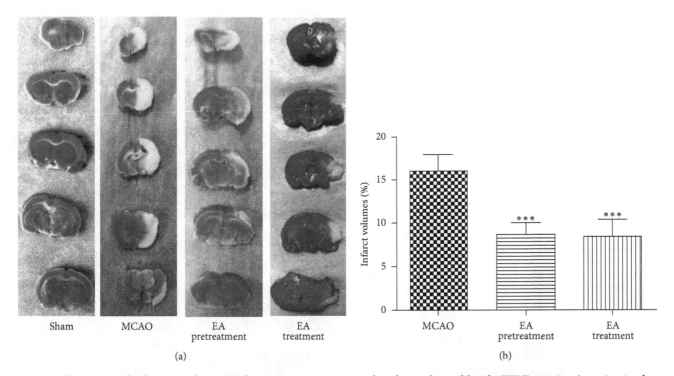

FIGURE 2: Observation of infarction volume: (a) the representative 2,3,5-triphenyltetrazolium chloride (TTC) staining ($n = 6$ animals per group), ischemic area being white and intact area stained red. (b) Percentage of infarct volume of the cerebral infarct in the rat brain ($n = 6$ animals per group). Brain tissues displayed obvious infarction in MCAO group compared to Sham-operated group. Both EA pretreatment and EA treatment groups showed a tendency of decrease in infarction volume compared to MCAO group. Results are expressed as mean ± SEM. *** $P < 0.001$ versus MCAO.

subjected to MCAO (Figure 2(a)). Rats pretreated with EA and treated with EA had significantly smaller infarct volumes than those in the MCAO group ($P < 0.001$, Figure 2(b)), confirming the neuroprotective effect of EA against cerebral I/R injury.

3.3. EA Attenuates Cerebral Damage.

HE staining was performed to observe the morphological changes, as shown in Figure 3(a). In the Sham group, there was no obvious pathological change in cortex. The arrangement of pyramidal cells was close and orderly, neurons kept arranged well, the nuclei were centered with clear staining, and the cytoplasm was abundant. In contrast, the ischemic cortex in the MCAO was damaged seriously. Neurons were significantly degenerated and necrotic, and their arrangement was disordered and sparse. There was nerve cells loss, and edema and deformation were visible with nuclear pyknosis, deep staining, and unclear nucleolus. However, EA pretreatment and EA treatment can obviously decrease the extent of damage induced by MCAO, and an edema and loss and deformation of the nerve cells were alleviated in cortex of rats. In addition, the number of normal neurons was markedly increased as well.

The neuroprotective effect of EA against cerebral ischemic damage was also supported by TEM. As shown in Figure 3(b), in the Sham group, the pyramidal cells were featured by elliptical cell nucleus, even chromatin, clear nucleolus, and cytoplasm. Moreover, there were many Golgi bodies, rough endoplasmic reticulum, and mitochondria with intact cristae in pyramidal cells. The vascular endothelial cells had smooth and flat surfaces, and the endothelia, basement membranes, and foot processes were in close contact. In contrast to Sham group, the pyramidal cells and astrocytes in MCAO showed shrunken nucleus, swollen cell organelles, chromatin condensation, and marginalization and formation of apoptotic bodies. Edema vacuoles around the minute vessels were observed outside the cells. The endothelial cells were swollen, and the thickened basement membrane was not well organized. In the treatment group, the damage to the neurons was alleviated compared to the model group. In EA pretreatment and treatment group, the presence of edema in organelle, cytoplasm, and vascular anomaly was obviously reduced, and the shrunken nucleus in nerve cells and astrocytes were alleviated. The vascular endothelial cells and the basement membrane exhibited smooth and intact surfaces with clear layers.

3.4. EA Inhibits Apoptosis following Cerebral I/R.

The protooncoproteins (Bcl-2 and Bax) are key regulators of the mitochondrial apoptotic pathway initiated by a variety of extracellular and intracellular stressors. To investigate whether EA could attenuate apoptosis in the hippocampal tissues after ischemia-reperfusion, we analyzed the protein expression status of Bax and Bcl-2 by immunohistochemistry staining. As shown in Figures 4(a) and 4(b), the number of Bcl-2-positive cells decreased in the ischemic hippocampal

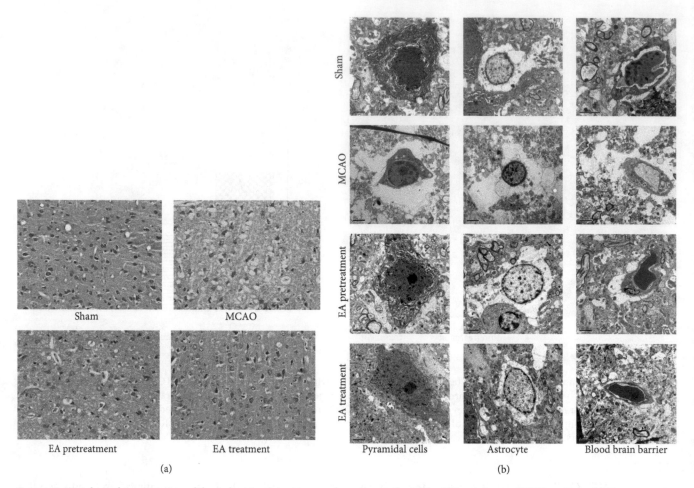

FIGURE 3: Histological examination of the ischemic cortex tissues of rats was evaluated by HE staining and TEM analysis. (a) Representative images of HE staining performed on sections from the ischemic cortex at 24 h after reperfusion in Sham, MCAO, EA pretreatment, and EA treatment groups ($n = 6$ animals per group). Ischemic cortex sections obtained from injured cerebral hemispheres were stained with haematoxylin and eosin and observed using Olympus microscope ($\times 400$). (b) Ultrastructure changes by transmission electron microscope ($\times 5800$). Graphs showing the ultrastructural changes of pyramidal cells, astrocyte, and blood brain barrier (BBB) in different groups ($n = 6$ animals per group).

CA1 region of the MCAO rats compared with the Sham group. However, the number of Bcl-2-positive cells was significantly higher in EA pretreatment rats relative to MCAO ($P < 0.001$). Conversely, the number of Bax-positive cells markedly decreased in the EA pretreatment group compared to MCAO group ($P < 0.001$, Figures 4(a) and 4(c)). These data indicate that EA pretreatment could balance the expression of apoptosis related proteins Bcl-2 and Bax and prevent the neuronal apoptosis in hippocampus.

3.5. EA Promotes the Expression of Nrf2 and GCS. Nrf2 is a key transcription factor that regulates antioxidant genes as an adaptive response to oxidative stress. To identify whether Nrf2/GCS signaling is involved in the neuroprotective effect of EA, we analyzed the expression of Nrf2 in ischemic hippocampal tissues by immunohistochemistry staining. Results showed that EA pretreatment induced a remarkable upregulation of Nrf2-positive cells in hippocampal CA1 region when compared with the MCAO group counterparts ($P <$

0.001, Figures 5(a) and 5(b)). Real-time PCR analysis at 24 h following reperfusion showed, in the ischemic hippocampal CA1 region in EA pretreatment and treatment rats, a significantly higher expression of Nrf2 mRNA level in comparison with that of MCAO animals ($P < 0.01$, Figure 5(c)).

GCS, a heterodimer consisting of heavy (GCSh) and light (GCSl) subunits, is regulated by Nrf2 [24]. It catalyzes the rate-limiting *de novo* biosynthesis of GSH, an abundant physiological antioxidant that plays important roles in regulating oxidative stress. Here, we found that there was remarkable increase in *GCSh* and *GCSl* mRNA levels in rats treated with EA pretreatment and treatment, compared with MCAO group ($P < 0.05$, Figures 5(d) and 5(e)).

3.6. EA Upregulates Endogenous Antioxidant Systems following I/R. To further understand the effect of EA on Nrf2 downstream antioxidant enzymes, we detected the activities of GSH and GSH-Px in rats' serum to examine the oxidative response at 24 h after ischemia. The activities of GSH

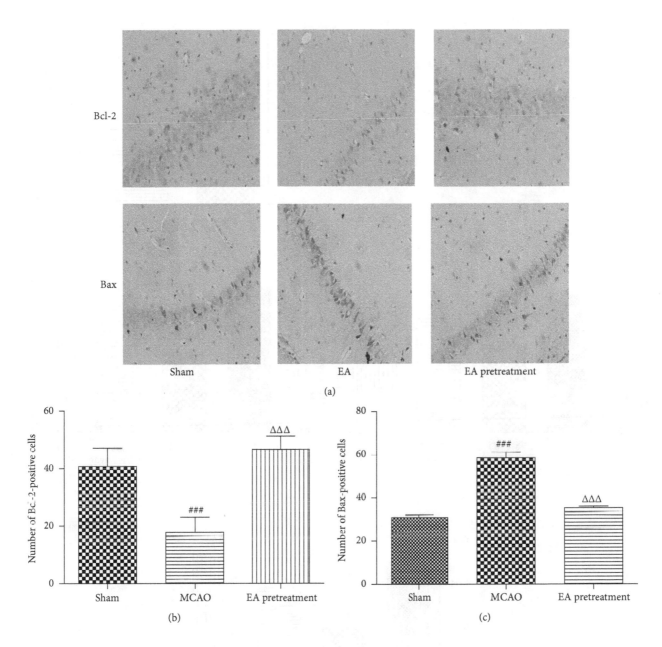

FIGURE 4: Effects of EA on the expression of Bax and Bcl-2 were investigated by immunohistochemistry assay after MCAO. (a–c) Immunohistochemistry staining for Bax or Bcl-2-positive cells in hippocampal CA1 region in different groups ($n = 6$ animals per group) (×400). Data represent mean ± SEM. $^{###}P < 0.001$ versus Sham and $^{\Delta\Delta\Delta}P < 0.001$ versus MCAO.

and GSH-Px were significantly lower in the MCAO group compared with the Sham group, which was restored by EA pretreatment and treatment ($P < 0.01$, Figure 6).

3.7. Effects of EA on the Levels of TNF-α, IL-1β, and IL-6 in Ischemic Cortex and Serum after MCAO. To explore whether EA could induce an anti-inflammatory pattern, we examined proinflammatory mediators in the ischemic cortex and serum after 24 h of reperfusion. Real-time PCR analysis showed a significant increase in *TNF-α* and *IL-6* in ischemic cortex 24 h after MCAO ($P < 0.05$, Figures 7(a) and 7(b)). EA treatment markedly suppressed ischemia-induced

upregulation of *TNF-α*, *IL-1β*, and *IL-6* in ischemic cortex ($P < 0.05$, $P < 0.05$, and $P < 0.01$, Figures 7(a), 7(b), and 7(c)). In addition, EA pretreatment also significantly reduced the expression of *IL-1β* and *IL-6* in ischemic cortex ($P < 0.05$, Figures 7(a), 7(b), and 7(c)). Consistent with the inhibitory effect of EA pretreatment on mRNA expression, the protein concentrations of TNF-α and IL-6 in serum 24 h after MCAO were measured by ELISA, and the results showed a similar trend to those observed in the real-time PCR analysis (Figures 7(d) and 7(e)). EA treatment also significantly inhibited the protein concentrations of TNF-α and IL-6 induced by MCAO (Figures 7(d) and 7(e)).

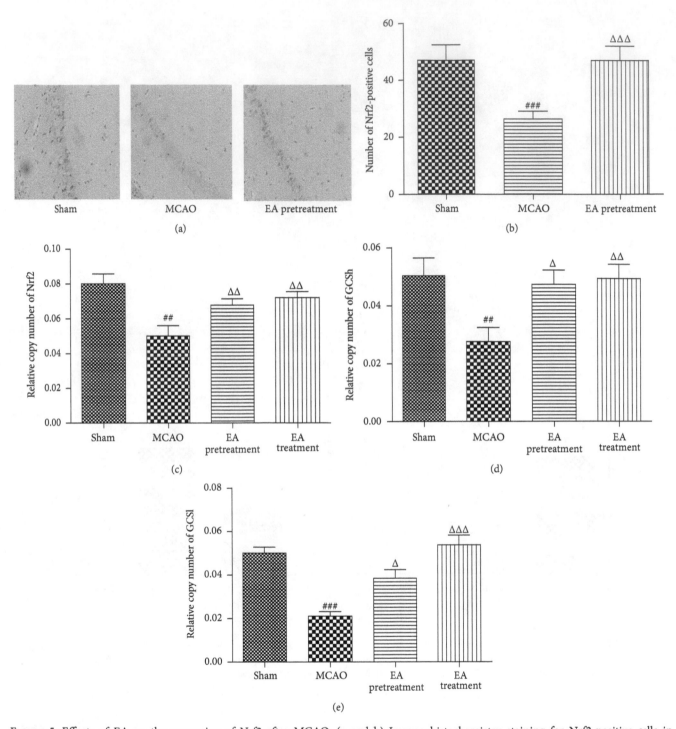

FIGURE 5: Effects of EA on the expression of Nrf2 after MCAO. (a and b) Immunohistochemistry staining for Nrf2-positive cells in hippocampal CA1 region in different groups (n = 6 animals per group) (×400). (c–e) Analysis of *Nrf2*, *GCSh*, and *GCSl* mRNA expression levels in cortex by real-time PCR. GAPDH was used as an internal control (n = 8 animals per group). Data represent mean ± SEM. ## $P < 0.01$, and ### $P < 0.001$ versus Sham and △ $P < 0.05$, △△ $P < 0.01$, and △△△ $P < 0.001$ versus MCAO.

3.8. Effects of EA on the Expression of NR2A and NR2B in Hippocampus. One of the major hallmarks of cerebral ischemia is excitotoxicity. The N-methyl-d-aspartate (NMDA) receptors (NMDARs) are considered to be largely responsible for excitotoxic injury due to their high Ca^{2+} permeability. In the hippocampus and cortex, NMDARs are most prominently

composed of combinations of two N1 subunits and two N2A (NR2A) and/or N2B (NR2B) subunits. However, the differential role of NR2A and NR2B subunits in excitotoxic injury was still controversial [25]. To identify the effects of EA on NR2A and NR2B, we analyzed the expression of NR2A and NR2B in hippocampal CA1 region by immunohistochemistry

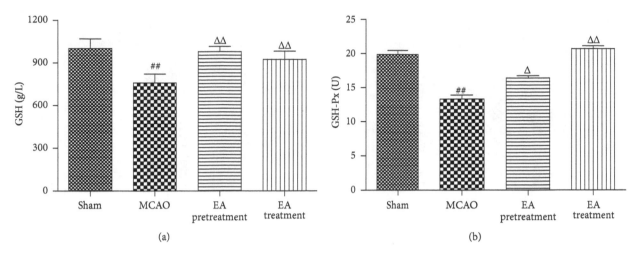

FIGURE 6: Effects of EA on the activities of GSH and GSH-Px. Treatment with EA significantly increased GSH (a) and GSH-Px (b) activities in serum compared with the MCAO group ($n = 8$ animals per group). Data represent mean ± SEM. $^{\#\#}P < 0.01$ versus Sham and $^{\Delta}P < 0.05$ and $^{\Delta\Delta}P < 0.01$ versus MCAO.

staining. Compared with Sham group, the numbers of NR2A-positive cells were significantly lower and the numbers of NR2B-positive cells were significantly higher in MCAO group (Figures 8(a), 8(b), and 8(c)). However, EA treatment induced a remarkable upregulation of NR2A-positive cells and downregulation of NR2B-positive cells in hippocampal CA1 region when compared with the MCAO group counterparts (Figures 8(a), 8(b), and 8(c)). In this regard, EA may alleviate the excitotoxicity which was medicated by NMDAR and attenuate I/R injury via affecting the whole activity of NMDARs complex (NR2A/NR2B).

4. Discussion

The present study analyzed the preventive and therapeutic potential of EA and its underlying mechanisms. Notably, we found that neuroprotective effect of EA was associated with the inhibition of apoptosis, preservation of antioxidative enzymes, reduction of inflammatory mediators, and alleviation of excitotoxicity. Taken together, these results indicated that EA could be a promising tool for complementary therapy in stroke.

Acupuncture represents an integral part of the traditional Chinese medical system. It could regulate body homeostasis and induce enormous physiological potential with minority energy stimulation. As evidences given by recent extensive reports, the beneficial effects of EA on brain ischemic damage in vivo or in vitro mainly focus on antiapoptotic [26], anti-inflammatory [27], and neuron protection [28]. Our study indicates that the underlying mechanism of EA against cerebral I/R injury is a multiple interaction which may involve the inhibition of apoptosis, preservation of antioxidative system, reduction of inflammatory response, and attenuation of excitotoxicity in MCAO rats.

Apoptosis is one of the major causes of cerebral I/R injury. Neuronal death or survival is dependent on the balance between proapoptotic (Bax) and antiapoptotic (Bcl-2)

proteins during cerebral ischemia [29, 30]. It is well known that the increase in brain damage is associated with increased apoptosis as indicated by increased levels of Bax and decreased levels of Bcl-2. A variety of evidences showed that induction of Bcl-2 expression was believed to be protective against ischemic insult. For example, antisense knockdown of endogenous Bcl-2 mRNA exacerbated cerebral ischemic injury in rats and blocked the neuroprotection afforded by ischemic preconditioning [31, 32]. In the present study, we found that the brains of MCAO rats showed obvious apoptotic morphology with dramatically decreased levels of Bcl-2 and increased levels of Bax. This is consistent with previous reports regarding the production of apoptosis [33, 34]. EA could decrease the number of apoptotic cells, upregulate Bcl-2, and downregulate Bax in the ischemic brain. Further studies are required to dissect the detailed mechanisms underlying the regulation of apoptosis.

Extensive studies have been carried out to investigate the immune mechanism of cerebral ischemia. Experiments indicated that inflammatory reactions played crucial roles in brain damage after cerebral I/R injury [35]. During cerebral ischemia, proinflammatory mediators such as TNF-α, IL-1β, and IL-6 are excessively produced by a variety of activated cell types, including microglia, endothelial cells, astrocytes, and neuron cells, which finally exacerbated neuronal injury [36]. Therefore, it is reasonable to speculate that pharmacological alleviation of inflammatory response may be a beneficial choice for stroke therapy [37]. EA has been reported to exert anti-inflammatory effects in several infectious and noninfectious disease models, such as passive endotoxemia, cutaneous anaphylaxis, spinal cord injury, and amyotrophic lateral sclerosis [38–41]. Lan et al. observed that EA decreased the levels of TNF-α, IL-1β, and IL-6 through the suppression of the toll-like receptor 4 and nuclear factor-kappa B (TLR4/NF-κB) signaling pathway in cerebral I/R injured rats [42]. In our study, we also found that EA decreased the expression of TNF-α, IL-1β, and IL-6 in serum and brain tissues. Our

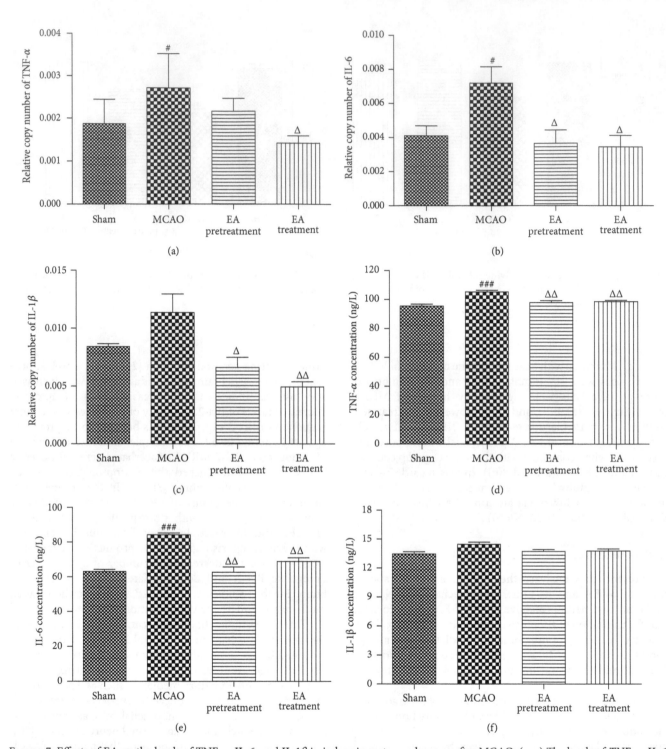

FIGURE 7: Effects of EA on the levels of TNF-α, IL-6, and IL-1β in ischemic cortex and serum after MCAO. (a–c) The levels of *TNF-α*, *IL-6*, and *IL-1β* mRNA in cortex were determined by real-time PCR (n = 8 animals per group). GAPDH was used as an internal control. (d–f) Protein concentrations of TNF-α, IL-6, and IL-1β in the serum in different groups (n = 8 animals per group). Data represent mean ± SEM. $^{###}P < 0.001$ versus Sham and $^{\Delta}P < 0.05$ and $^{\Delta\Delta}P < 0.01$ versus MCAO. $^{#}P < 0.05$ versus Sham.

study revealed that EA could modulate the systemic and local inflammatory reaction in MCAO rats.

The role of oxidative stress in pathogenesis of neuronal death after cerebral ischemia has emerged as an attractive field [43]. Nrf2 is a key regulator of antioxidant and

antioxidative genes including γ-GCS, heme oxygenase 1 (HO-1), and superoxide dismutase (SOD) which plays a vital role in antagonizing oxidative stress [44]. More importantly, Nrf2 is becoming a promising therapeutic target for neuroprotection [45]. In addition, EA could exert antioxidant properties to

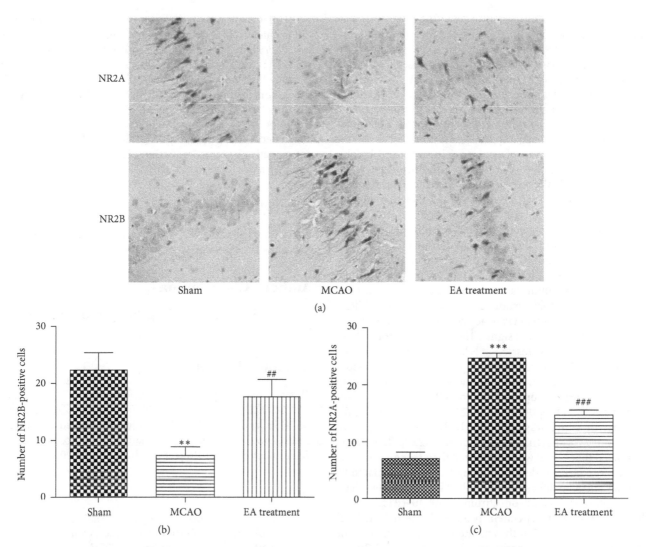

FIGURE 8: Effects of EA on expression of NR2A and NR2B after MCAO. (a–c) Immunohistochemistry staining for NR2A- and NR2B-positive cells in hippocampal CA1 region in different groups (×400) (n = 6 animals per group). Data represent mean ± SEM. $^{**}P$ < 0.01 and $^{***}P$ < 0.001 versus Sham and $^{##}P$ < 0.01 and $^{###}P$ < 0.001 versus MCAO.

counteract the oxidative stress in Parkinson's disease through activation of Nrf2 pathway [13]. Recent studies also reported that intervention of Nrf2 defense pathway could facilitate ischemic brain injury alleviation [46, 47]. In this study, EA significantly increased the expression of Nrf2 in hippocampus at 24 h after MCAO. Our study also demonstrated that EA treatment could upregulate γ-GCS, the rate-limiting enzyme in GSH biosynthesis. Given that these genes were regulated by Nrf2, we deduced that neuroprotective effect of EA might be associated with the upregulation of Nrf2 and GCS.

GSH-Px, GSH, and SOD, indicators of the rate and extent of oxidative stress, could provide first line of protection from ischemic cerebral injury [48]. EA induced neuroprotection against cerebral ischemia through reducing oxidative stress, which may provide new mechanisms [49, 50]. To explore the possible mechanism of EA on the relief of oxidative stress induced by I/R injury, we also investigated the EA-dependent effects on GSH-Px and GSH in MCAO rats. In the present

study, increased activity of antioxidant enzymes can be found in MCAO rats. In this regard, our results have provided evidence for EA's antioxidative activity after cerebral I/R.

Since EA has several advantages, such as economy, convenience, and few side effects, it has been widely applied in stroke patients and in animal stroke models [16, 51]. Preconditioning or pretreatment, potent endogenous protective response, activates several endogenous signaling pathways that result in tolerance against ischemia [52]. Recently, numerous studies have shown that EA pretreatment reduced focal cerebral ischemia in a manner mimicking the ischemia pretreatment [51, 53, 54]. Our study demonstrated that EA pretreatment at *Baihui* (GV20) and *Dazhui* (GV14) for 30 min a day for five days could reduce infarct volumes and improve neurological function after 24 h occlusion. These findings indicate that EA pretreatment could also induce tolerance to cerebral ischemic insult. Meanwhile, the design of EA pretreatment in our study embodies the academic theory of "preventive treatment of disease," which provides enormous guidance for disease preventions. Although it has been known that EA pretreatment can induce tolerance to ischemic brain injury [17, 55], the molecular mechanisms that contribute to brain ischemia tolerance by EA pretreatment remain poorly understood. In this study, we found that EA pretreatment attenuated cerebral ischemia and reperfusion injury in MCAO rat via modulation of apoptosis, inflammation, and oxidative stress.

Excitotoxicity, a kind of neurotoxicity mediated by glutamate, provides link between ischemia and neuronal death, and intervention of the relevant molecules that result in excitotoxicity can prevent stroke damage [56]. Glutamate exerts its function by activating the NMDAR which has been shown to be a critical factor in neuronal damage following ischemia-reperfusion insults [57]. NR2A is predominantly located at synapses, whereas NR2B is mainly found at extrasynaptic locations. However, there was an opposing action of the NR2A and NR2B subunits in mediating cell death and cell survival [58–60]. These evidences indicate that the NR2A subunit produces prosurvival activity, whereas the NR2B subunit leads to a prodeath signal. There are few reports about the effects of EA on expression of NMDAR in stroke. Reports showed that EA reversed the high NR1 subunit expression in a MCAO rat [61, 62]. Our data showed that EA treatment induced a remarkable upregulation of NR2A and downregulation of NR2B in hippocampus. Hence, EA may alleviate the excitotoxicity which was medicated by NMDAR and attenuate I/R injury via affecting the activity of NR2A/NR2B. Sun et al. reported that NR2B was more lethal than those containing NR2A. Moreover, prodeath signaling pathways mediated by neuronal nitric oxide synthase (nNOS), phosphatase and tensin homolog located on chromosome 10 (PTEN), and calcium/calmodulin-dependent protein kinase II (CaMKII) have been linked to NR2B activation [59]. Therefore, the effects of the signaling pathways that activated NR2B are worthy of consideration.

Several studies have shown that EA stimulation potentially provided neuroprotection effects against cerebral I/R injury at different acupoints and at various frequencies. For instance, experimental studies in rats have shown that EA stimulation at the *Baihui* acupoint (2/15 Hz) displayed antiapoptotic effects by increasing the Bcl-2 expression [63, 64]. Tian et al. demonstrated that EA stimulation at the *Baihui*, *Mingmen*, and *Zusanli* acupoints (30/50 Hz) provided neuroprotection in MCAO rats [65]. Moreover, Kim et al. have reported that EA at *Baihui* and *Dazhui* acupoints elicited neuroprotection against cerebral I/R injury [66]. In this study, we chose the *Baihui* and *Dazhui* acupoints according to our practice experience. *Baihui* could affect nerve and periosteum efficiency, dredge and activate *Du* meridian, and revive brain. *Dazhui* could activate blood circulation to dissipate blood stasis and also activate brain function to cause resuscitation. Our findings thus suggest that EA stimulation at *Baihui* and *Dazhui* acupoints, at a frequency of 2/15 Hz, exerts neuroprotective effects against cerebral I/R injury.

Recently, Tao et al. reported that EA alleviated neurological deficits possibly by promoting the proliferation and differentiation of nerve stem cells (NSC) [67]. Extra experiments are required to confirm the influence of EA on the proliferation and differentiation of NSC and neurogenesis. Moreover, additional targets of EA may be relevant for stroke. Future studies need to knock down these targets to evaluate their relevance for protection.

In conclusion, the present results indicate that EA pretreatment or treatment may induce a neuroprotection in transient MCAO rats. The underlying mechanisms were associated with the inhibition of apoptosis, preservation of antioxidative systems, reduction of inflammatory mediators, and alleviation of excitotoxicity.

Competing Interests

The authors declare that they have no competing interests regarding the publication of this paper.

Authors' Contributions

Mei-hong Shen and Chun-bing Zhang contributed equally to this work.

Acknowledgments

This study was supported by grants from the National Natural Science Foundation of China (nos. 81373748, 81171659, 11574156, and 81403136); 333 Project of Jiangsu Province in China (no. BRA2014341); and Jiangsu Province Science and Technology Support Project in China (no. BE2010769).

References

[1] C.-F. Tsai, B. Thomas, and C. L. M. Sudlow, "Epidemiology of stroke and its subtypes in Chinese vs white populations," *Neurology*, vol. 81, no. 3, pp. 264–272, 2013.

[2] L. B. Goldstein, R. Adams, K. Becker et al., "Primary prevention of ischemic stroke: a statement for healthcare professionals from the stroke council of the American Heart Association," *Stroke*, vol. 32, no. 1, pp. 280–299, 2001.

[3] C. L. Allen and U. Bayraktutan, "Oxidative stress and its role in the pathogenesis of ischaemic stroke," *International Journal of Stroke*, vol. 4, no. 6, pp. 461–470, 2009.

[4] B. R. S. Broughton, D. C. Reutens, and C. G. Sobey, "Apoptotic mechanisms after cerebral ischemia," *Stroke*, vol. 40, no. 5, pp. e331–e339, 2009.

[5] C. Iadecola and J. Anrather, "The immunology of stroke: from mechanisms to translation," *Nature Medicine*, vol. 17, no. 7, pp. 796–808, 2011.

[6] P. Lipton, "Ischemic cell death in brain neurons," *Physiological Reviews*, vol. 79, no. 4, pp. 1431–1568, 1999.

[7] B. Zhang, X.-J. Sun, and C.-H. Ju, "Thrombolysis with alteplase 4.5-6 hours after acute ischemic stroke," *European Neurology*, vol. 65, no. 3, pp. 170–174, 2011.

[8] Z. Tan, X. Li, R. C. Turner et al., "Combination treatment of r-tPA and an optimized human apyrase reduces mortality rate and hemorrhagic transformation 6h after ischemic stroke in aged female rats," *European Journal of Pharmacology*, vol. 738, pp. 368–373, 2014.

[9] Y.-J. Zeng, S.-Y. Tsai, K.-B. Chen, S.-F. Hsu, J. Y.-R. Chen, and Y.-R. Wen, "Comparison of electroacupuncture and morphine-mediated analgesic patterns in a plantar incision-induced pain model," *Evidence-Based Complementary and Alternative Medicine*, vol. 2014, Article ID 659343, 12 pages, 2014.

[10] F. Guo, W. Song, T. Jiang et al., "Electroacupuncture pretreatment inhibits NADPH oxidase-mediated oxidative stress in diabetic mice with cerebral ischemia," *Brain Research*, vol. 1573, pp. 84–91, 2014.

[11] J.-W. Choi, S.-Y. Kang, J.-G. Choi et al., "Analgesic effect of electroacupuncture on paclitaxel-induced neuropathic pain via spinal opioidergic and adrenergic mechanisms in mice," *The American Journal of Chinese Medicine*, vol. 43, no. 1, pp. 57–70, 2015.

[12] J.-B. Yu, J. Shi, L.-R. Gong et al., "Role of Nrf2/ARE pathway in protective effect of electroacupuncture against endotoxic shock-induced acute lung injury in rabbits," *PLoS ONE*, vol. 9, no. 8, Article ID e104924, 2014.

[13] E. Lv, J. Deng, Y. Yu et al., "Nrf2-ARE signals mediated the anti-oxidative action of electroacupuncture in an MPTP mouse model of Parkinson's disease," *Free Radical Research*, vol. 49, no. 11, pp. 1296–1307, 2015.

[14] A. J. Liu, J. H. Li, H. Q. Li et al., "Electroacupuncture for acute ischemic stroke: a meta-analysis of randomized controlled trials," *The American Journal of Chinese Medicine*, vol. 43, no. 8, pp. 1541–1566, 2015.

[15] X. Li, P. Luo, Q. Wang, and L. Xiong, "Electroacupuncture pretreatment as a novel avenue to protect brain against ischemia and reperfusion injury," *Evidence-Based Complementary and Alternative Medicine*, vol. 2012, Article ID 195397, 12 pages, 2012.

[16] Q. Wang, X. Li, Y. Chen et al., "Activation of epsilon protein kinase c-mediated anti-apoptosis is involved in rapid tolerance induced by electroacupuncture pretreatment through cannabinoid receptor type 1," *Stroke*, vol. 42, no. 2, pp. 389–396, 2011.

[17] F. Zhou, J. Guo, J. Cheng, G. Wu, and Y. Xia, "Electroacupuncture increased cerebral blood flow and reduced ischemic brain injury: dependence on stimulation intensity and frequency," *Journal of Applied Physiology*, vol. 111, no. 6, pp. 1877–1887, 2011.

[18] Q. Wang, F. Wang, X. Li et al., "Electroacupuncture pretreatment attenuates cerebral ischemic injury through α7 nicotinic acetylcholine receptor-mediated inhibition of high-mobility group box 1 release in rats," *Journal of Neuroinflammation*, vol. 9, article 24, 2012.

[19] M. H. Shen, X. R. Xiang, Y. Li, J. L. Pan, C. Ma, and Z. R. Li, "Effect of electroacupuncture on expression of gamma-glutamylcysteine synthetase protein and mRNA in cerebral cortex in rats with focal cerebral ischemia-reperfusion," *Zhen Ci Yan Jiu*, vol. 37, no. 1, pp. 25–30, 2012.

[20] Z.-R. Li and L. Cui, "Application of TC index location on Longa's animal model of regional experimental cerebral ischemia and reperfusion," *Zhongguo Zhong Xi Yi Jie He Za Zhi*, vol. 26, supplement, pp. 18–20, 2006.

[21] J. H. Garcia, S. Wagner, K.-F. Liu, and X.-J. Hu, "Neurological deficit and extent of neuronal necrosis attributable to middle cerebral artery occlusion in rats. Statistical validation," *Stroke*, vol. 26, no. 4, pp. 627–635, 1995.

[22] A. Mdzinarishvili, C. Kiewert, V. Kumar, M. Hillert, and J. Klein, "Bilobalide prevents ischemia-induced edema formation in vitro and in vivo," *Neuroscience*, vol. 144, no. 1, pp. 217–222, 2007.

[23] B. P. Walcott, K. T. Kahle, and J. M. Simard, "Novel treatment targets for cerebral edema," *Neurotherapeutics*, vol. 9, no. 1, pp. 65–72, 2012.

[24] R. T. Mulcahy, M. A. Wartman, H. H. Bailey, and J. J. Gipp, "Constitutive and β-naphthoflavone-induced expression of the human γ-glutamylcysteine synthetase heavy subunit gene is regulated by a distal antioxidant response element/TRE sequence," *The Journal of Biological Chemistry*, vol. 272, no. 11, pp. 7445–7454, 1997.

[25] M. M. Vieira, J. Schmidt, J. S. Ferreira et al., "Multiple domains in the C-terminus of NMDA receptor GluN2B subunit contribute to neuronal death following in vitro ischemia," *Neurobiology of Disease*, vol. 89, pp. 223–234, 2016.

[26] J.-H. Chung, E.-Y. Lee, M.-H. Jang et al., "Acupuncture decreases ischemia-induced apoptosis and cell proliferation in dentate gyrus of gerbils," *Neurological Research*, vol. 29, supplement 1, no. 1, pp. S23–S27, 2007.

[27] F. Zhou, J. Guo, J. Cheng, G. Wu, J. Sun, and Y. Xia, "Electroacupuncture and brain protection against cerebral ischemia: specific effects of acupoints," *Evidence-Based Complementary and Alternative Medicine*, vol. 2013, Article ID 804397, 14 pages, 2013.

[28] K. A. Kang, E. S. Shin, J. Hur et al., "Acupuncture attenuates neuronal cell death in middle cerebral artery occlusion model of focal ischemia," *Neurological Research*, vol. 32, supplement 1, pp. 84–87, 2010.

[29] M. Sun, Y. Gu, Y. Zhao, and C. Xu, "Protective functions of taurine against experimental stroke through depressing mitochondria-mediated cell death in rats," *Amino Acids*, vol. 40, no. 5, pp. 1419–1429, 2011.

[30] Y. Zhu, J. H. M. Prehn, C. Culmsee, and J. Krieglstein, "The β2-adrenoceptor agonist clenbuterol modulates Bcl-2, Bcl-xl and Bax protein expression following transient forebrain ischemia," *Neuroscience*, vol. 90, no. 4, pp. 1255–1263, 1999.

[31] J. Chen, R. P. Simon, T. Nagayama et al., "Suppression of endogenous bcl-2 expression by antisense treatment exacerbates ischemic neuronal death," *Journal of Cerebral Blood Flow and Metabolism*, vol. 20, no. 7, pp. 1033–1039, 2000.

[32] S. Shimizu, T. Nagayama, K. L. Jin et al., "bcl-2 Antisense treatment prevents induction of tolerance to focal ischemia in the rat brain," *Journal of Cerebral Blood Flow and Metabolism*, vol. 21, no. 3, pp. 233–243, 2001.

[33] P. Jie, Z. Hong, Y. Tian et al., "Activation of transient receptor potential vanilloid 4 induces apoptosis in hippocampus through downregulating PI3K/Akt and upregulating p38 MAPK signaling pathways," *Cell Death and Disease*, vol. 6, Article ID e1775, 2015.

[34] W. Chen, B. Xu, A. Xiao et al., "TRPM7 inhibitor carvacrol protects brain from neonatal hypoxic-ischemic injury," *Molecular Brain*, vol. 8, article 11, 2015.

[35] C. Iadecola and M. Alexander, "Cerebral ischemia and inflammation," *Current Opinion in Neurology*, vol. 14, no. 1, pp. 89–94, 2001.

[36] M. Lalancette-Hbert, D. Phaneuf, G. Soucy, Y. C. Weng, and J. Kriz, "Live imaging of toll-like receptor 2 response in cerebral ischaemia reveals a role of olfactory bulb microglia as modulators of inflammation," *Brain*, vol. 132, no. 4, pp. 940–954, 2009.

[37] P. M. Madsen, B. H. Clausen, M. Degn et al., "Genetic ablation of soluble tumor necrosis factor with preservation of membrane tumor necrosis factor is associated with neuroprotection after

focal cerebral ischemia," *Journal of Cerebral Blood Flow & Metabolism*, 2015.

[38] D. C. Choi, J. Y. Lee, Y. J. Moon, S. W. Kim, T. H. Oh, and T. Y. Yune, "Acupuncture-mediated inhibition of inflammation facilitates significant functional recovery after spinal cord injury," *Neurobiology of Disease*, vol. 39, no. 3, pp. 272–282, 2010.

[39] J. H. Jiang, E. J. Yang, M. G. Baek, S. H. Kim, S. M. Lee, and S.-M. Choi, "Anti-inflammatory effects of electroacupuncture in the respiratory system of a symptomatic amyotrophic lateral sclerosis animal model," *Neurodegenerative Diseases*, vol. 8, no. 6, pp. 504–514, 2011.

[40] P.-D. Moon, H.-J. Jeong, S.-J. Kim et al., "Use of electroacupuncture at ST36 to inhibit anaphylactic and inflammatory reaction in mice," *NeuroImmunoModulation*, vol. 14, no. 1, pp. 24–31, 2007.

[41] G. Gu, Z. Zhang, G. Wang et al., "Effects of electroacupuncture pretreatment on inflammatory response and acute kidney injury in endotoxaemic rats," *Journal of International Medical Research*, vol. 39, no. 5, pp. 1783–1797, 2011.

[42] L. Lan, J. Tao, A. Chen et al., "Electroacupuncture exerts antiinflammatory effects in cerebral ischemia-reperfusion injured rats via suppression of the TLR4/NF-κB pathway," *International Journal of Molecular Medicine*, vol. 31, no. 1, pp. 75–80, 2013.

[43] T. Sugawara and P. H. Chan, "Reactive oxygen radicals and pathogenesis of neuronal death after cerebral ischemia," *Antioxidants and Redox Signaling*, vol. 5, no. 5, pp. 597–607, 2003.

[44] W.-W. Ma, C.-Q. Li, H.-L. Yu et al., "The oxysterol 27-hydroxycholesterol increases oxidative stress and regulate Nrf2 signaling pathway in astrocyte cells," *Neurochemical Research*, vol. 40, no. 4, pp. 758–766, 2015.

[45] Y. Ding, M. Chen, M. Wang, Y. Li, and A. Wen, "Posttreatment with 11-keto-β-boswellic acid ameliorates cerebral ischemia–reperfusion injury: Nrf2/HO-1 pathway as a potential mechanism," *Molecular Neurobiology*, vol. 52, no. 3, pp. 1430–1439, 2014.

[46] A. Alfieri, S. Srivastava, R. C. M. Siow et al., "Sulforaphane preconditioning of the Nrf2/HO-1 defense pathway protects the cerebral vasculature against blood-brain barrier disruption and neurological deficits in stroke," *Free Radical Biology and Medicine*, vol. 65, pp. 1012–1022, 2013.

[47] Y. Ding, M. Chen, M. Wang et al., "Neuroprotection by acetyl-11-keto-β-boswellic acid, in ischemic brain injury involves the Nrf2/HO-1 defense pathway," *Scientific Reports*, vol. 4, article 7002, 2014.

[48] S. K. Min, J. S. Park, L. Luo et al., "Assessment of C-phycocyanin effect on astrocytes-mediated neuroprotection against oxidative brain injury using 2D and 3D astrocyte tissue model," *Scientific Reports*, vol. 5, article 14418, 2015.

[49] C.-Y. Cheng, J.-G. Lin, N.-Y. Tang, S.-T. Kao, and C.-L. Hsieh, "Electroacupuncture-like stimulation at the Baihui (GV20) and Dazhui (GV14) acupoints protects rats against subacute-phase cerebral ischemia-reperfusion injuries by reducing S100B-mediated neurotoxicity," *PLoS ONE*, vol. 9, no. 3, Article ID e91426, 2014.

[50] S. Sun, X. Chen, Y. Gao et al., "Mn-SOD upregulation by electroacupuncture attenuates ischemic oxidative damage via CB1R-mediated STAT3 phosphorylation," *Molecular Neurobiology*, vol. 53, no. 1, pp. 331–343, 2016.

[51] H. Dong, Y.-H. Fan, W. Zhang, Q. Wang, Q.-Z. Yang, and L.-Z. Xiong, "Repeated electroacupuncture preconditioning attenuates matrix metalloproteinase-9 expression and activity after focal cerebral ischemia in rats," *Neurological Research*, vol. 31, no. 8, pp. 853–858, 2009.

[52] N. E. Stagliano, M. A. Pérez-Pinzón, M. A. Moskowitz, and P. L. Huang, "Focal ischemic preconditioning induces rapid tolerance to middle cerebral artery occlusion in mice," *Journal of Cerebral Blood Flow and Metabolism*, vol. 19, no. 7, pp. 757–761, 1999.

[53] Q. Wang, Y. Peng, S. Chen et al., "Pretreatment with electroacupuncture induces rapid tolerance to focal cerebral ischemia through regulation of endocannabinoid system," *Stroke*, vol. 40, no. 6, pp. 2157–2164, 2009.

[54] J. Du, Q. Wang, B. Hu et al., "Involvement of ERK 1/2 activation in electroacupuncture pretreatment via cannabinoid CB1 receptor in rats," *Brain Research*, vol. 1360, pp. 1–7, 2010.

[55] S. Zhang, G. Li, X. Xu, M. Chang, C. Zhang, and F. Sun, "Acupuncture to point Baihui prevents ischemia-induced functional impairment of cortical GABAergic neurons," *Journal of the Neurological Sciences*, vol. 307, no. 1-2, pp. 139–143, 2011.

[56] T. W. Lai, S. Zhang, and Y. T. Wang, "Excitotoxicity and stroke: identifying novel targets for neuroprotection," *Progress in Neurobiology*, vol. 115, pp. 157–188, 2014.

[57] Z.-Q. Shi, C. R. Sunico, S. R. McKercher et al., "S-nitrosylated SHP-2 contributes to NMDA receptor-mediated excitotoxicity in acute ischemic stroke," *Proceedings of the National Academy of Sciences of the United States of America*, vol. 110, no. 8, pp. 3137–3142, 2013.

[58] M. Chen, T.-J. Lu, X.-J. Chen et al., "Differential roles of NMDA receptor subtypes in ischemic neuronal cell death and ischemic tolerance," *Stroke*, vol. 39, no. 11, pp. 3042–3048, 2008.

[59] Y. Sun, L. Zhang, Y. Chen, L. Zhan, and Z. Gao, "Therapeutic targets for cerebral ischemia based on the signaling pathways of the GluN2B C terminus," *Stroke*, vol. 46, no. 8, pp. 2347–2353, 2015.

[60] Y. Liu, P. W. Tak, M. Aarts et al., "NMDA receptor subunits have differential roles in mediating excitotoxic neuronal death both in vitro and in vivo," *Journal of Neuroscience*, vol. 27, no. 11, pp. 2846–2857, 2007.

[61] N. Sun, X. Zou, J. Shi, X. Liu, L. Li, and L. Zhao, "Electroacupuncture regulates NMDA receptor NR1 subunit expression via PI3-K pathway in a rat model of cerebral ischemia-reperfusion," *Brain Research*, vol. 1064, no. 1-2, pp. 98–107, 2005.

[62] Y.-W. Lin and C.-L. Hsieh, "Electroacupuncture at Baihui acupoint (GV20) reverses behavior deficit and long-term potentiation through N-methyl-D-aspartate and transient receptor potential vanilloid subtype 1 receptors in middle cerebral artery occlusion rats," *Journal of Integrative Neuroscience*, vol. 9, no. 3, pp. 269–282, 2010.

[63] X. Zhu, J. Yin, L. Li et al., "Electroacupuncture preconditioning-induced neuroprotection may be mediated by glutamate transporter type 2," *Neurochemistry International*, vol. 63, no. 4, pp. 302–308, 2013.

[64] H. Zhou, Z. Zhang, H. Wei et al., "Activation of STAT3 is involved in neuroprotection by electroacupuncture pretreatment via cannabinoid CB1 receptors in rats," *Brain Research*, vol. 1529, pp. 154–164, 2013.

[65] W.-Q. Tian, Y. G. Peng, S.-Y. Cui, F.-Z. Yao, and B.-G. Li, "Effects of electroacupuncture of different intensities on energy metabolism of mitochondria of brain cells in rats with cerebral ischemia-reperfusion injury," *Chinese Journal of Integrative Medicine*, vol. 21, no. 8, pp. 618–623, 2015.

[66] J. H. Kim, K. H. Choi, Y. J. Jang et al., "Electroacupuncture preconditioning reduces cerebral ischemic injury via BDNF

and SDF-1α in mice," *BMC Complementary and Alternative Medicine*, vol. 13, article 22, 2013.

[67] J. Tao, X.-H. Xue, L.-D. Chen et al., "Electroacupuncture improves neurological deficits and enhances proliferation and differentiation of endogenous nerve stem cells in rats with focal cerebral ischemia," *Neurological Research*, vol. 32, no. 2, pp. 198–204, 2010.

Garlic Attenuates Plasma and Kidney ACE-1 and AngII Modulations in Early Streptozotocin-Induced Diabetic Rats: Renal Clearance and Blood Pressure Implications

Khaled K. Al-Qattan, Martha Thomson, Divya Jayasree, and Muslim Ali

Department of Biological Sciences, Faculty of Science, Kuwait University, P.O. Box 5969, 13060 Safat, Kuwait

Correspondence should be addressed to Martha Thomson; mmtkuniv@gmail.com

Academic Editor: Khalid Rahman

Raw garlic aqueous extract (GE) has ameliorative actions on the renin-angiotensin system in type-1 diabetes mellitus (DM); however its effects on plasma and kidney angiotensin I converting enzyme type-1 (ACE-1) and angiotensin II (AngII) require further elucidation. This study investigated the effect of GE on plasma and kidney ACE-1 and AngII concentrations and in relation to systemic and renal clearance indicators significant to blood pressure (BP) homeostasis in early streptozotocin- (STZ-) induced type-1 DM. Normal rats ($n = 10$) received 0.5 mL normal saline (NR/NS), diabetic rats ($n = 10$) received 0.5 mL NS (DR/NS), and treated diabetic rats ($n = 10$) received 50 mg/0.1 mL/100 g body weight GE (DR/GE) as daily intraperitoneal injections for 8 weeks. Compared to NR/NS, DR/NS showed a significant increase in plasma ACE-1 and AngII and conversely a decrease in kidney ACE-1 and AngII. These changes were associated with an increase in BP and clearance functions. Alternatively and compared to DR/NS, DR/GE showed normalization or attenuation in plasma and kidney ACE-1 and AngII. These GE induced rectifications were associated with moderation in BP elevation and renal clearance functions. Garlic attenuates modulations in plasma and kidney ACE-1 and AngII, in addition to BP and renal clearance function in type-1 DM.

1. Introduction

The endocrinal renin-angiotensin system (RAS) was initially described as follows: upon stimulation, renin, a protease, is released by both kidneys to the general circulation. In the plasma, renin acts on angiotensinogen, an α-globulin synthesized by the liver, to liberate a decapeptide known as angiotensin I (AngI). While passing through the pulmonary circulation, AngI is cleaved by a dipeptidyl dipeptidase known as angiotensin I converting enzyme (ACE-1) to free an octapeptide called angiotensin II (AngII) [1]. Recently, it has been asserted that the kidneys produce all components of the RAS [2, 3].

ACE-1 is the second rate limiting enzyme that controls the liberation of AngII: the most active component of the RAS [4]. AngII has numerous biological activities, including vasoconstriction, antinatriuresis, and antidiuresis, actions which are closely affiliated with renal clearance functions and

BP regulation [5]. It is most probable that under physiological conditions renally and systemically produced AngII work synergistically, where renal AngII acts as the principle paracrine regulator of the kidneys' clearance function determinants, including renal hemodynamics, glomerular filtration rate (GFR), and tubular handling of electrolytes and water [6]. Alternatively, systemically produced AngII operates as the main telocrine modulator of, firstly, general and, secondly, peripheral vascular resistance [7]. The fine tuning of the AngII-mediated actions is achieved by AngII binding to and activating either/or both of its two major receptor types: AT_1 and AT_2 [8, 9]. Specifically, AT_1 receptor facilitates the AngII known actions of general and peripheral vasoconstriction, renal antinatriuresis and antidiuresis, and cell growth and proliferation [10], while the AT_2 receptor mediates the suggested AngII vasodilatation, natriuresis and diuresis, apoptosis, and antiproliferation, actions that antagonize those evoked by the AT_1 receptor type [11].

Dysregulation in the RAS associated with AngII AT_1/AT_2 receptors expression imbalance is major factors in the initiation and progression of tissue remodeling and refunctioning in biochemical-physiological pathologies [8, 10, 12, 13] including diabetes mellitus (DM) [14]. DM is a progressive disease that entails dynamic phase-changing, structural-functional characteristics. In an attempt to elucidate the nature of RAS modulations in insulin-dependent type-1 DM [15], the findings of previous studies led to the formulation of two major conflicting views.

A group of studies have suggested an increase in the RAS activity and consequently ACE-1 and AngII bioavailability especially in renal tissue and nephronal structures. This view was supported by findings that inhibitors of different RAS components and AngII receptor blockers were effective in partially diminishing DM abnormalities [12, 14]. An augmented RAS activity most likely occurs at later stages of DM when molecular/cellular transformations collectively lead to severe renal-nephronal injuries; in particular glomerulotubular sclerosis, which impedes kidney clearance function leading to the end-stage renal failure that is characteristic of advanced DM [16–18]. A hypoinsulinemic-hyperglycemic provoked high AngII concentration and stimulation of overexpressed AT_1 receptors lead to the following events in the kidneys: sodium transport and retention, vascular resistance, glomerular capillary pressure, mechano-stretch-induced reactive oxygen species production, and tubulointerstitial cell hypertrophy and hyperplasia associated with extracellular mesangial matrix production [19, 20]. This AngII/AT_1 scenario is exacerbated by downregulation of intrarenal AT_2 receptor expression [21] and subsequent minimization of its mediated alleviating responses including inhibition of Na^+-K^+-ATPase activity [22], sodium pump action in renal proximal tubules [23], antinatriuresis [24], vasoconstriction [11], cell hypertrophy, and renal glomerular and tubular remodeling [8, 10, 25].

Other studies have reported opposite findings and variations in the activity of plasma and renal RAS components, particularly ACE-1 and AngII, in early DM. In 4 weeks after streptozotocin- (STZ-) induced type-1 DM rats, it was reported that the RAS is downregulated at the level of mRNA expression [26]. Furthermore, renal ACE content [27] as well as AngII concentration [28] was reduced. In addition, a further decline in AngII concentration was suggested to result from an increase in degradation by the enzyme angiotensinase A [29]. In a review, Copper et al. [30] argued that RAS activation is controversial as different animal-molecular studies reported conflicting results. In particular, it was suggested that in early DM the indices of RAS are lower and the concentrations of renal AngII and its receptor AT_1 are reduced leading to hyperfiltration. An increased GFR, which can be monitored by measuring creatinine clearance in live subjects [31], with a suggested lower AngII type AT_1 receptor-mediated activation of sodium retention leads to higher sodium and water clearance. This excretory behavior causes polyuria, in addition to albuminuria, and necessary, however futile, polydipsia: a myriad of symptoms that are typically observed at the early stages of DM.

Garlic has long been used in traditional medicine as an easily available and accessible natural medicine [32] to control BP and sugar in general [33] and when affiliated with DM complications [34]. Within the past two decades, garlic, either as an aqueous extract (GE) or isolated organosulfur constituents, has been the focus of intensive studies in the STZ-induced experimental model of type-1 DM [35] showing several interesting and well documented ameliorative actions [36]. Among these actions is garlic's ability to induce several biochemical-physiological measures at the systemic level; particularly, serum insulin elevation [37, 38], blood glucose reduction [38, 39], serum ACE activity diminution and suggested reduced AngII generation [40], and, therefore, hypotension [36]. The induced hypotension may be mediated, in part, through a reduced AngII concentration resulting in lower vasoconstrictive action and/or indirectly through an increase in the amounts and actions of vasodilatory agents [41]. More recently, our group has also shown that GE treatment in early STZ-DM improved kidney clearance functions [42], in addition to preserving the normal expression and balance of the two AngII receptors types [43, 44].

To further elucidate garlic's ameliorative mechanism related to RAS in early type-1 DM, this study investigated the effect of GE on DM-induced changes in plasma and renal ACE-1 and AngII concentrations. The effects of GE on ACE-1 and AngII were correlated to simultaneous modulations in BP and systemic and renal indicators of clearance function.

2. Materials and Methods

2.1. Materials. The materials used in this study, unless otherwise stated, were obtained accordingly: analysis kits as indicated in this section, Thiopental Sodium from May & Baker (England) and STZ, chemicals, and reagents from Sigma-Aldrich (USA).

2.2. Preparation of Raw Garlic Aqueous Extract. The GE (50 mg/0.1 mL) used in this study was prepared from locally purchased, peeled fresh garlic cloves (*Allium sativum L.*) as previously described [45]. The prepared GE was immediately stored as 1 mL aliquots in 1.5 mL self-capping, inert-plastic freeze-durable Eppendorf tubes at −20°C. The required volume of GE was thawed daily to ambient temperature before administration and following use any remaining amount was discarded. GC-MS comparative analysis of the GE after different times of freeze-storage showed similar composition and concentration of components [42, unpublished data].

2.3. Animals. The animals used in this study were male Sprague-Dawley rats (ancestors origin: Harland Lab, Oxfordshire, England) having an initial body weight of 150–200 grams. Before and during the study, the rats were kept in adequate-size separate cages and housed in an Animal Care Facility under standard ambient conditions ($23 \pm 2°C$, natural day/night cycle). The rats were provided with standard rodent diet (170 mmol Na^+/kg) and tap water *ad libitum*.

The care and use of all rats used in this study was in full compliance with the Guide for the Care and Use of Laboratory Animals, National Research Council [46].

2.4. Induction of Type-1 Diabetes. The type-1 DM rats used in this study were produced by intraperitoneally injecting each of a sufficient number of overnight fasting rats with a single dose of STZ (6 mg/100 g body weight) dissolved in citrate buffer (0.3 mL, 0.01 M, pH 4.5) as described previously [39]. After 5 days, STZ-injected rats with a blood glucose concentration ≥16 mmol/L measured in a drop of tail-blood (One Touch UltraEasy Glucometer, UK) under mild ether sedation were deemed diabetic ($n = 20$) and used in the study.

2.5. Rats' Groups and Treatments. At day 7 after STZ injection, DM rats were divided into two groups and treated for 8 weeks with either a single daily intraperitoneal injection of 0.1 mL of normal saline/100-gram body weight (DR/NS, $n = 10$) or 50 mg/100-gram body weight/0.1 mL of GE (DR/GE, $n = 10$). For reference, normal rats, injected initially with 0.3 mL of only citrate buffer and having normal blood glucose ≤8 mmol/L ($n = 10$), received a single daily intraperitoneal injection of 0.1 mL/100-gram body weight of normal saline (NR/NS, $n = 10$) also for 8 weeks.

2.6. Measurements of Blood Glucose, Blood Pressure, Water Intake, and Urine Output. The following parameters were measured for all rats in each group as follows: blood glucose before and at weeks 4 and 8 of respective treatment; BP at weeks 1 and 8 of respective treatment as an average of 3 readings for each rat using the tail-cuff method (Harvard Apparatus, England); water intake and urine output before and at weeks 1, 4, and 8 of respective treatment for 24 h and calculated for 1 h.

2.7. Collection of Blood and Preparation of Plasma and Serum Samples. At the end of the 8-week treatment period, each rat was anesthetized with an intraperitoneal injection of Thiopental Sodium (4–6 mg/100 g). Within 2-3 minutes, blood was collected via cardiac puncture from each rat as 3 separate portions of 2 mL each into 3 × 15 mL inert-plastic tubes (Falcon, USA) and treated accordingly: (1) 2 mL blood in a tube containing 0.4 mL of a peptidase inhibitor cocktail (0.2 mL trisodium citrate (0.1 M), 0.05 mL O-phenanthroline (0.44 mM), 0.05 mL pepstatin (0.12 mM), 0.05 mL EDTA (0.6 M), and 0.05 mL P-hydroxymercuribenzoic acid (1 mM)) for plasma preparation used for AngII concentration determination, which was done immediately as described below; (2) 2 mL blood in a tube containing 0.2 mL EDTA for plasma preparation used for ACE-1 concentration estimation; (3) 2 mL blood in a tube for serum collection used for insulin, albumin, and creatinine measurement. Collected plasma (except for AngII analysis) and serum samples were stored as approximately 0.5 mL aliquots in Eppendorf tubes at −40°C for later analysis.

2.8. Preparation of Kidneys' Homogenate and Collection of Supernatant Samples. Following collection of blood and

within 30–45 seconds, the left kidney of each rat was excised and while bathing in the peptidase inhibitor cocktail decapsulated cut into 4-5 portions and placed separately in 10 mL, capped inert-glass vials containing 3 mL of the inhibitor. Also, within 30–45 seconds, the right kidney was excised and while bathing in Tris-HCl (0.05 M, pH = 7.6) buffer decapsulated, cut into 4-5 portions, and placed separately in a 10 mL vial containing 3 mL of the buffer. Afterwards, each kidney was homogenized, allowed to stand on ice for few minutes, and then centrifuged for 15 minutes at 8000 ×g at 4°C. The supernatant of each right kidney was stored separately as 0.5 mL aliquots in Eppendorf tubes at −40°C for later analysis, while the supernatant of the left kidney was assayed immediately for AngII and protein concentrations as described below.

2.9. Determination of Insulin, Angiotensin Converting Enzyme I, Angiotensin II, Albumin, and Creatinine Concentrations. These parameters were quantitated using analysis kits supplied as indicated and following the manufacturers' instructions: serum insulin was measured by the ELISA method using kits from SPIbio (France); plasma and kidney ACE-1 concentration were also determined by the ELISA method using kits acquired from Uscn Life Sciences Inc. (China); plasma and kidney AngII were measured by the immunoassay procedure using kits from RayBiotech (USA); serum and urine albumin were determined by a colorimetric technique using kits from BioAssay Systems (USA); and finally, serum and urine creatinine levels were estimated by a colorimetric method using kits from Randox (USA).

2.10. Number of Experimentation Cycles Carried Out. All procedures stated above were carried out through the necessary number of experimental cycles to replace rats that did not develop typical symptoms of DM after STZ injection or died during the different treatment protocols. The rate of success of the first cycle was very high.

2.11. Statistical Analysis. The data are presented in bar graphs as the mean ± SEM of the absolute values of the measured and calculated parameters. Statistical differences between the 3 groups were calculated using *One-Way ANOVA* (SPSS, V 22, IBM) with LSD post hoc test at $P < 0.05$ indicating significance. Differences between the 3 groups at each corresponding stage of the experiment are also presented in percentage values in Results.

3. Results

3.1. Effect of Garlic Extract on Blood Glucose, Body Weight, Water Intake, Urine Output, and Blood Pressure. At day 6 after STZ injection and before commencing the treatment protocol, the blood glucose level of both diabetic rats groups was significantly higher by 195% compared to that of the NR/NS group (Figure 1). The elevated blood glucose was sustained in the DR/NS group during the 8-week treatment period. Alternatively, at week 4 and week 8 of treatment, the DR/GE group had blood glucose levels that were significantly

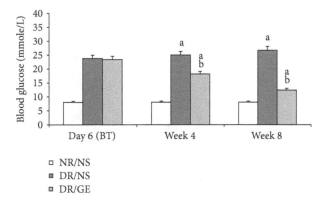

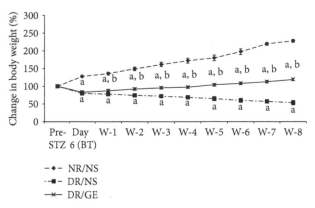

FIGURE 1: GE treatment decreased blood glucose of diabetic rats. Blood glucose was measured at day 6 after STZ injection and at the end of weeks 4 and 8 of the treatment period. NR/NS: normal rats/normal saline treated; DR/NS: diabetic rats/normal saline treated; DR/GE: diabetic rats/garlic extract treated; BT: before treatment; [a]significantly different compared to NR/NS; [b]significantly different compared to DR/NS.

FIGURE 2: GE treatment increased body weight of diabetic rats. GE was administered IP to diabetic rats for 8 weeks abbreviated at DR/GE. Diabetic control rats (DR/NS) and normal control rats (NR/NS) were given normal saline. The animals were weighed before STZ injection (pre-STZ), 6 days after STZ injection (day 6 (BT)), and weekly for the 8-week treatment period. Weights are plotted as percentiles with the starting weights all standardized to 100%. Pre-STZ: before streptozotocin administration; BT: before treatment; w: week; [a]significantly different compared to NR/NS; [b]significantly different compared to DR/NS.

less by 27 and 54%, respectively, compared to the DR/NS group; however, these levels were significantly higher than those of NR-NS group by 128% at week 4 and 55% at week 8 (Figure 1).

The initial body weight average of the rats for each group was similar among the 3 groups. However, as the study proceeded, the average body weight started to shift at day 6 after STZ injection, where the NR/NS body weight started to increase, while both diabetic groups' body weight started, slightly but significantly, to decline compared to their and the NR/NS initial weight. As the treatment proceeded, the NR/NS weight increased steadily, while the DR/NS weight decreased continuously. Alternatively, the DR/GE weight picked up from the initial drop and even showed a slight gain at the last 2-3 weeks compared to their starting weight. At the end of the treatment protocol, the 3 groups of rats showed the following changes in body weight: NR/NS gained 135%; DR/NS lost 54%; DR/GE gained 18% (Figure 2).

Again, at day 6 after STZ injection and before starting the treatment protocol, the measured water intake and urine output of both diabetic groups were significantly higher by an average of 381 and 900%, respectively, compared to the water intake and urine output measured for the NR/NS group. The NR/NS group's water intake and urine output did not change significantly when measured at week 4 and week 8. As far as the DR/NS group is concerned, not only did these rats' elevated water intake and urine output remain significantly higher, but their water intake even increased steadily to higher levels at week 4 and week 8 of the treatment period. As for the DR/GE group, although these rats water intake and urine output were still significantly higher than the measured values of the NR/NS at week 4 and week 8 by an average of 323 and 555%, respectively, the values of these parameters at these same weeks for the GE-treated diabetic group were significantly less by an average of 29 and 20%, respectively, compared to the values of the DR/NS group (Figure 3).

At week 1 of the treatment period, the NR/NS group BP was within normal range and remained at that level when measured at week 8. Alternatively and at week 1, both the DR/NS and DR/GE groups had a significantly higher BP by an average of 65% compared to the NR/NS group. Although this elevated BP was still evident for both of the DR/NS and DR/GE groups at week 8, it was slightly but significantly less in the DR/GE group by an average of 10% compared to both this group's reading at week 1 and the DR/NS group reading at week 8 (Figure 4).

3.2. Effect of Garlic Extract on Insulin, Angiotensin Converting Enzyme-1, Angiotensin II, Albumin, and Creatinine. At the end of the 8-week treatment period, the serum insulin level for the DR/NS group was significantly less by 89% compared to the insulin value measured for the NR/NS group. In the DR/GE group, although the insulin level was still less than for the NR/NS by 54%, it was significantly higher by 331% compared to the insulin level measured for the DR/NS group (Figure 5).

The plasma and kidney levels of ACE-1 in the NR/NS group were 550 pg/mL and 1917 pg/mg protein, respectively. In the DR/NS group, and compared to the NR/NS, ACE-1 levels showed opposite, yet significant changes, where the plasma ACE-1 was higher by 37% and the kidney ACE-1 was lower by 48%. In the DR/GE group, the plasma and kidney ACE-1 values, with only minor but significant difference of 14%, were almost comparable to those measured in the NR/NS group (Figure 6).

In the DR/NS and DR/GE rats, the observed changes in the plasma and kidney AngII levels showed parallel behaviors to those quantitated for their respective ACE-1 concentrations. More precisely, the plasma AngII level was

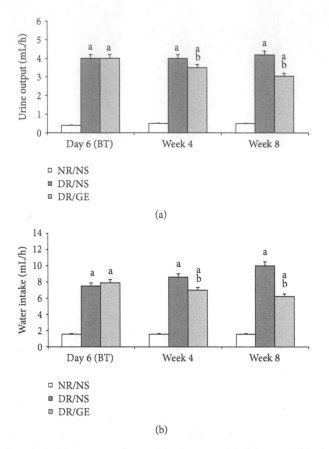

(a)

(b)

FIGURE 3: GE treatment decreased urine output and water intake of diabetic rats. (a) Urine output (mL/h) and (b) water intake (mL/h) were measured before treatment (BT) and after 4 and 8 weeks of treatment. NR/NS: normal rats/normal saline treated; DR/NS: diabetic rats/normal saline treated; DR/GE: diabetic rats/garlic extract treated; BT: before treatment; [a]significantly different compared to NR/NS; [b]significantly different compared to DR/NS.

significantly higher by 25% in the DR/NS group compared to that in the NR/NS group and less by 29% in the DR/GE group than in the DR/NS group. As for the kidney AngII concentration, it was significantly less by 57% in the DR/NS group than in the NR/NS group and higher by 92% in the DR/GE group than in the DR/NS group. Although the plasma and kidney AngII levels in the DR/GE group were almost comparable to those in the NR/NS, they were still significantly different by 10 and 22%, respectively, in a manner almost similar to that observed for the ACE-1 (Figure 7).

The concentration of serum albumin was significantly less by 55% in the DR/NS group than in the NR/NS group. On the other hand, in the DR/GE group, the level of serum albumin was significantly higher by 56% than in the DR/NS group and less by 31% compared to that in the NR/NS group. The urine albumin showed opposite concentration patterns to those measured for the serum in the three rat groups. The level of urine albumin was considerably higher by 147% in the DR/NS group compared to the NR/NS group and was less by 69% in the DR/GE group than in the DR/NS group, which was less by 24% than in the NR/NS group (Figure 8).

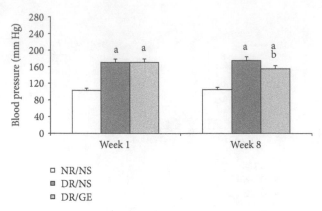

FIGURE 4: GE treatment lowers blood pressure of diabetic rats. Systolic blood pressure (mm Hg) was measured after STZ (week 1) and at the end of the treatment period (week 8). NR/NS: normal rats/normal saline treated; DR/NS: diabetic rats/normal saline treated; DR/GE: diabetic rats/garlic extract treated; [a]significantly different compared to NR/NS; [b]significantly different compared to DR/NS.

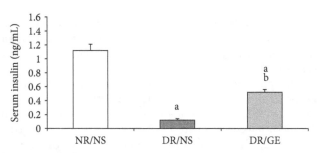

FIGURE 5: GE treatment increased serum insulin of diabetic rats. Serum insulin was quantitated at the end of the treatment period (week 8). NR/NS: normal rats/normal saline treated; DR/NS: diabetic rats/normal saline treated; DR/GE: diabetic rats/garlic extract treated; [a]significantly different compared to NR/NS; [b]significantly different compared to DR/NS.

The magnitude of serum creatinine was significantly higher by 41% in the DR/NS group compared to the NR/NS group, while in the DR/GE group the serum creatinine level was significantly less by 22% than in the DR/NS group and higher by 9.6% compared to that measured in the NR/NS group (Figure 9(a)). The urine creatinine levels showed similar pattern of change to that observed in the serum of the diabetic groups. Notably, the urine creatinine level was considerably higher by 908% in the DR/NS group compared to that quantified for the NR/NS group and less by 43% in the DR/GE group compared to that in the DR/NS group. Furthermore, the urine creatinine level remained higher by 471% in the DR/GE group than in the NR/NS group (Figure 9(b)). As for creatinine clearance, it was significantly higher by 240% in the DR/NS group than in the NR/NS group. Conversely, in the DR/GE rats, although the creatinine clearance was still higher by 98% than the level calculated for the NR/NS, it was less by 42% compared to the magnitude estimated for the DR/NS group (Figure 9(c)).

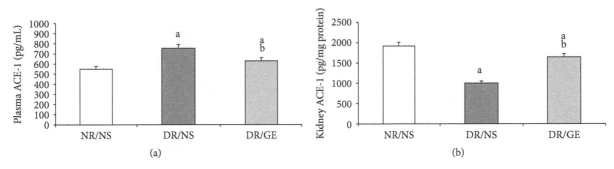

Figure 6: GE treatment decreased plasma ACE-1 and increased kidney ACE-1 in diabetic rats. ACE-1 was quantitated in both (a) plasma (pg/mL) and (b) kidney (pg/mg) at the end of the treatment period (week 8). NR/NS: normal rats/normal saline treated; DR/NS: diabetic rats/normal saline treated; DR/GE: diabetic rats/garlic extract treated; [a]significantly different compared to NR/NS; [b]significantly different compared to DR/NS.

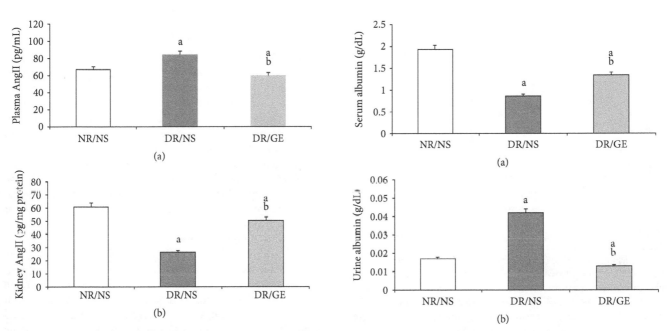

Figure 7: GE treatment decreased plasma AngII and increased kidney AngII in diabetic rats. AngII was quantitated in both (a) plasma (pg/mL) and (b) kidney (pg/mg) at the end of the treatment period (week 8). NR/NS: normal rats/normal saline treated; DR/NS: diabetic rats/normal saline treated; DR/GE: diabetic rats/garlic extract treated; [a]significantly different compared to NR/NS; [b]significantly different compared to DR/NS.

Figure 8: GE treatment reversed albuminuria of diabetic rats. Serum albumin (a) and urine albumin (b) were determined (g/dL) at the end of the treatment period (week 8). NR/NS: normal rats/normal saline treated; DR/NS: diabetic rats/normal saline treated; DR/GE: diabetic rats/garlic extract treated; [a]significantly different compared to NR/NS; [b]significantly different compared to DR/NS.

4. Discussion

Diabetes mellitus is one of the most morbid medical conditions that aggressively afflict a growing number of the world's population [47]. Type-1 DM results from a reduction in insulin secretion that can vary and accordingly determines the severity of this condition. This form of DM can be induced in rats by chemically destroying their pancreatic insulin-producing β-cells using the drug STZ. Experimentally produced STZ-type-1 DM rats develop most of the signature symptoms that are manifested in "naturally" afflicted diabetic humans [48]. It is well known that type-1 DM is a progressive disease that exhibits chronologically varied characteristics

dependent on the time of commencement and aggressiveness of the different pathobiochemical-physiological mechanisms. The arguments presented in this section relate to the renal ACE-1 and AngII findings of this study and pertain to a certain transient stage in the life of STZ-induced DM rats.

In this study and at week 8 following the induction of type-1 DM, the DR/NS showed all the expected symptoms of the early stages of the condition. Many of the early typical abnormalities targeted and observed here included severe hypoinsulinemia (Figure 5), hyperglycemia (Figure 1), body weight loss (Figure 2), water intake (Figure 3(b)), urine output (Figure 3(a)), serum albumin decline (Figure 8(a)) with

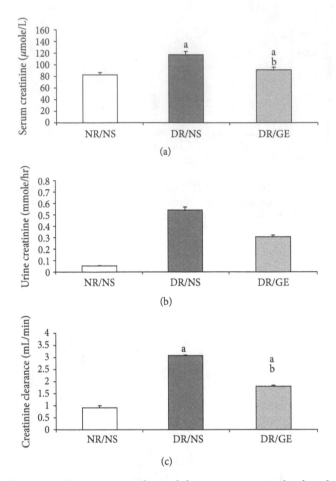

FIGURE 9: GE treatment ameliorated changes in creatinine levels and creatinine clearance of diabetic rats. Creatinine levels in (a) serum (μmole/L) and (b) urine (mmole/hr) were determined at the end of the treatment period (week 8). (c) Creatinine clearance (mL/min) was calculated from these values. NR/NS: normal rats/normal saline treated; DR/NS: diabetic rats/normal saline treated; DR/GE: diabetic rats/garlic extract treated; [a]significantly different compared to NR/NS; [b]significantly different compared to DR/NS.

albuminuria (Figure 8(b)), and elevation in serum and urine creatinine concentration and creatinine clearance (Figure 9), in addition to moderate hypertension (Figure 4). Most of these symptoms have been reported previously in a review by Eleazu et al. [49]. The currently observed pathological rise in water, albumin, and creatinine clearance, as indicators of diseased renal functioning, that is, hyperfiltration and reduced tubular reabsorption, can be taken as evidence of nephronal structural remodeling including glomerular and tubular injury, which have been observed in our laboratory as well as others in early DM [37, 41, 50]. This renal injurious structural remodeling, hence refunctioning, could be the result of increased oxidative stress [51], which, in addition to causing many basic structural deformities [8, 16, 20], leads to abnormal receptor expression of advanced glycation end product (AGEs) [52] that could be partly responsible for glomerular glycation [53]. In addition, the augmented renal clearance function could result from a reduction in the

intrarenal AngII concentration, and therefore a decline in this octapeptide stimulated absorptive power, as discussed next.

One of the focal objectives of this study was investigating the nature of modulations occurring in the levels of plasma and kidney ACE-1 and AngII in the early stages of STZ-induced DM. The ACE-1 observations of DR/NS (Figure 6) in the current study are in line with the view that ACE-1 concentration increases in the plasma and decreases in the kidney [30]. Furthermore, the levels of AngII show that the changes in this octapeptide concentration are in parallel with those of ACE-1, where the systemically measured ACE-1 and AngII increased simultaneously (Figures 6(a) and 7(a)), while the renally measured ACE-1 and AngII decreased simultaneously (Figures 6(b) and 7(b)). What supports the present study's systemic and renal AngII findings are the following measured physical parameters: first, the detected elevation in BP (Figure 4), which could be the result of a rise in the general vascular resistance induced by an increased vasoactivity caused by increased systematic levels of AngII (Figure 7) [7] and second, the observed tremendous increase in renal clearance of water, albumin, and creatinine (Figures 3, 8, and 9), which could possibly have resulted from a reduction in the renal conservation power of the decreased kidney AngII (Figure 7). This possibility is supported by previous studies by our group and others that showed an increase in the kidney's AT_1 receptors in DM [16, 44, 54] indicating a reduction in renal AngII concentration and hence its induced biological effects. This form of dynamic reciprocal change between AngII and its AT_1 receptor represents a classical ligand-receptor relationship that strives to maintain a proper physiological sensitization.

As far as BP is concerned, examination of previous studies carried out on STZ-induced type-1 DM may suggest the existence of two conflicting views. On one hand, a group of studies have reported no change [55] or even a decrease [56, 57] in the exhibited BP. Alternatively, more recent studies, in agreement with the current observation, reported hypertension in the majority [58–60] or a good percentage of the diabetic rats [61]. This view is even supported by the findings of a human study on the same type of diabetes [62]. It is highly conceivable that these differences in the reported BP findings could have been due to the fact that those studies in which observations are inconsistent with the current view were carried out on different rat gender [55], time of measurement and BP model [56], and/or method of measurement [57].

Exploring the GE effect on DM rats' plasma and kidney ACE-1 and AngII concentrations revealed a further dimension to the corrective actions of this natural product. First and as reported here earlier, DR/GE exhibited a significantly higher level of serum insulin (Figure 5), which was associated with more than 50% lower blood glucose (Figure 1), thus providing further support to the suggested hyperinsulinemic-hypoglycemic mechanism of the corrective action of GE reported in the STZ-DM model [37, 39, 41]. Second, and in relationship to another main objective of this study, the corrections in the levels of insulin and glucose by GE were associated with restorations of plasma and renal ACE-1 and AngII concentrations, specifically, a decrease in the plasma

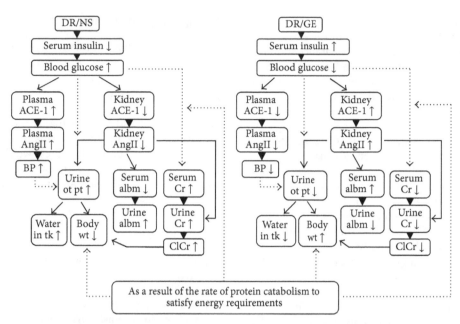

FIGURE 10: Endocrinal, biochemical, and physiological changes in DR/NS (compared to NR/NS) and DR/GE (compared to DR/NS). The schematic suggests that in early STZ-induced hypoinsulinemia the ensuing hyperglycemia leads to an increase in plasma ACE-1 and, as a result and simultaneously, plasma AngII with a concomitant decrease in kidney ACE-1 and, hence, kidney AngII. As a result of these modulations, BP, water intake, serum creatinine, and renal clearance of water, albumin, and creatinine increased significantly; in addition body weight and serum albumin decreased significantly. Conversely and as seen in the DR/GE group, treatment with GE significantly attenuated and counteracted the modulations observed in the DR/NS. DR/NS: diabetic rats treated with normal saline; DR/GE: diabetic rats treated with garlic extract; ACE-1: angiotensin converting enzyme type-1; AngII: angiotensin II; BP: blood pressure; body wt: body weight; urine ot pt: urine output; serum albm: serum albumin; urine Cr: urine creatinine; water in tk: water intake; ClCr: clearance of creatinine; ↑: increase in concentration or amount; ↓: decrease in concentration or amount; ▼/↓: leads to; straight-lined-arrows: suggestions made depending on the data of this study; dotted-lined-arrows: scientific facts.

AngII concentration associated with a reduction in plasma ACE-1 (Figures 6 and 7) and, at the same time, an increase in renal AngII concentration associated with a rise in renal ACE-1 concentration (Figures 6 and 7). The reduction in the systemic AngII generation correlated nicely to the lower BP measured in response to GE treatment (Figure 4), while the increase in renal AngII availability correlated well with the documented effect of GE on restoring normal AT_1/AT_2 balance that is distorted in DM [43, 44]. Furthermore, the increase in renal AngII concentration, in spite of the reported reduction in AT_1 receptor expression [43], suggests an increase in the antidiuretic processes and a reduction in renal albumin and creatinine clearance, which was observed here in the DR/GE. The reduction in these clearance variables also could have been mediated by the attenuation of oxidative stress processes [50], decreased AGE formation [63], and most importantly the reduction of glomerular glycation [53], in addition to actions which presumably delay the progression of diabetic nephropathy. In this study, the observed changes in the concentration of plasma and kidney ACE-1 and AngII and their effects on BP and renal clearance function are in agreement with earlier reports [5–7, 12].

In this study, the observed concurrent rise in both serum and urine creatinine concentrations presents a different perspective regarding the diabetic kidney clearance function of this variable in the early stages of type-1 DM. Typically,

it is suggested that the diabetic kidney GFR declines as a result of glomerulonephritis leading to a fall in creatinine clearance and consequently a rise in its serum concentration [64]. This sort of creatinine handling materializes towards the late stages of DM and the beginning of renal failure. However, during the early onset of DM and when renal clearance function is exaggerated, a greater clearance of creatinine is expected as observed in this study. In connection, the most plausible interpretation for the current rise in urine creatinine, as suggested by the schematic in Figure 10, is the following metabolic cascade: (1) the development of a higher steady-state rate of protein catabolism as an alternative source of energy [65] to compensate for the decline in cellular uptake of glucose due to hypoinsulinemia [66]. This suggestion is supported by the finding in this study that DR/NS were abnormally lean and showed a continuous pathological decline in body weight compared to NR/NS, as well as DR/GE. As expected and consequent to this elevated protein catabolism is a surge in plasma creatinine load and (2) highly elevated GFR in this early stage of DM. This prediction is supported by the increase in creatinine excretion observed in this study, as well as polyuria and glycosuria reported here and elsewhere [67], all of which are classical symptoms of an early diabetic kidney.

Finally, it is worth stating the following: because DM is a progressive disease, the changes in its physiobiochemical mechanisms, associated with developing structural modifications, are also progressive. Therefore and in the early stages, type-1 DM starts with an increase in renal clearance functions permitted by "appropriate" nephronal and renal mechanistic and structural modifications, which shift to a gradual decline in renal clearance function, again, facilitated by "appropriate" nephronal and renal mechanistic and structural alterations, ultimately leading to the classical end-stage case of renal failure. In support, Kikkawa et al. [68] suggested that hypoinsulinemia-induced hyperglycemia causes a biphasic alteration of RAS due to volume depletion and later due to volume expansion. The control DM rats' data in this study, in particular the renal ACE-1 and AngII changes, support the excretory behavior that is noticed here and is well known to occur at the early stages of type-1 DM. The data of this study also suggest a strong correlation between changes in ACE-1 and AngII and insulin and glucose concentrations in DM rats. A relationship between AngII production and glucose concentration, although opposite to what was observed in this study, was shown by Singh et al. [69] in culture studies. Irrespective of the nature of change in AngII generation, the current observations in DR/GE give further support the view that the GE corrective actions on the ACE-1 and AngII concentration are closely mediated via the insulin-glucose pathway. Accordingly, it is highly probable that, whatever the stage of DM, GE may be effective in slowing down distortion of mechanisms, especially those related to ACE-1 and AngII concentration modulation that affect renal structure and function.

5. Conclusion

The findings of this study suggest that the ameliorative action of garlic on the elevated BP and renal clearance functions in early STZ-induced type-1 DM may be partially mediated through attenuating modulations in plasma and renal ACE-1 and AngII concentrations.

Abbreviations

ACE-1: Angiotensin I converting enzyme type-1
AGE: Advanced glycation end product
AngI: Angiotensin I
AngII: Angiotensin II
AT_1:   Angiotensin type-1 receptor
AT_2:   Angiotensin type-2 receptor
BP: Blood pressure
DM: Diabetes mellitus
DR/GE: Diabetic rats/garlic extract
DR/NS: Diabetic rats/normal saline
GC-MS: Gas chromatography-mass spectroscopy
GE: Garlic extract
GFR: Glomerular filtration rate
LSD: Least significant difference
NR/NS: Normal rats/normal saline
RAS: Renin-angiotensin system
SEM: Standard error mean
STZ: Streptozotocin.

Competing Interests

No competing interests, financial or otherwise, are declared by the authors.

Acknowledgments

The authors would like to thank the Research Sector at Kuwait University for funding this project (Research Grant no. SL09/10). In particular, they would sincerely like to acknowledge the major contribution of their late colleague and friend Professor Mohamed H. Mansour, who passed away during the final stages of preparing this paper.

References

[1] M. J. Peach, "Renin-angiotensin system: biochemistry and mechanisms of action," *Physiological Reviews*, vol. 57, no. 2, pp. 313–370, 1977.

[2] M. Paul, A. P. Mehr, and R. Kreutz, "Physiology of local renin-angiotensin systems," *Physiological Reviews*, vol. 86, no. 3, pp. 747–803, 2006.

[3] H. Kobori, M. Nangaku, L. G. Navar, and A. Nishiyama, "The intrarenal renin-angiotensin system: from physiology to the pathobiology of hypertension and kidney disease," *Pharmacological Reviews*, vol. 59, no. 3, pp. 251–287, 2007.

[4] L. G. Navar, K. D. Mitchell, L. M. Harrison-Bernard, H. Kobori, and A. Nishiyama, "Intrarenal angiotensin II levels in normal and hypertensive states," *Journal of the Renin-Angiotensin-Aldosterone System*, vol. 2, no. 1, pp. S176–S184, 2001.

[5] P. S. Leung, "The peptide hormone angiotensin II: its new functions in tissues and organs," *Current Protein and Peptide Science*, vol. 5, no. 4, pp. 267–273, 2004.

[6] L. G. Navar and A. Nishiyama, "Why are angiotensin concentrations so high in the kidney?" *Current Opinion in Nephrology and Hypertension*, vol. 13, no. 1, pp. 107–115, 2004.

[7] M. Burnier, "Angiotensin II type 1 receptor blockers," *Circulation*, vol. 103, no. 6, pp. 904–912, 2001.

[8] H. M. Siragy, "AT_1 and AT_2 receptor in the kidney: role in health and disease," *Seminars in Nephrology*, vol. 24, no. 2, pp. 93–100, 2004.

[9] M. de Gasparo, K. J. Catt, T. Inagami, J. W. Wright, and T. Unger, "The angiotensin II receptors," *Pharmacological Reviews*, vol. 52, no. 3, pp. 415–472, 2000.

[10] E. Kaschina and T. Unger, "Angiotensin AT_1/AT_2 receptors: regulation, signalling and function," *Blood Pressure*, vol. 12, no. 2, pp. 70–88, 2003.

[11] R. M. Carey, "Update on the role of the AT_2 receptor," *Current Opinion in Nephrology and Hypertension*, vol. 14, no. 1, pp. 67–71, 2005.

[12] U. C. Brewster and M. A. Perazella, "The renin-angiotensin-aldosterone system and the kidney: effects on kidney disease," *American Journal of Medicine*, vol. 116, no. 4, pp. 263–272, 2004.

[13] G. Wolf, "Molecular mechanisms of angiotensin II in the kidney: emerging role in the progression of renal disease: beyond haemodynamics," *Nephrology Dialysis Transplantation*, vol. 13, no. 5, pp. 1131–1142, 1998.

[14] A. Ribeiro-Oliveira Jr., A. I. Nogueira, R. M. Pereira, W. W. Vilas Boas, R. A. Souza dos Santos, and A. C. Simões e Silva, "The renin-angiotensin system and diabetes: an update," *Vascular Health and Risk Management*, vol. 4, no. 4, pp. 787–803, 2008.

[15] K. G. Alberti and P. Z. Zimmet, "Definition, diagnosis and classification of diabetes mellitus and its complications. Part 1: diagnosis and classification of diabetes mellitus," *Provisional Report of a WHO Consultation*, vol. 15, no. 7, pp. 535–622, 1998.

[16] H. M. Siragy, A. Awad, P. Abadir, and R. Webb, "The angiotensin II type 1 receptor mediates renal interstitial content of tumor necrosis factor-α in diabetic rats," *Endocrinology*, vol. 144, no. 6, pp. 2229–2233, 2003.

[17] D. J. Kelly, J. L. Wilkinson-Berka, T. J. Allen, M. E. Cooper, and S. L. Skinner, "A new model of diabetic nephropathy with progressive renal impairment in the transgenic (mRen-2)27 rat (TGR)," *Kidney International*, vol. 54, no. 2, pp. 343–352, 1998.

[18] G. M. London, S. J. Marchais, A. P. Guerin, F. Metivier, and H. Adda, "Arterial structure and function in end–stage renal disease," *Nephrology Dialysis Transplantation*, vol. 17, no. 10, pp. 1713–1724, 2002.

[19] L. G. Navar, G. Saccomani, and K. D. Mitchell, "Synergistic intrarenal actions of angiotensin on tubular reabsorption and renal hemodynamics," *American Journal of Hypertension*, vol. 4, no. 1 I, pp. 90–96, 1991.

[20] A. A. Banday and M. F. Lokhandwala, "Oxidative stress-induced renal angiotensin AT1 receptor upregulation causes increased stimulation of sodium transporters and hypertension," *American Journal of Physiology—Renal Physiology*, vol. 295, no. 3, pp. F698–F706, 2008.

[21] G. J. Wehbi, J. Zimpelmann, R. M. Carey, D. Z. Levine, and K. D. Burns, "Early streptozotocin-diabetes mellitus downregulates rat kidney AT_2 receptors," *American Journal of Physiology—Renal Physiology*, vol. 280, no. 2, pp. F254–F265, 2001.

[22] A. C. Hakam and T. Hussain, "Angiotensin II AT_2 receptors inhibit proximal tubular Na^+-K^+-ATPase activity via a NO/cGMP-dependent pathway," *American Journal of Physiology—Renal Physiology*, vol. 290, no. 6, pp. F1430–F1436, 2006.

[23] A. C. Hakam and T. Hussain, "Angiotensin II type 2 receptor agonist directly inhibits proximal tubule sodium pump activity in obese but not in lean Zucker rats," *Hypertension*, vol. 47, no. 6, pp. 1117–1124, 2006.

[24] A. C. Hakam, A. H. Siddiqui, and T. Hussain, "Renal angiotensin II AT_2 receptors promote natriuresis in streptozotocin-induced diabetic rats," *American Journal of Physiology—Renal Physiology*, vol. 290, no. 2, pp. F503–F508, 2006.

[25] H. M. Siragy, "The angiotensin II type 2 receptor and the kidney," *Journal of the Renin-Angiotensin-Aldosterone System*, vol. 11, no. 1, pp. 33–36, 2010.

[26] L. A. Cassis, "Downregulation of the renin-angiotensin system in streptozotocin-diabetic rats," *American Journal of Physiology—Endocrinology and Metabolism*, vol. 262, no. 1, pp. E105–E109, 1992.

[27] S. Anderson, F. F. Jung, and J. R. Ingelfinger, "Renal renin-angiotensin system in diabetes: functional, immunohistochemical, and molecular biological correlations," *American Journal of Physiology—Renal Physiology*, vol. 265, no. 4, pp. F477–F486, 1993.

[28] V. Vallon, L. M. Wead, and R. C. Blantz, "Renal hemodynamics and plasma and kidney angiotensin II in established diabetes mellitus in rats: effect of sodium and salt restriction," *Journal of the American Society of Nephrology*, vol. 5, no. 10, pp. 1761–1767, 1995.

[29] F. Thaiss, G. Wolf, N. Assad, G. Zahner, and R. A. K. Stahl, "Angiotensinase A gene expression and enzyme activity in isolated glomeruli of diabetic rats," *Diabetologia*, vol. 39, no. 3, pp. 275–280, 1996.

[30] M. E. Cooper, R. E. Gilbert, D. F. Kelly, and T. Allen, *Chronic Complications in Diabetes: Animal Models and Chronic Complications*, Harwood Academic Publishers: Glycemic Control and Diabetic Nephropathy, Newark, NJ, USA, 2000.

[31] B. J. Nankivell, "Creatinine clearance and the assessment of renal function," *Australian Prescriber*, vol. 24, no. 1, pp. 15–17, 2001.

[32] R. S. Rivlin, "Historical perspective on the use of garlic," *Journal of Nutrition*, vol. 131, no. 3, pp. 951S–954S, 2001.

[33] E. Ayaz and H. C. Alpsoy, "Garlic (*Allium sativum*) and traditional medicine," *Türkiye Parazitolojii Dergisi*, vol. 31, no. 2, pp. 145–149, 2007.

[34] W. L. Li, H. C. Zheng, J. Bukuru, and N. De Kimpe, "Natural medicines used in the traditional Chinese medical system for therapy of diabetes mellitus," *Journal of Ethnopharmacology*, vol. 92, no. 1, pp. 1–21, 2004.

[35] M. Wei, L. Ong, M. T. Smith et al., "The streptozotocin-diabetic rat as a model of the chronic complications of human diabetes," *Heart Lung and Circulation*, vol. 12, no. 1, pp. 44–50, 2003.

[36] S. K. Banerjee and S. K. Maulik, "Effect of garlic on cardiovascular disorders: a review," *Nutrition Journal*, vol. 1, article 1, 2002.

[37] K. Al-Qattan, M. Thomson, and M. Ali, "Garlic (*Allium sativum*) and ginger (*Zingiber officinale*) attenuate structural nephropathy progression in streptozotocin-induced diabetic rats," *e-SPEN Journal*, vol. 3, no. 2, pp. e62–e71, 2008.

[38] G. Saravanan and P. Ponmurugan, "S-allylcysteine improves streptozotocin-induced alterations of blood glucose, liver cytochrome P450 2E1, plasma antioxidant system, and adipocytes hormones in diabetic rats," *International Journal of Endocrinology and Metabolism*, vol. 11, no. 4, article e10927, 2013.

[39] M. Thomson, Z. M. Al-Amin, K. K. Al-Qattan, L. H. Shaban, and M. Ali, "Anti-diabetic and hypolipidaemic properties of garlic (*Allium sativum*) in streptozotocin-induced diabetic rats," *International Journal of Diabetes & Metabolism*, vol. 15, no. 3, pp. 108–115, 2007.

[40] M. Hosseini, S. M. Shafiee, and T. Baluchnejadmojarad, "Garlic extract reduces serum angiotensin converting enzyme (ACE) activity in nondiabetic and streptozotocin-diabetic rats," *Pathophysiology*, vol. 14, no. 2, pp. 109–112, 2007.

[41] M. A. Vazquez-Prieto, R. E. González, N. F. Renna, C. R. Galmarini, and R. M. Miatello, "Aqueous garlic extracts prevent oxidative stress and vascular remodeling in an experimental model of metabolic syndrome," *Journal of Agricultural and Food Chemistry*, vol. 58, no. 11, pp. 6630–6635, 2010.

[42] M. Thomson, K. K. Al-Qattan, J. S. Divya, and M. Ali, "Ameliorative actions of garlic (*Allium sativum*) and ginger (*Zingiber officinale*) on biomarkers of diabetes and diabetic nephropathy in rats: comparison to aspirin," *International Journal of Pharmacology*, vol. 9, no. 8, pp. 501–512, 2013.

[43] M. H. Mansour, K. K. Al-Qattan, M. Thomson, and M. Ali, "Garlic (*Allium sativum*) modulates the expression of angiotensin II AT_2 receptor in adrenal and renal tissues of streptozotocin-induced diabetic rats," *Advances in Biological Chemistry*, vol. 1, pp. 93–102, 2011.

[44] M. H. Mansour, K. Al-Qattan, M. Thomson, and M. Ali, "Garlic (*Allium sativum*) down-regulates the expression of angiotensin II AT1 receptor in adrenal and renal tissues of streptozotocin-induced diabetic rats," *Inflammopharmacology*, vol. 21, no. 2, pp. 147–159, 2013.

[45] M. Ali and S. Y. Mohammed, "Selective suppression of platelet thromboxane formation with sparing of vascular prostacyclin synthesis by aqueous extract of garlic in rabbits," *Prostaglandins, Leukotrienes and Medicine*, vol. 25, no. 2-3, pp. 139–146, 1986.

[46] *Guide for the Care and Use of Laboratory Animals*, Institute of Laboratory Animal Resources: Commission on Life Sciences: National Research Council: National Academy Press, Washington, Wash, USA, 1996.

[47] S. A. Tabish, "Is diabetes becoming the biggest epidemic of the twenty-first century?" *Internal Journal of Health Sciences*, vol. 1, no. 2, pp. 5–8, 2007.

[48] A. J. F. King, "The use of animal models in diabetes research," *British Journal of Pharmacology*, vol. 166, no. 3, pp. 877–894, 2012.

[49] C. O. Eleazu, K. C. Eleazu, S. Chukwuma, and U. N. Essien, "Review of the mechanism of cell death resulting from streptozotocin challenge in experimental animals, its practical use and potential risk to humans," *Journal of Diabetes and Metabolic Disorders*, vol. 12, article 60, 2013.

[50] J. Pedraza-Chaverrí, D. Barrera, P. D. Maldonado et al., "S-allylmercaptocysteine scavenges hydroxyl radical and singlet oxygen in vitro and attenuates gentamicin-induced oxidative and nitrosative stress and renal damage in vivo," *BMC Clinical Pharmacology*, vol. 4, pp. 5–18, 2004.

[51] H. Drobiova, M. Thomson, K. Al-Qattan, R. Peltonen-Shalaby, Z. Al-Amin, and M. Ali, "Garlic increases antioxidant levels in diabetic and hypertensive rats determined by a modified peroxidase method," *Evidence-Based Complementary and Alternative Medicine*, vol. 2011, Article ID 703049, 8 pages, 2011.

[52] K. K. Al-Qattan, M. H. Mansour, M. Thomson, and M. Ali, "Garlic decreases liver and kidney receptor for advanced glycation end products expression in experimental diabetes," *Pathophysiology*, vol. 23, no. 2, pp. 135–145, 2016.

[53] K. K. Al-Qattan, M. Thomson, M. Ali, and M. H. Mansour, "Garlic (*Allium sativum*) attenuate glomerular glycation in streptozotocin-induced diabetic rats: a possible role of insulin," *Pathophysiology*, vol. 20, no. 2, pp. 147–152, 2013.

[54] L. Brown, D. Wall, C. Marchant, and C. Sernia, "Tissue-specific changes in angiotensin II receptors in streptozotocin- diabetic rats," *Journal of Endocrinology*, vol. 154, no. 2, pp. 355–362, 1997.

[55] L. Kohler, N. Boillat, P. Lüthi, J. Atkinson, and L. Peters-Haefeli, "Influence of streptozotocin-induced diabetes on blood pressure and on renin formation and release," *Naunyn-Schmiedeberg's Archives of Pharmacology*, vol. 313, no. 3, pp. 257–261, 1980.

[56] D. Susic, A. K. Mandal, D. J. Jovovic, G. Radujkovic, and D. Kentera, "Streptozotocin-induced diabetes mellitus lowers blood pressure in spontaneously hypertensive rat," *Clinical and Experimental Hypertension*, vol. 12, no. 6, pp. 1021–1035, 1990.

[57] M. J. Katovich, K. Hanley, G. Strubbe, and B. E. Wright, "Effects of streptozotocin-induced diabetes and insulin treatment on blood pressure in the male rat," *Biological Research for Nursing*, vol. 208, no. 3, pp. 300–306, 1995.

[58] S. Raghunathan, P. Tank, S. Bhadada, and B. Patel, "Evaluation of buspirone on streptozotocin induced type 1 diabetes and its associated complications," *BioMed Research International*, vol. 2014, Article ID 948427, 9 pages, 2014.

[59] R. D. Bunag, T. Tomita, and S. Sasaki, "Streptozotocin diabetic rats are hypertensive despite reduced hypothalamic responsiveness," *Hypertension*, vol. 4, no. 4, pp. 556–565, 1982.

[60] X. Si, P. Li, Y. Zhang, W. Lv, and D. Qi, "Renoprotective effects of olmesartan medoxomil on diabetic nephropathy in streptozotocininduced diabetes in rats," *Biomedical Reports*, vol. 2, no. 1, pp. 24–28, 2014.

[61] S. Chen, C. M. Yuan, F. J. Haddy, and M. B. Pamnani, "Effect of administration of insulin on streptozotocin-induced diabetic hypertension in rat," *Hypertension*, vol. 23, no. 6, part 2, pp. 1046–1050, 1994.

[62] E. Matteucci, C. Consani, M. C. Masoni, and O. Giampietro, "Circadian blood pressure variability in type 1 diabetes subjects and their nondiabetic siblings—influence of erythrocyte electron transfer," *Cardiovascular Diabetology*, vol. 9, article 61, 2010.

[63] M. S. Ahmad and N. Ahmed, "Antiglycation properties of aged garlic extract: possible role in prevention of diabetic complications," *Journal of Nutrition*, vol. 136, no. 3, pp. 796S–799S, 2006.

[64] M. Wyss and R. Kaddurah-Daouk, "Creatine and creatinine metabolism," *Physiological Reviews*, vol. 80, no. 3, pp. 1107–1213, 2000.

[65] N. Møller and K. S. Nair, "Diabetes and protein metabolism," *Diabetes*, vol. 57, no. 1, pp. 3–4, 2008.

[66] J. M. Olefsky and M. Kobayashi, "Ability of circulating insulin to chronically regulate the cellular glucose transport system," *Metabolism*, vol. 27, no. 12, supplement 2, pp. 1917–1929, 1978.

[67] R. Sharma, V. Dave, S. Sharma, P. Jain, and S. Yadav, "Experimental models on diabetes: a comprehensive review," *International Journal of Advances in Pharmaceutical Sciences*, vol. 4, pp. 1–8, 2013.

[68] R. Kikkawa, E. Kitamura, Y. Fujiwara, M. Haneda, and Y. Shigeta, "Biphasic alteration of renin-angiotensin-aldosterone system in streptozotocin-diabetic rats," *Renal Physiology*, vol. 9, no. 3, pp. 187–192, 1986.

[69] R. Singh, N. Alavi, A. K. Singh, and D. J. Leehey, "Role of angiotensin II in glucose-induced inhibition of mesangial matrix degradation," *Diabetes*, vol. 48, no. 10, pp. 2066–2073, 1999.

7

Stress and Fatigue Management Using Balneotherapy in a Short-Time Randomized Controlled Trial

Lolita Rapolienė,[1,2] Artūras Razbadauskas,[3,4] Jonas Sąlyga,[2,3] and Arvydas Martinkėnas[5]

[1]Klaipeda Seamen's Health Care Center, Taikos Street 46, LT-91213 Klaipėda, Lithuania
[2]Department of Nursing of Klaipeda University, H. Manto Street 84, LT-92294 Klaipėda, Lithuania
[3]Klaipeda Seamen's Hospital, Liepojos Street 45, LT-92288 Klaipėda, Lithuania
[4]Faculty of Health Science, Klaipėda University, H. Manto Street 84, LT-92294 Klaipėda, Lithuania
[5]Department of Statistics, Klaipėda University, H. Manto Street 84, LT-92294 Klaipėda, Lithuania

Correspondence should be addressed to Lolita Rapolienė; lolita.rapoliene@inbox.lt

Academic Editor: Antonella Fioravanti

Objective. To investigate the influence of high-salinity geothermal mineral water on stress and fatigue. *Method.* 180 seamen were randomized into three groups: geothermal (65), music (50), and control (65). The geothermal group was administered 108 g/L salinity geothermal water bath for 2 weeks five times a week. Primary outcome was effect on stress and fatigue. Secondary outcomes were the effect on cognitive function, mood, and pain. *Results.* The improvements after balneotherapy were a reduction in the number and intensity of stress-related symptoms, a reduction in pain and general, physical, and mental fatigue, and an improvement in stress-related symptoms management, mood, activation, motivation, and cognitive functions with effect size from 0.8 to 2.3. In the music therapy group, there were significant positive changes in the number of stress symptoms, intensity, mood, pain, and activity with the effect size of 0.4 to 1.1. The researchers did not observe any significant positive changes in the control group. The comparison between the groups showed that balneotherapy was superior to music therapy and no treatment group. *Conclusions.* Balneotherapy is beneficial for stress and fatigue reduction in comparison with music or no therapy group. Geothermal water baths have a potential as an efficient approach to diminish stress caused by working or living conditions.

1. Introduction

Stress is an important contributing factor to an individual's quality of life, and high levels of stress, if not managed, can negatively affect an individual's emotions, health, and implicit well-being [1–3]. Stress is linked to the six leading causes of death: heart disease, accidents, cancer, liver disease, lung ailments, and suicide [1]. It is also associated with an individual's absenteeism from work, increased medical expenses, loss of productivity, insomnia, fatigue, cognitive impairment, depression, and other mental or neurological illnesses, hypertension, arthritis, ulcers, asthma, migraines, immune system disturbances, skin diseases, aggression and relational conflict, and substance abuse and increases the negative effects of aging [3–6].

Stress can be caused by noise, vibrations, heat, improper lighting, and rapid acceleration in an individual's work pace,

anxiety, fatigue, frustration, and anger [1, 2]. Stress is the second most frequently reported work-related health problem after musculoskeletal diseases, affecting 22% of workers in the European Union (EU) and accounting for 50–60% of all lost working days, with an annual cost of 20 billion Euro in 2002 (EU-15) [7]. Stress is widespread among health care and education workers and among other white-collar workers and seafarers [7–10]. Seafaring is a dangerous and challenging profession worldwide and is associated with a high level of work-related stress [11–13]. In the EU, prevention of work-related stress is one of the most important new strategies for health and safety at work [14].

Stress has a direct association with fatigue and health [2]. The prevalence of fatigue in the general working population has been estimated to be as high as 22%, and this fatigue is associated with pain, tiredness, nervous system mechanisms, and environmental stimuli in individuals who experience the effects [1, 15]. The effects of fatigue are multifaceted and complex, overlapping various biological areas such as performance, physiology, cognition, and emotion [1].

Health promotion and disease prevention are more important than ever in societies with increasing life expectancy and growing stress levels. Health promotion measures can help prevent the onset of a disease and may have a beneficial effect on the course of the disease, thus contributing to healthy aging with good quality of life [16]. Numerous approaches are available for stress and fatigue management that can decrease patients' suffering from stress and fatigue and enhance their quality of life, but no single approach fits for all individuals. Stress model demonstrates the favorable effects exhibited by sleep, recovery, and social support [2]. It has been proven that relaxation techniques such as behavioral therapy, meditation, yoga, breathing techniques, reflexology, massage, Reiki, water therapy, and others are beneficial for stress reduction [11, 17–21]. Specifically, a technique called music therapy involves the use of music therapeutically to address physical, psychological, cognitive, and/or social functioning for patients of all ages. According to researchers, music therapy improves human psychological conditions, reduces symptoms of anxiousness and depression, and treats long-term stress-related physical ailments [12, 17, 19].

Balneotherapy (lat. balneum – bath + gr. therapeia – treatment, nursing) involves using natural mineral spring water for the prevention and cure of disease. The World Health Organization recognizes the therapeutic impact of medicinal mineral waters, thermal or nonthermal [20]. Natural mineral water is a general term applied to both spring and other underground continental waters (from deep-seated water-wells). Because of high temperature and mineralization, geothermal water can serve people from various economical areas for improving health during balneotherapy procedures [13, 22]. Natural mineral water has been considered a curative tool for millennia, having well-known healing properties in terms of prevention, treatment, and rehabilitation of skin, musculoskeletal, cardiovascular, endocrine, nervous, and other human body systems [11, 16, 20, 23–28]. During the last 30 years, a number of controlled trials have demonstrated the efficacy of balneotherapy in treating certain diseases, mostly musculoskeletal conditions [16, 25, 27, 29].

The essence of balneotherapy effects (including antistress) are local changes caused by the direct influence of mechanical, thermal, and chemical factors through the skin and mucous membranes and complex adjustment reactions as a result of neuroreflexive, humoral mechanisms, caused by stimulation of mechano-, thermo-, baro-, and chemoreceptors by biochemical active substances during the balneoprocedure [21, 30–36].

Researchers in balneotherapy studies commonly used mineral water of 0.6–31.9 g/L total mineralization, excluding studies in the Dead Sea [22, 23, 25, 28, 33–35, 37–39]. We performed the study with 108 g/L TDS in order to increase the effectiveness for the general working population. To our knowledge, there have not been any trials with such a high salinity of thermal water. This study may be the first published in English applying such a highly concentrated brine application in which the mineral age of the water is not less than 1 million years.

The objective of our study was to investigate the influence of high-salinity geothermal mineral water from artificial sources on seamen's stress and fatigue and to find an effective measure of health protection and restoration for individuals working in highly stressful occupations.

2. Patients and Methods

This prospective open-label randomized controlled parallel-group biomedical trial was implemented in observance of the rules of good clinical practice; our research protocol was approved by the Kaunas Regional Biomedical Research Ethics Committee (Approval number BE-2-31/2012). All subjects were informed about the purpose, conditions, and course of the study prior to the inclusion and signed a participant's agreement.

This study was conducted in Klaipėda, Lithuania, during September–November, 2012. The target population consisted of working seamen from Klaipėda region (Lithuania), recruited and examined by a trained independent general practitioner (GP) during a medical examination at a Sea Center in the Seamen's Hospital and Seamen's Health Care Center in Klaipėda city. Out of the 220 seamen, 180 met inclusion criteria and agreed to participate in the study and were subject to a randomization procedure. Inclusion criteria were as follows: male seamen, aged 25–64, and working at sea for more than 5 years, stress and fatigue intensity level more than 2 (visual analogue scale (VAS) from 0 to 10). Our exclusion criteria were related to the following symptoms: acute organic neurological deficit, neoplastic or inflammatory lesion, decompensated cardiovascular disease, unstable metabolic disorders, febrile infections, and cutaneous suppuration.

After the completion of survey for sociodemographic, work-related, and clinical data, 180 subjects were randomized into three groups: the balneotherapy group (65), the music therapy group (50), and the control group (65). The disposition of the participants is shown in Figure 1. The randomization was simple, with generation of random numbers. The generation of random number order was performed by a professional using the SPSS v. 21 software package. The independent professional performing the statistical analysis was aware of the randomization. The enrolled patients completed the balneotherapy and music therapy treatments as outpatients, with no change in their daily routine or work attendance. The same instructions were made for the participants of the control group. The side effects of balneotherapy were supposed to be evaluated by the physician supervising the treatments by means of an observational sheet, side effects of music therapy, in self-administered observational sheets.

The numbers of participants included in the analysis were as follows: in the geothermal group, 55 subjects were analyzed in order to determine the influence of the therapy on stress and fatigue, as well as its effect on the cardiopulmonary system, mood, and pain; in the music therapy group, data from 35 subjects were studied, and, in the control group, 50 participants were analyzed.

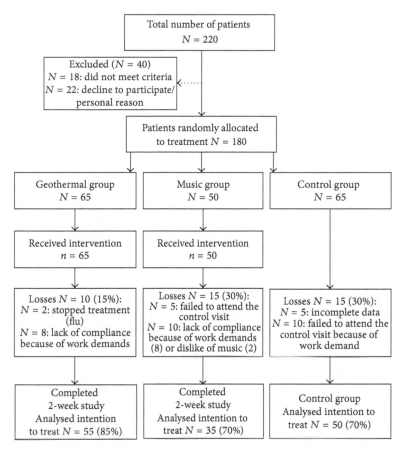

FIGURE 1: Disposition of the study participants.

The balneotherapy group was administered a head-out immersion bath with naturally warm (34.6°C on average) highly mineralized (108 g/L) geothermal Na-Cl-Ca-Mg-SO$_4$ mineral water with a pH 6.07 from a "Geoterma2P" borehole (1135 m depth, Lower Devonian layer, mineral age of more than 1 million years). Volumetric activity of radon in the water was 29 ± 5 Bq/L. The water chemical composition is shown in Table 1.

The subjects underwent balneotherapy sessions for 15 min daily, five times a week, for 2 weeks, and were monitored continuously during the treatment sessions by trained personnel. Each participant was told to move slightly in the bathtub during the procedure. After the baths, participants were recommended to gently dry the skin with a towel and not to shower for about one hour to prolong the effects of the procedure [20]. The study protocol required that participants attend at least 60% of treatments or a minimum of 6 balneotherapy sessions. We performed ten procedures of music therapy at home with Peter Huebner's Medical Resonance Therapy Music© (RRR 932 General Stress) [40]. We used the receptive intervention of music therapy, which asks participants to listen to music, allowing them to become recipients of the musical experience. We used standardized music therapy procedures approved by the Rehabilitation Department of Klaipėda Seamen's Hospital and recommended by Medical Resonance Therapy Music, which involve treatment through the following process: 20 minutes of

sitting or lying down with closed eyes and earphones and avoiding disturbances from outside noise. The participants were trained for the music therapy procedure and for blood pressure and heart rate measurement. They were given self-observational protocols and were asked to record any changes in their general feelings after the procedure. Adherence to the self-administered music therapy protocol was controlled by daily telephone calls.

Baseline and posttherapy assessments of all three groups were performed by a trained GP. The GP's evaluation consisted of overall reported health, medication use, evaluation of pain using visual analogue scale (VAS) from 0 to 10 (0 = no pain; 10 = worst imaginable pain), mood according to Likert's 5-point scale ((1) bad, (2) satisfactory, (3) good, (4) very good, and (5) perfect mood), systolic and diastolic blood pressure (mmHg), and heart and respiratory rates (time/min) as changes in feelings and side effects. Stress and fatigue were assessed by the self-administered general symptoms distress scale (GSDS) [41], the Multidimensional Fatigue Inventory (MFI) [42], and the Cognitive Failures Questionnaire (CFQ) [43].

The primary outcome measures were as follows. (1) First is the change of distress level in the GSDS between baseline and posttreatment evaluations. The GSDS (T. Badger, Arizona, USA) was chosen due to its adequate internal consistency, reliability, good constructional and prognostic validity, and good correlation with depression and positive and negative

TABLE 1: The mineral composition of geothermal water.

Element	Concentration, mg/L
Cl^-	66930
Na^+	27580
Ca^{2+}	8990
Mg^{2+}	2630
SO_4^{2-}	1330
K^+	690
HCO_3^-	74
Br	60.62
N	22
Fe	12.14
B	6.501
Si^{4+}	4.886
Li^+	1.2
Cr	1
F^-	0.91
Mn^{2+}	0.501
H_2S	0.33
Cu^{2+}	0.167
Zn^{2+}	0.062
Total amount of dissolved mineral substances (TDS), mg/L	**108334**

affects [41]. This short psychometric tool allows for assessing specific distress symptoms and evaluating their intensity and control on a 10-point scale. (2) Second is the changes in fatigue scores (MFI). The MFI is a 20-item self-report instrument designed to measure fatigue. It covers the following dimensions: general fatigue, physical fatigue, mental fatigue, reduced motivation, and reduced activity. The use of this instrument offers the opportunity to obtain a profile of fatigue [42]. The secondary outcome measures of the study included such self-assessment scales as CFQ, mood and pain scales, changes in the cardiopulmonary system (blood pressure, heart rate, and respiration rate), and medication use.

The sample size was estimated using the IBM SPSS Sample Power Release software v. 3 for the stress outcome using the general symptoms distress scale (GSDS). We examined mean differences between balneotherapy and the control groups. We estimated that the sample size in both groups should be 32 subjects, with the power of 81.7% to achieve a statistically significantly different result. This computation assumes that the mean difference in the general symptoms distress between the balneotherapy and the control or the music therapy groups would be not less than 0.8, and the standard deviation within the groups would be 1.1. This effect was selected as the least significant effect of detectable importance; any smaller effect would not be of clinical or substantive significance. We assumed that the influence of balneotherapy and music therapy on the difference in the mean values of the variables is valid because such changes during the procedures are fully probable in this field of

research. The mean difference of the observed variables of 0.8 (1.1) would be presented with a 95% CI of 0.25 to 1.35.

3. Statistical Analysis

A descriptive analysis (mean, standard deviation (SD), frequencies, and percentages) was used to examine the participants' background, demographic variables, and treatments. Data were presented with mean (SD). Data distribution was assessed by applying the Kolmogorov-Smirnov test.

We used the parametric criteria and Student's t-test to determine mean differences between two groups; the ANOVA with Bonferroni difference test was applied for multiple comparisons if equal variances were assumed, and Tamhane's T^2 multiple comparison test was used if equal variances were not assumed between the three groups. Due to the nonnormality of the distribution of the variables, nonparametric methods (the Mann-Whitney test) were used in statistical analyses. The categorical variables between the groups were compared using the chi-squared (χ^2) and Fisher's exact test. p-values less than 0.05 were interpreted as statistically significant.

Paired effect sizes before and after the treatment in the groups were estimated with a 95% confidence interval (CI).

The results were evaluated by applying the intention-to-treat analysis (ITT).

The data were analyzed using SPSS (version 21.0; SPSS Inc., Chicago, IL, USA) software.

4. Results

The subjects' sociodemographic and clinical characteristics and health-related issues are shown in Table 2. All three groups were similar concerning sociodemographic characteristic, working conditions, stress, fatigue, and pain frequency and intensity, the perceived health status, and harmful addictions. Lower body mass indices and lower medication usage, yet higher morbidity, were found in the geothermal group. All groups were similar concerning neurological diseases, and a significantly bigger morbidity in musculoskeletal, gastrointestinal, and urological and ear, nose, and throat (ENT) diseases was seen in the geothermal group (Table 2).

After a 2-week treatment, patients receiving geothermal water therapy showed a significant therapeutic response compared to the control and music therapy groups (Table 3).

The inside-the-group analysis showed significant positive changes in primary and secondary (CFQ, mood, and pain) outcome measures with the large effect size from 0.78 to 2.25 ($p < 0.001$). The biggest effect was observed for decreasing stress symptoms, pain, stress intensity, and general fatigue (Table 3).

A significant positive effect of music therapy was seen in the reduction of stress symptoms (large effect) and the intensity of stress (medium effect) and pain (medium effect), as well as an increase in activity (small effect) and mood (medium effect).

During the inside-the-group analysis, the participants of the control group showed significant negative changes

TABLE 2: Sociodemographic and clinical characteristic of the participants in groups.

	Geothermal ($n = 55$)	Music group ($n = 35$)	Control ($n = 50$)	p value
Age, years, mean (SD)[a]	47.5 (10.6)	47.6 (10.7)	46.2 (9.3)	0.733
Education, N (%)[b]				
Secondary school	10 (19.2)	4 (11.8)	4 (8.3)	
College	26 (41.9)	10 (29.4)	21 (43.8)	0.304
Higher education	20 (32.3)	18 (52.9)	21 (43.8)	
Marital status, N (%)[b]				
Single	8 (15.1)	4 (11.4)	2 (4.1)	0.590
Married	36 (67.9)	27 (77.1)	40 (81.6)	
Work experience, years, mean (SD)[a]	22.5 (11.4)	23.1 (11.5)	22.4 (9.9)	0.950
Working hours per day, N (%)[b]				
8–12 hours	32 (58.2)	19 (54.3)	34 (68.0)	
13–15 hours	21 (38.2)	11 (31.4)	12 (24.0)	0.302
16–18 hours	1 (1.8)	3 (8.6)	3 (6.0)	
>18 hours	1 (1.8)	2 (5.7)	0	
Resting hours in 24 hours, N (%)[b]				
10 hours	12 (21.8)	3 (8.6)	8 (16)	
8 hours	17 (30.9)	15 (42.9)	12 (24)	0.366
6 hours	20 (36.4)	14 (40.0)	21 (42)	
<6 hours	6 (10.9)	3 (8.6)	9 (18)	
Leading work position, N (%)[b]	19 (35.2)	14 (46.7)	21 (43.8)	0.433
Frequent stress, N (%)[b]	15 (27.3)	10 (28.6)	14 (28.0)	0.405
Frequent fatigue, N (%)[b]	20 (36.4)	9 (25.7)	10 (20.8)	0.149
Frequent pain, N (%)[b]	4 (7.3)	1 (2.9)	4 (8.0)	0.100
Stress intensity, VAS, cm, mean (SD)[a]	3.8 (1.6)	3.7 (1.9)	3.6 (1.7)	0.820
Pain intensity, VAS, cm, mean (SD)[a]	3.1 (1.7)	2.9 (1.7)	2.4 (1.6)	0.131
Fatigue intensity (0–7), cm, mean (SD)[a]	3.4 (1.3)	3.3 (1.1)	3.3 (1.0)	0.746
Insufficient sleep, N (%)[b]	17 (30.9)	8 (22.9)	12 (24.5)	0.848
BMI, mean (SD)[a]	27.1 (3.0)	28.9 (3.0)	26.7 (5.1)	0.040
Morbidity, N (%)[b]	51 (94.4)[c]	28 (80.0)[d]	34 (68.0)[d]	0.002
Cardiovascular diseases	28 (50.9)	12 (34.4)	16 (32.0)	0.103
Musculoskeletal diseases	48 (87.3)[c]	19 (54.3)[d]	29 (58.0)[d]	0.001
Gastrointestinal diseases	24 (43.6)[c]	11 (31.4)[c]	6 (12.0)[d]	0.002
Neurological diseases	27 (49.1)	14 (40.0)	20 (40.0)	0.571
Respiratory diseases	9 (16.4)	4 (11.4)	4 (8.0)	0.419
ENT diseases	10 (18.2)[c]	1 (2.9)[c]	3 (6.0)[d]	0.031
Urological diseases	19 (34.5)[c]	2 (5.7)[d]	6 (12.0)[d]	0.001
Medication usage, N (%)[b]	19 (29.7)	20 (57.1)	23 (46.9)	0.021
Amount of cigarettes per day, units, mean (SD)[a]	13.5 (6.2)	10.4 (6.3)	14.1 (9.3)	0.399
Amount of alcohol units* per week, mean (SD)[a]	3.75 (3.1)	4.45 (5.84)	3.25 (2.35)	0.384
Good health state, N (%)[b]	32 (58.1)	20 (57.1)	30 (60)	0.332

[a]ANOVA test with Bonferroni correction, [b]chi-squared (χ^2) test, and [c,d]z-test, between proportions from each other $p < 0.05$.
*1 unit = 0.5 pint of beer/lager or a small glass of wine or a pub measure of spirits or a small glass of sherry or port.

in health status concerning stress management, all fatigue dimensions, and cognitive function. No positive changes were seen after 2 weeks (Table 3).

Group comparison is as follows. The changes in the intervention groups (G versus M) were significant in lowering the number of stress symptoms (medium effect size 0.5, 95% CI −0.9 to −0.05 (bias corrected by Hedges)), decreasing pain intensity (large effect size 0.95, 95% CI −1.4 to −0.5), and improving of mood (medium effect size 0.6, 95% CI 0.17 to 1.03) (Table 3). No significant differences were found in other stress items as well as some fatigue dimensions between groups because of significant differences in baseline data.

The comparison between the geothermal and the control groups showed a significant positive therapeutic effect in geothermal group on all primary (stress and fatigue) and secondary (mood and pain) outcomes despite certain

TABLE 3: The effect of changes stress, fatigue, and pain, follow-up compared with baseline; comparison of changes and of treatment groups.

Item	Geothermal, n = 55 Baseline After Mean (SD)	Changes compared to the baseline Mean 95% CI	Effect size[a] 95% CI	p value	Music group, n = 35 Baseline After Mean (SD)	Changes compared to the baseline Mean 95% CI	Effect size[a] 95% CI	p value	Control group, n = 50 Baseline After Mean (SD)	Changes compared to the baseline Mean 95% CI	Effect size[a] 95% CI	p value	Group comparison G-M p_B	G-M p_A	G-C p_B	G-C p_A
Stress symptoms	4.35 (1.85) / 1.71 (1.38)	-2.64 (-2.98 to -2.30)	2.25 (1.94 to 2.55)	<0.001	3.09 (1.58) / 2.37 (1.37)	-0.71 (-0.94 to -0.49)	1.13 (0.79 to 1.48)	<0.001	3.32 (1.77) / 3.38 (1.31)	0.06 (-0.28 to 0.40)	-0.05 (-0.36 to 0.25)	0.722	0.003	0.029	0.010	<0.001
Stress intensity	5.41 (1.78) / 3.16 (1.95)	-2.25 (-2.71 to -1.78)	1.31 (0.96 to 1.66)	<0.001	3.54 (1.72) / 3.00 (1.63)	-0.54 (-0.81 to -0.28)	0.70 (0.30 to 1.09)	<0.001	3.82 (1.83) / 3.80 (1.29)	-0.02 (-0.32 to 0.28)	0.02 (-0.29 to 0.33)	0.894	<0.001	0.681	<0.001	0.050
Stress management	5.64 (1.99) / 7.62 (2.21)	1.98 (1.33 to 2.64)	-0.82 (-1.21 to -0.43)	<0.001	6.77 (2.57) / 7.17 (2.16)	0.40 (-0.25 to 1.05)	-0.22 (-0.77 to 0.34)	0.221	6.44 (2.05) / 6.00 (1.68)	-0.44 (-0.84 to 0.04)	0.32 (-0.05 to 0.69)	0.033	0.050	0.348	0.179	<0.001
General fatigue	46.36 (26.34) / 22.61 (17.45)	-23.75 (-29.43 to -18.07)	1.22 (-2.95 to 5.40)	<0.001	34.64 (22.86) / 31.43 (25.79)	-3.21 (-7.85 to 1.42)	0.24 (-5.47 to 5.95)	0.168	35.38 (19.75) / 40.50 (15.94)	5.1 (2.60 to 7.65)	-0.63 (-4.15 to 2.89)	<0.001	0.064	0.056	0.051	<0.001
Physical fatigue	37.62 (25.54) / 20.83 (18.85)	-16.78 (-22.25 to -11.32)	0.88 (-3.32 to 5.07)	<0.001	34.29 (21.30) / 29.64 (24.92)	-4.64 (-11.46 to 2.17)	0.24 (-5.19 to 5.67)	0.175	27.63 (17.99) / 33.50 (15.14)	5.88 (3.80 to 7.95)	-0.87 (-4.13 to 2.39)	<0.001	1.000	0.061	0.053	<0.001
Reduced activity	44.43 (20.86) / 25.11 (16.99)	-19.32 (-23.89 to -14.75)	1.17 (-2.39 to 4.72)	<0.001	35.99 (18.75) / 29.74 (24.26)	-6.25 (-12.22 to -0.28)	0.39 (-4.69 to 5.47)	0.041	34.88 (18.60) / 39.38 (14.79)	4.50 (2.47 to 6.53)	-0.74 (-4.04 to 2.55)	<0.001	0.196	0.297	0.040	<0.001
Reduced motivation	40.28 (19.97) / 21.41 (16.31)	-18.87 (-23.82 to -13.91)	1.06 (-2.35 to 4.46)	<0.001	28.22 (17.34) / 25.57 (19.10)	-2.65 (-8.92 to 3.62)	0.15 (-4.12 to 4.42)	0.395	28.63 (18.17) / 32.00 (16.25)	3.38 (1.57 to 5.18)	-0.56 (-3.93 to 2.82)	<0.001	0.013	0.283	0.007	0.001
Mental fatigue	33.9 (23.3) / 19.9 (17.6)	-15.34 (-20.53 to -10.15)	0.78 (-3.08 to 4.63)	<0.001	24.46 (20.30) / 24.46 (21.08)	0.0 (-5.13 to 5.13)	0.00 (-4.85 to 4.85)	1.000	23.38 (16.41) / 28.38 (13.55)	5.00 (2.94 to 7.06)	-0.75 (-3.70 to 2.20)	<0.001	0.051	0.268	0.011	0.007
CFQ	31.52 (11.45) / 24.54 (10.40)	-6.98 (-8.76 to -5.21)	1.09 (-0.96 to 3.13)	<0.001	26.59 (13.79) / 22.94 (9.79)	-3.65 (-8.26 to 0.97)	0.28 (-2.52 to 3.09)	0.117	26.02 (9.50) / 27.32 (7.36)	1.3 (0.42 to 2.18)	-0.58 (-2.25 to 1.08)	0.005	0.172	0.476	0.054	0.121
Mood	2.52 (0.87) / 3.62 (0.59)	1.10 (0.49 to 0.94)	-1.03 (-1.16 to -0.89)	<0.001	2.94 (0.54) / 3.29 (0.46)	0.34 (0.16 to 0.53)	-0.65 (-0.77 to -0.54)	0.001	3.08 (0.53) / 3.06 (0.32)	-0.02 (-0.16 to 0.12)	0.05 (-0.04 to 0.13)	0.766	0.031	0.033	<0.001	<0.001
VAS	4.10 (2.74) / 0.71 (1.06)	-3.38 (-4.42 to -2.4)	1.95 (1.56 to 2.34)	<0.001	2.24 (2.02) / 2.03 (1.77)	-0.21 (-0.35 to -0.06)	0.64 (0.19 to 1.08)	0.006	2.06 (1.61) / 1.98 (1.33)	-0.8 (-0.28 to 0.11)	0.13 (-0.16 to 0.42)	0.399	0.004	0.001	0.001	<0.001

VAS: Visual Analog Scale (0–10 cm). CFQ: sum of overall cognitive failures;

G: geothermal, M: music, and C: control groups.

Baseline (B): state before treatment and after (A): state after treatment; [a] 95% CI: 95% confidence interval.

baseline clinical differences between the groups, which were unfavorable to the geothermal group (Tables 2 and 3). Large effect sizes between G versus C groups were found in lowering the stress symptoms (1.2, 95% CI −1.65 to −0.81), pain (1.05, 95% CI −1.46 to −0.65), and general fatigue (1.06, 95% CI −1.47 to −0.65) and in increasing stress management (0.8, 95% CI 0.42 to 1.21), activity (−0.89, 95% CI −1.29 to −0.48), and mood (1.16, 95% CI 0.74 to 1.57); a medium effect size was seen in reducing physical (0.73, 95% CI 1.13 to −0.34) and mental fatigue (0.53, 95% CI −0.92 to −0.14) and increasing motivation (0.65, 95% CI −1.04 to −0.25); and a small effect size was observed for reducing stress intensity (0.38, 95% CI −0.77 to 0.01).

After 2 weeks of balneotherapy treatment, changes in other study secondary outcomes—cardiopulmonary system parameters—were seen: a reduction of systolic (from 136.4 to 129.5 mmHg; mean difference, 7 mmHg; CI 3.03 to 11.7; $p = 0.001$) and diastolic (from 84.3 to 78 mmHg; mean difference, 6 mmHg; CI 3.22 to 8.06; $p < 0.001$) blood pressure, heart rate (from 87.3 to 72.4 bpm; mean difference, 15 bpm; CI 1.03 to 5.0; $p = 0.004$), and respiratory rate (from 15.7 to 14.3 times/min; mean difference, 1.4 times/min; CI 0.47 to 1.7; $p = 0.001$), while in the music therapy group, only the respiratory rate was significantly reduced (from 15.6 to 14.7 times/min; mean difference, 0.9 times/min; CI 0.23 to 1.49; $p = 0.009$). No significant changes were seen in the control group. The differences between the groups were significant ($p < 0.001$).

In the geothermal therapy group, less medication use was observed ($p = 0.047$, $z = 2.0$); no significant changes were observed in the music therapy or the control groups.

Adverse events during balneotherapy were assessed and registered by a GP; they were mild and transient: skin irritation (redness, rash), 4.6% (3), and exacerbation of psoriasis, 1.5% (1). However, no patients had to discontinue treatments because of adverse events. The side effects of music therapy included headaches (3%) (1) and annoyance due to the dislike of the music (3%) (1).

5. Discussion

The results of the study demonstrated that the 2-week geothermal bath had a positive effect on stress, fatigue, mood, pain, and cognitive function, as cardiopulmonary function. Compared to music therapy, balneotherapy showed a more significant effect in reducing stress symptoms and pain and in improving the mood of the participants. When counting large-medium effect sizes, geothermal water treatment was more effective in relieving stress- and fatigue-related symptoms and pain, compared to the results of the control groups. Our study proved the safety of geothermal very high-salinity water as a treatment for the general working population.

A number of trials exploring the benefits of balneotherapy to humans have been conducted [16, 20, 23, 25, 27]. The combined effects of balneotherapy have been shown to result in positive outcomes related to rheumatic, skin, cardiovascular, pulmonary, endocrine, and mental diseases and in the improvement of public health [22–29, 37–39, 44–47]. However, spa medicine is not yet sufficiently recognized in psychiatry [23]. The effect of relaxation, a sense of well-being,

and a reduction of stress are associated with changes in hormones like cortisol or endogenous opiates [21, 35]. Our trial results correlate with positive effects of balneotherapy related to relieving stress, pain, feelings of depression, and burnout and improving the quality of life, sleep, psychoemotional well-being, and mental activity [18, 25, 37, 45–49]. Dubois et al. provided the first research-based proof that balneotherapy was effective and well-suited for the treatment of generalized anxiety disorder. The mean change in Hamilton's total score after 8 weeks was significantly greater in the balneotherapy than in the paroxetine group (−12 versus −8.7; $p < 0.001$); the change in the Montgomery-Asberg Depression Rating Scale was bigger in the balneotherapy group (−8.4 versus −7; $p = 0.04$) [44]. The 3-week trial with Lintong mineral spring water demonstrated a positive effect on tension (from 4.75 to 2.17), anger (from 2.09 to 0.88), fatigue (from 3.46 to 1.12), confusion (from 3.36 to 1.17), and vigor (from 15.87 to 21.71) mood scores ($p < 0.05$), and the mood state of depression-dejection also showed a decreasing trend (from 0.5 to 0.36) [37]. Positive results of a 3-week spa therapy were also observed by Blasche in patients with breast cancer (improved mood and the quality of life) and occupational burnout (reduced general fatigue, distress, and increased motivation) [46]. Compared to resting and progressive muscle relaxation, balneotherapy was more beneficial with regard to subjective effects of relaxation and similarly effective with regard to a decrease in salivary cortisol levels [48]. According to the results of a study by Latorre-Román et al., 12-day balneotherapy had a positive effect on pain, mood, sleep quality, and depression in healthy older people: pain decreased by 1.2 on VAS ($p = 0.001$), depression by 0.18 ($p = 0.03$), anxiety by 0.38 ($p = 0.001$), tension by 0.37 ($p = 0.001$), and fatigue by 0.35 ($p = 0.001$), whereas vigor increased by 0.18 ($p = 0.049$) [49].

There is a strong association between stress and pain [2, 10], and the analgesic effect of thermal water is well-known and confirmed in meta-analyses and systematic reviews [23–25, 27, 50]. Naumann and Sadaghiani conducted a systematic review and meta-analysis of randomized trials on hydrotherapy and balneotherapy in fibromyalgia patients, which showed moderate evidence for a significant reduction of pain at the end of the balneotherapy treatment (standard mean difference (SMD) −0.84; $p = 0.002$) and for a medium improvement in the quality of life (SMD −0.78; $p < 0.0001$); there was no significant effect on depressive symptoms (SMD −0.87; $p = 0.07$) [50]. All the reviewed studies on lower back pain reported that balneotherapy was superior in long term to tap water therapy in relieving pain and improving function and that spa therapy combining balneotherapy with mud pack therapy and/or exercise therapy, physiotherapy, and/or education was effective in the management of low back pain and superior or equally effective to the control treatments in short and long terms [51]. The various articles are exploring the importance and significance of traditional/alternative way of pain treatment with conclusion that pain is best controlled using coordinated efforts of both traditional and alternate measures [52]. Our trial demonstrated that after 2 weeks of procedures, systolic (by 7 mmHg) and diastolic (by 6 mmHg) blood pressure, as well as heart rate (15 bpm) and respiratory rate (1 time/min) lowered among our subjects. This finding is in line with the results of a study conducted by Xu et al., demonstrating improved cardiopulmonary function after thermal baths [38] and safety of the therapy for participants with mild to moderate hypertension [33, 34, 39, 47]. Becker et al. have revealed hydrotherapy effects on lowering blood pressure, 12 mmHg in systolic blood pressure and 26 mmHg in diastolic blood pressure [31]; other scientists found that one mineral bath is lowering systolic blood pressure 2–15 mmHg and reducing heart rate 5-6 t/min [53].

The ability to rest, relax, and recuperate is a form of self-treatment and an important aspect in combating the harmful effects of cumulative stress [17]. Since each person responds to stress differently, there is no single effective stress reduction strategy. Individuals may successfully achieve work- or life-related stress reduction through multidisciplinary work utilizing an integrated approach [7, 14]: organizational risk prevention [5, 8], changing one's mindset from "stress-is-debilitating" to "stress-is-enhancing" (which can profoundly influence psychological, behavioral, and physiological outcomes) [17], living a healthy lifestyle, and using interventions to balance or minimize stress intensity [54] with the help of population-based wellness strategies. Balneotherapy using geothermal water may be a valuable strategy to use [23, 29, 46, 48, 49].

To our knowledge, this study is the first to explore the effect and safety of geothermal mineral water therapy with very high-salinity water. Our results showing big promises for relieving psychoneurological conditions in humans might be related to water mineralization or its origin. The limitations of our study are significant differences in certain scale dimensions between the groups that emerged during the initial stages of the study, the evaluation of the effect of the therapy on the representatives of a single profession and by a single GP, subjective measures of stress and fatigue, administration of music therapy at home, open-label trial, and no follow-up. The challenge for the future will be to carry out well designed studies in larger patient population with different water mineralization levels and follow-up. The results of our study results demonstrate a need for further research in balneotherapy using geothermal waters as a stress-reducing tool as well as a separate tool for disease prevention and treatment.

6. Conclusions

(1) Geothermal water baths reduce stress, fatigue, and pain, improve mood, stress management and cognitive functions, and have a positive effect on the cardiopulmonary system.

(2) Balneotherapy using geothermal water proved to be more efficient for relieving stress and pain than music therapy was, whereas, for all stress- and fatigue-related conditions, it was more efficient than no therapy.

(3) Balneotherapy could be an effective measure for stress prevention and health restoration as an integral part of a multimodal work-related stress-reducing program.

Ethical Approval

Approval was obtained from Kaunas Regional Biomedical Research Ethics Committee, no. BE-2-31/2012 (Lithuania).

Competing Interests

There are no competing interests regarding this paper.

References

[1] J. L. McLauglin, *Stress, fatigue and workload: determining the combined effect on human performance [Doctor Dissertation]*, University of Central Florida, Orlando, Fla, USA, 2007.

[2] S. Maghout-Juratli, J. Janisse, K. Schwartz, and B. B. Arnetz, "The causal role of fatigue in the stress-perceived health relationship: a MetroNet study," *Journal of the American Board of Family Medicine*, vol. 23, no. 2, pp. 212–219, 2010.

[3] B. M. Kudielka and S. Wüst, "Human models in acute and chronic stress: assessing determinants of individual hypothalamus-pituitary-adrenal axis activity and reactivity," *Stress*, vol. 13, no. 1, pp. 1–14, 2010.

[4] T. Rosenthal and A. Alter, "Occupational stress and hypertension," *Journal of the American Society of Hypertension*, vol. 6, no. 1, pp. 2–22, 2012.

[5] European Commission and Directorate for Employment-Social Affairs and Inclusion, *Guidance on Work-Related Stress—Spice of Life or Kiss of Death?* Office for Official Publications of the European Communities, Luxembourg City, Luxembourg, 2000, http://bookshop.europa.eu/is-bin/INTERSHOP.enfinity/WFS/EU-Bookshop-Site/en_GB/-/EUR/ViewPublication-Start?PublicationKey=CE2599851.

[6] How to measure human stress, Center for studies on human stress, Ferrnand-Sequin Research Center, Canada, 2007.

[7] European Agency for Safety and Health at Work, *OSH in Figures: Stress at Work. Facts and Figures*, European Agency for Safety and Health at Work, Bilbao, Spain, 2009.

[8] R. Kuodytė-Kazėlienė, I. Užaitė, R. Palinauskienė, A. Kuznikovas, L. Šerytė, and R. Ulianskienė, "Prevalence of stress, depression and anxiety in healthcare and education workers in Panevezystawn," *Medicinosteorijairpraktika* , vol. 13, no. 4, pp. 479–484, 2007.

[9] R. T. B. Iversen, "The mental health of seafarers," *International Maritime Health*, vol. 63, no. 2, pp. 78–89, 2012.

[10] J. Sąlyga, "Lifestyle of Lithuanian seamen at the sea: fatigue, stress and related factors," *Sveikatos Mokslai*, vol. 2, pp. 1664–1669, 2008.

[11] N. A. Lysov, V. V. Goryachev, and V. Goryachev, *Resort Medicine: Monography*, NSEI HPE Medical Institute REAVIZ, 2013.

[12] L. Bernardi, C. Porta, G. Casucci et al., "Dynamic interactions between musical, cardiovascular, and cerebral rhythms in humans," *Circulation*, vol. 119, no. 25, pp. 3171–3180, 2009.

[13] HydroGlobe, "Definition of a global framework for hydrotherapy A FEMTEC—FoRSTjoint project with the cooperation of ISMH and the technical support oh WHO," *Essentials from the Final Report*, 2013, http://termasworld.com/documentos/hydroglobe.pdf.

[14] J. Burton, *WHO Healthy Workplace Framework and Model: Background and Supporting Literature and Practices*, World Health Organization, Geneva, Switzerland, 2010, https://osha.europa.eu/en/tools-and-publications/publications/reports/priorities-for-occupational-safety-and-health-research-in-europe-2013-2020.

[15] A. Smith, P. Allen, and A. Wadsworth, *Seafarer Fatigue: The Cardiff Research Programme*, Cardiff University, Centre for Occupational and Health Psychology, Cardiff, UK, 2006.

[16] M. Stier-Jarmer, S. Kus, D. Frisch, C. Sabariego, and A. Schuh, "Health resort medicine in non-musculoskeletal disorders: is there evidence of its effectiveness?" *International Journal of Biometeorology*, vol. 59, no. 10, pp. 1523–1544, 2015.

[17] A. J. Crum, P. Salovey, and S. Achor, "Rethinking stress: the role of mindsets in determining the stress response," *Journal of Personality and Social Psychology*, vol. 104, no. 4, pp. 716–733, 2013.

[18] M. Sekine, A. Nasermoaddeli, H. Waqng, H. Kanayma, and S. Kagamimori, "Spa resort use and health-related quality of life, sleep, sickness absence and hospital admission: the Japanese civil servants study," *Complementary Therapiesin Medicine*, vol. 14, no. 2, pp. 133–143, 2006.

[19] R. McCaffrey, "Music listening: its effects in creating a healing environment," *Journal of Psychosocial Nursing and Mental Health Services*, vol. 46, no. 10, pp. 39–44, 2008.

[20] VŠĮ Lithuanian Resort Research Center, *Standardized Recommendation for Mineral Water Use in Resorts for Wellness, Prevention, Treatment and Rehabilitation*, VŠĮ Lithuanian Resort Research Center, Druskininkai, Lithuania, 2008.

[21] M. Toda, K. Morimoto, S. Nagasawa, and K. Kitamura, "Change in salivary physiological stress markers by spa bathing," *Biomedical Research*, vol. 27, no. 1, pp. 11–14, 2006.

[22] M. Gudmundsóttir, A. Brynjólfsdóttir, and A. Albertsson, "The history of the blue lagoon in Svartsengi," in *Proceedings of the World Geothermal Congress*, Bali, Indonesia, April 2010.

[23] F. Maraver and Z. Karagulle, *Medical Hydrology and Balneology: Environmental Aspects*, vol. 6 of *Serie de Monografias*, 2012.

[24] A. Fraioli, G. Mennuni, M. Grassi et al., "SPA treatments of diseases pertaining to internal medicine," *Clinica Terapeutica*, vol. 161, no. 2, pp. e63–e79, 2011.

[25] M. E. Falagas, E. Zarkadoulia, and P. I. Rafailidis, "The therapeutic effect of balneotherapy: evaluation of the evidence from randomised controlled trials," *International Journal of Clinical Practice*, vol. 63, no. 7, pp. 1068–1084, 2009.

[26] A. Françon and R. Forestier, "Spa therapy in rheumatology. Indications based on the clinical guidelines of the French National Authority for health and the European League Against Rheumatism, and the results of 19 randomized clinical trials," *Bulletin de l'Academie Nationale de Medecine*, vol. 193, no. 6, pp. 1345–1356, 2009.

[27] A. Nassermoaddeli and A. Kagamimori, "Balneotherapy in medicine: a review," *Environmental Health and Preventive Medicine*, vol. 10, no. 4, pp. 171–179, 2005.

[28] K. Horváth, Á. Kulisch, A. Németh, and T. Bender, "Evaluation of the effect of balneotherapy in patients with osteoarthritis of the hands: a randomized controlled single-blind follow-up study," *Clinical Rehabilitation*, vol. 26, no. 5, pp. 431–441, 2012.

[29] T. Bender, G. Bálint, Z. Prohászka, P. Géher, and I. K. Tefner, "Evidence-based hydro- and balneotherapy in Hungary—a systematic review and meta-analysis," *International Journal of Biometeorology*, vol. 58, no. 3, pp. 311–323, 2014.

[30] S. Tenti, A. Fioravanti, G. M. Guidelli, N. A. Pascarelli, and S. Cheleschi, "New evidence on mechanisms of action of spa therapy in rheumatic diseases," *TANG Humanitas Medicine*, vol. 4, no. 1, p. e3, 2014.

[31] B. E. Becker, K. Hildenbrand, R. K. Whitcomb, and J. P. Sanders, "Biophysiologic effects of warm water immersion," *International Journal of Aquatic Research and Education*, vol. 3, pp. 24–37, 2009.

[32] M. Vitale, "Basic sciences and balneology," in *Proceedings of the European Thermal Meeting*, Enghien-les-Bains, France, November 2013, http://www.europeanspas.eu/press/Post_conference_News_European_Thermal_Meeting.

[33] M. Oláh, A. Koncz, J. Fehér et al., "The effect of balneotherapy on C-reactive protein, serum cholesterol, triglyceride, total antioxidant status and HSP-60 levels," *International Journal of Biometeorology*, vol. 54, no. 3, pp. 249–254, 2011.

[34] M. Oláh, Á. Koncz, J. Fehér et al., "The effect of balneotherapy on antioxidant, inflammatory, and metabolic indices in patients with cardiovascular risk factors (hypertension and obesity)—a randomised, controlled, follow-up study," *Controlled Clinical Trials*, vol. 32, no. 6, pp. 793–801, 2011.

[35] S. Baroni, D. Marazziti, G. Concoli, M. Piccheti, M. Catena-Dell'osso, and A. Galassi, "Modulation of the platelet serotonin transporter by thermal balneotherapy: a study in healthy subjects," *European Review for Medical and Pharmacological Sciences*, vol. 16, pp. 589–593, 2012.

[36] K. Yamamoto, Y. Aso, S. Nagata, K. Kasugai, and S. Maeda, "Autonomic, neuro-immunological and psychological responses to wrapped warm footbaths—a pilot study," *Complementary Therapies in Clinical Practice*, vol. 14, no. 3, pp. 195–203, 2008.

[37] L. Xu, R. Shi, B. Wang et al., "Effect of 3 weeks of balneotherapy on immunological parameters, trace metal elements and mood states in pilots," *Journal of Physical Therapy Science*, vol. 25, no. 1, pp. 51–54, 2013.

[38] L. Xu, R. Shi, B. Wang et al., "21-day balneotherapy improves cardiopulmonary function and physical capacity of pilots," *Journal of Physical Therapy Science*, vol. 25, no. 1, pp. 109–112, 2013.

[39] A. Kapetanovic, S. Hodžic, and D. Advic, "The effect of mineral radon water applied in the form of full baths on blood pressure in patients with hypertension," *Journal of Health Sciences*, vol. 3, no. 1, pp. 38–40, 2013.

[40] P. Hubner, "Medical Resonance Therapy Music," General Stress Symptoms Medical Music Program, http://www.dynamicspacestereophony.com/ScientificResearch/science.php?track=10001099.

[41] T. A. Badger, C. Segrin, and P. Meek, "Development and validation of an instrument for rapidly assessing symptoms: the general symptom distress scale," *Journal of Pain and Symptom Management*, vol. 41, no. 3, pp. 535–548, 2011.

[42] A. J. Dittner, S. C. Wessely, and R. G. Brown, "The assessment of fatigue. A practical guide for clinicians and researchers," *Journal of Psychosomatic Research*, vol. 56, no. 2, pp. 157–170, 2004.

[43] D. E. Broadbent, P. F. Cooper, P. FitzGerald, and K. R. Parkes, "The cognitive failures questionnaire (CFQ) and its correlates," *British Journal of Clinical Psychology*, vol. 21, no. 1, pp. 1–16, 1982.

[44] O. Dubois, R. Salamon, C. Germain et al., "Balneotherapy versus paroxetine in the treatment of generalized anxiety

disorder," *Complementary Therapies in Medicine*, vol. 18, no. 1, pp. 1–7, 2010.

[45] M. Secher, M. Soto, S. Gillette et al., "Balneotherapy, prevention of cognitive decline and care the Alzheimer patient and his family: Outcome of a multidisciplinary workgroup," *Journal of Nutrition, Health and Aging*, vol. 13, no. 9, pp. 797–806, 2009.

[46] G. Blasche, "Association of spa therapy with improvement of psychological symptoms of occupational burnout," *Forschende Komplementärmedizin*, vol. 17, no. 3, pp. 132–136, 2010.

[47] L. M. Iashina, L. E. Shatrova, K. S. Zhdanova, and T. A. Kuznetsova, "The influence of radon baths on the lipid profi le of patients with cardiovascular diseases and dyslipidemia," *Voprosy Kurortologii, Fizioterapii, I Lechebnoĭ Fizicheskoĭ Kultury*, no. 2, pp. 3–4, 2011.

[48] F. Matzer, E. Nagele, B. Bahadori, K. Dam, and C. Fazekas, "Stress-relieving effects of short-term balneotherapy—a randomized controlled pilot study in healthy adults," *Forschende Komplementarmedizin*, vol. 21, no. 2, pp. 105–110, 2014.

[49] P. Á. Latorre-Román, M. Rentero-Blanco, J. A. Laredo-Aguilera, and F. García-Pinillos, "Effect of a 12-day balneotherapy programme on pain, mood, sleep, and depression in healthy elderly people," *Psychogeriatrics*, vol. 15, no. 1, pp. 14–19, 2015.

[50] J. Naumann and C. Sadaghiani, "Therapeutic benefit of balneo therapy and hydro therapyinthe management of fibromyalgia syndrome: a qualitative systematic reviewand meta-analysis of randomized controlledtrials," *Arthritis Research & Therapy*, vol. 16, no. 4, article R141, 2014.

[51] M. Karagülle and M. Z. Karagülle, "Effectiveness of balneotherapy and spa therapy for the treatment of chronic low back pain: a review on latest evidence," *Clinical Rheumatology*, vol. 34, no. 2, pp. 207–214, 2015.

[52] H. Khan, B. Eto, V. De Feo, and A.-U.-H. Gilani, "Evidence based alternative medicines in pain management," *Evidence-Based Complementary and Alternative Medicine*, vol. 2015, Article ID 313821, 2 pages, 2015.

[53] E. V. Vladimirsky and T. N. Filtsagina, "The problems of anti-hypertensive balneotherapy," *Voprosy Kurortologii, Fizioterapii, I Lechebnoĭ Fizicheskoĭ Kultury*, no. 5, pp. 40–45, 2013.

[54] L. O. Fjorback, "Mindfulness and bodily distress," *Danish Medical Journal*, vol. 59, no. 11, Article ID B4547, 2012.

8

The Effects of Xiangqing Anodyne Spray on Treating Acute Soft-Tissue Injury Mainly Depend on Suppressing Activations of AKT and p38 Pathways

Shudong Wang,[1] Tao Li,[2] Wei Qu,[2] Xin Li,[2] Shaoxin Ma,[2] Zheng Wang,[1] Wenya Liu,[1] Shanshan Hou,[2] and Jihua Fu[3]

[1]*Department of Pharmaceutics, Jinling Hospital, Nanjing University School of Medicine, Nanjing 210002, China*
[2]*China Pharmaceutical University, Nanjing 211198, China*
[3]*Department of Physiology, China Pharmaceutical University, 639 Long Mian Road, Nanjing, Jiangsu 211198, China*

Correspondence should be addressed to Jihua Fu; jihua_fu@cpu.edu.cn

Academic Editor: Ki-Wan Oh

Objectives. In the present study we try to elucidate the mechanism of Xiangqing anodyne spray (XQAS) effects on acute soft-tissue injury (STI). *Methods.* Acute STI model was established by hammer blow in the rat hind leg muscle. Within 8 hours, instantly after modeling and per 2-hour interval repeated topical applications with or without XQAS, CP or IH ethanol extracts spray (CPS and IHS) were performed, respectively; muscle swelling rate and inflammation-related biochemical parameters, muscle histological observation, and mRNA and protein expression were then examined. *Results.* XQAS dose-dependently suppressed STI-caused muscle swelling, proinflammatory mediator productions, and oxidative stress as well as severe pathological changes in the injured muscle tissue. Moreover, CPS mainly by blocking p38 activation while IHS majorly by blocking AKT activation led to cytoplastic IκBα degradation with NF-κB p65 translocated into the nucleus. There are synergistic effects between CP and IH components in the XQAS on preventing from acute STI with suppressing IκBα degradation, NF-κB p65 translocation, and subsequent inflammation and oxidative stress-related abnormality. *Conclusion.* Marked effects of XQAS on treating acute STI are ascribed to strong anti-inflammatory and antioxidative actions with a reasonable combination of CP active components, blocking p38-NF-κB pathway activated, and IH active components, blocking AKT-NF-κB pathway activated.

1. Introduction

There are many ancient archives for treatment of soft-tissue injury (STI) using Traditional Chinese Medicine. STI care can be traced back to early civilizations, and many of these treatments were based on the use of herbal remedies. The report showed that approximately one-third of all traditional medicines in use are for the treatment of wounds and soft-tissue disorders, compared to only 1%–3% of modern drugs [1]. Xiangqing anodyne spray (XQAS) is a spray formulation by topical administration, which is a mixture of two ethanol extracts that were extracted, respectively, from equal-mass crude of two Traditional Chinese Medicines, *Cynanchum paniculatum* (CP) and *Illicium henryi* (IH), with additional penetration enhancers. In previous study, we have found that

XQAS effects on treating neuralgia and postherpetic neuralgia in clinical application were prominent and superior to the ethanol extract of IH or CP treatment alone [2, 3]. In the modern medicine, the ethanol or water-soluble extracts of CP have been demonstrated to relieve various pains, such as rheumatic arthralgia, lumbago, pain due to traumatic injuries, abdominal pain, and toothache, which were also used to treat skin diseases such as eczema, rubella, and neurodermatitis [4]; the water-soluble extracts of IH have also been applied clinically as an analgesic agent by intramuscular injection in China [5]. We found that paeonol and quercetin may be the major active compounds in CP and IH (see Section 2), respectively. Paeonol effects on anti-inflammatory, antioxidant, and cardiovascular protective activities have been demonstrated [6], while antioxidant properties of quercetin associated with anti-inflammatory effects and so forth were also reported [7, 8].

The acute STI, majorly showing skeletal muscle injury, is mainly traumatic aseptic inflammation. When it occurs, the pathological changes include local tissue necrosis, blood capillary dilation, inflammatory cell infiltration with release of inflammatory mediators, and tissue edema [9]. Further, the secondary lesion growth is related to progressive microcirculatory and inflammatory reaction. Direct trauma to microvessels results in membrane damage, endothelial cell swelling, widely vascular hemorrhage, and uncontrolled clot formation, leading to additional local ischemia, which, in turn, induces further degradation of membrane phospholipids, accumulation of free radicals, and inflammation-induced oxidative stress [10, 11]. As the extension of injury process, severe muscle fibers degeneration and necrosis following marked collagen fiber hyperplasia, massive inflammatory cell infiltrates, and interstitial ecchymosed will emerge in the site of damaged tissue to create irreversible structural changes [12]. Hence, early diagnosis and treatment with rapid attenuating tissue swelling and inhibiting inflammation can improve functional results and diminish structural damage in the early and acute period of skeletal muscle injury, which is necessary for treatment of STI [13]. According to the mechanism of inflammatory production, nuclear factor-κB (NF-κB) directly participates in inflammation reaction [14], while both MAPK and AKT signaling activation, in turn, activates transcription factors, such as activator protein-1 and NF-κB, which promotes the gene and protein expressions of inflammation-correlated cytokines [14, 15].

Our previous study has indicated that repeated topical administration with XQAS in the STI site, which was modeled by hammer blow in the hind leg of rat, showed rapidly therapeutical effects on soft-tissue swelling and inflammatory mediators production, while repeated XQAS treatment for four days significantly suppressed STI-caused skeletal muscle necrosis and fibrosis, effectively recovering impaired muscle tissue in a dose-dependent manner. There is a synergistic effect between CP and IH in the XQAS [16]. XQAS effects were associated with suppression of activated NF-κB p65 gene expression in the impaired muscle tissue. However, the molecular mechanism of XQAS effects, especially the synergistic effect between CP and IH on rapidly treating STI, remains unclear. This study tries to elucidate the mechanism of prominent efficacy of XQAS on treating acute STI and the reason why the efficacy is superior to CP or IH alone. An acute STI model with mass-drop injury method, according to Stratton et al. introduction [17], was constructed in this study.

2. Material and Methods

2.1. Preparation of Xiangqing Anodyne Spray (XQAS). XQAS was prepared as previously described [16]. Briefly, the root barks of *Cynanchum paniculatum* (*CP*) or *Illicium henryi* (*IH*) were extracted by 75% ethanol, and penetration enhancers, which include Azone, peppermint oil, and PEG 400 borneol in the 75% ethanol, were added. The final XQAS contains 0.50 g (crude drug) *CP* and 0.50 g (crude drug) *IH* per milliliter, which contains 0.858 mg paeonol and 7.33 mg

quercetin per milliliter. XQAS was examined by high performance liquid chromatography analysis. Using the same method, the *Cynanchum paniculatum* spray (CPS) and *Illicium henryi* spray (IHS) were prepared, containing 1.0 g (crude drug)/mL *CP* or *IH*, respectively.

2.2. Animals. The animal experiment was performed in accordance with China state regulations on animal experimentation and approved by Animal Experimental Ethical Center of Southeast University (protocol number 20120023). Male Sprague-Dawley rats (250 to 300 g) were supplied by Suzhou Industrial Park, Matt Ireland Ltd. All animals were maintained on a standard 12 h light-dark cycle, in a temperature-controlled environment ($24 \pm 2°C$), with free access to water and chow. They were acclimatized for at least one week before initiating the experiments.

2.3. Acute Closed Soft-Tissue Injury (STI) Induction. Like the previously described method [16], the rats were anesthetized by ethyl ether, the inner hind thigh was epilated with depilatory Na_2S solvent in advance and fixed in lateral, and the thigh muscle was hit with a cylindrical hammer (200 g in weight, 1.0 cm in top diameter, and 1.5 cm in bottom diameter) by free falling vertically from inside of a hard smooth plastic tube (75 cm in length and 1.5 cm in inner diameter), only resulting in closed STI but not to cause femoral fracture, which was established by a drop-mass method, similar to the model first described by Stratton et al. [17].

2.4. Animal Experiments. The rats were randomly divided into six groups ($n = 8$ per group): control (Ctrl), model (Mod), high-dose XQAS treatment (HXQAS), low-dose XQAS treatment (LXQAS), CPS treatment (CPS), and IHS treatment (IHS). Except for Ctrl group, other-group rats were subject to two-time blows to hind leg muscle to model acute STI. After modeling, the rats were instantly applied topically with 150 μL/time penetration enhancers in the Ctrl and Mod group, XQAS in the HXQAS (containing 0.50 g (crude drug)/mL both *CP* and *IH*, resp.) and LXQAS (containing 0.25 g (crude drug)/mL both *CP* and *IH*, resp.) group, CPS (containing 1.0 g (crude drug)/mL *CP*), or IHS (containing 1.0 g (crude drug)/mL *IH*), respectively. Next, topical application was repeated with a 2-hour interval in a duration of 8 h after modeling, and the circumference located in the injured thigh muscle was measured at 0 (before modeling), 1, 2, 3, 4, 6, and 8 h; muscle swelling rate (MSR) was then calculated (MSR (%) $= (S/S_0 - 1) \times 100\%$, where S_0 represents the circumference at 0 h, while S represents the circumference at the different time point after making the model) [18]. At the end of experiment, rats were sacrificed after anesthetization with urethane (1.0 g/kg), and the injured thigh muscle in each rat was then divided into two parts: one was stored at $-80°C$ to be used to measure biochemical parameters and to detect gene or protein expressions; the other was fixed in neutral buffered formalin to be used to observe the morphological change.

2.5. Biochemical Analysis of the Muscle Tissue. The muscle tissue was homogenized in 0.02 M phosphate buffered solution (PBS, pH 7.4). The parameter was measured according to the protocols of respective kits. The levels of interleukin-1 beta (IL-1β), tumor necrosis factor-alpha (TNF-α), and prostaglandin-E2 (PGE-2) were measured by ELISA kits provided by Abcam (HK) Ltd. The contents of myeloperoxidase (MPO), nitric oxide (NO), malondialdehyde (MDA), and superoxide dismutase (SOD) were measured by spectrophotometer kits, respectively, provided by Nanjing Jiancheng Bioengineering Institute.

2.6. Reverse Transcription-Polymerase Chain Reaction (RT-PCR) Analysis.

2.6. Reverse Transcription-Polymerase Chain Reaction (RT-PCR) Analysis. The muscle tissue in six of the eight rats in each group was randomly chosen for RT-PCR assay. Total RNA was isolated from tissues using RNAiso plus Isolation Reagent (TAKARA, Otsu, Shiga, Japan). Total RNA solution was first reverse transcribed and then immediately amplified in a GeneAmp PCR system (Eppendorf). Primers used were NF-κB p65 (forward-GGG ACT ATG ACT TGA ATG CG; reverse-CAG GCT AGG GTC AGC GTA T), IL-1β (forward-GAT GAC GAC CTG CTA GTG T; reverse-CTT CTT CTT TGG GTA TTG TT), TNF-α (forward-TCC AGG CGG TTG CCT ATG T; reverse-GAG CGT GGT GGC CCC), and GAPDH (forward-ATG TAT CCG TTG TGG ATC TG; reverse-GAT GGT ATT CGA GAG AAG GG). The gel was photographed by GeneGenius automatic gel imaging and analysis system (Syngene, Cambridge, UK) and the bands on the film were scanned by densitometry for quantitation. To exclude variations due to RNA quantity and quality, the data for all genes were adjusted to GAPDH.

2.7. Western-Blot Analysis.

2.7. Western-Blot Analysis. Six randomly chosen injury muscle samples from each group were homogenized in lysis buffer (150 mM NaCl, 10 mM HEPES, pH 7.9, 1 mM EDTA, 0.6% NP-40, 0.5 mM PMSF, 1 μg/mL leupeptin, 1 μg/mL aprotonin, and 10 μg/mL trypsin inhibitor). Samples were then sonicated and incubated on ice for 15 minutes. Protein was extracted by Cytosol and Nucleus Protein Extraction Kit (KeyGEN Bio TECH). Protein concentration was determined by Bradford's method. Samples were separated by SDS-PAGE gel and electrophoretically transferred to nitrocellulose membrane. Nonspecific binding sites were blocked with Trisbuffered saline (TBS; 40 mM Tris, pH 7.6, 300 mM NaCl) containing 5% BSA for 12 h at 4°C. And the membranes were incubated with anti-NF-κB (p65), anti-COX-2, anti-iNOS, anti-IκBα, anti-phosphor-AKT (Ser^{473}), anti-AKT, anti-phosphor-p38 (Thr^{180}/Tyr^{182}), anti-p38, anti-phosphor-JNK (Thr^{183}/Tyr^{185}), anti-JNK, anti-β-actin, and anti-Lamin B1 antibodies (all from Signalway Antibody Co., Ltd., USA) at 1 : 1000 concentration overnight at 4°C. After being washed with TBST (TBS with 0.1% Tween-20), membranes were incubated with secondary antibody for 2 h at room temperature, which was conjugated to horseradish peroxidase (Santa Cruz Biotechnology, Inc., Santa Cruz, CA). Immunopositive bands were visualized by a chemiluminescent method (ECL, Tanon-5200).

2.8. Histological Observation of Muscle Tissue.

2.8. Histological Observation of Muscle Tissue. After fixation in neutral buffered formalin, the muscle was sectioned and processed routinely for hematoxylin-eosin (HE) staining for qualitative histological analysis. All histopathological examinations were performed by a trained pathologist. The muscle injury, including mainly muscle fibers degeneration and necrosis, interstitial ecchymosis, and inflammatory cell infiltrates, in each sample was assessed using the method reported by Bunn et al. [13].

2.9. Statistical Analysis.

2.9. Statistical Analysis. Results were expressed as mean ± standard deviation (SD). For statistical significance, except the MRS differences between groups which were tested using analysis of covariance (the baseline value in the control as a covariate), the other data were tested using one-way analysis of variance (ANOVA) followed by LSD's multiple comparison test. Differences were considered significant at $P < 0.05$ and extremely significant at $P < 0.01$.

3. Results

3.1. The Effects of XQAS on Muscle Swelling Rate (MSR) in Acute STI Model.

3.1. The Effects of XQAS on Muscle Swelling Rate (MSR) in Acute STI Model. The MSR in the hit hind leg of rats quickly elevated at 1 h after hitting and reached top extent at 2 h, which were in the top value always at 2 h to 8 h after hitting. XQAS treatment dose-dependently attenuated MSR with significant inhibition on MSR starting from 1 h after hitting in the HXQAS and LXQAS group, respectively. Either CPS or IHS treatment also attenuated MSR similarly to XQAS. However, the effect of HXQAS was obviously superior to both CPS effect at 2 h, 3 h, 4 h, and 6 h after hitting and IHS effect at 3 h, 4 h, and 6 h after hitting, exhibiting an effect with "one plus one more than two," suggesting a synergistic effect between *CP* and *IH* on inhibition of hit-induced acute traumatic swelling (Figure 1).

3.2. Evaluation of XQAS on Anti-Inflammatory Reaction and Antioxidative Stress in the Acute STI Model Induced by Hitting Hind Leg Muscle in Rats

3.2.1. Effects of XQAS on mRNA Expressions and Levels of TNF-α and IL-1β in the Injured Muscle Tissues.

3.2.1. Effects of XQAS on mRNA Expressions and Levels of TNF-α and IL-1β in the Injured Muscle Tissues. As inflammation is the most important reaction when acute STI occurs [19], we found that the mRNA expressions and levels of TNF-α and IL-1β in the damaged muscle tissue were markedly increased at 8 h after hitting hind leg muscle. XQAS treatment dose-dependently inhibited the overexpression of TNF-α and IL-1β mRNA and both levels increased in the acute injured muscle tissue. These effects were also observed in both CPS- and IHS-treated group but were significantly less than the HXQAS effects, indicating a synergistic effect between *CP* and *IH* (Figures 2(a) and 2(b)).

3.2.2. Effects of XQAS on Expressions of COX-2 and iNOS and Levels of PGE-2 and NO in the Injured Muscle Tissue.

3.2.2. Effects of XQAS on Expressions of COX-2 and iNOS and Levels of PGE-2 and NO in the Injured Muscle Tissue. The overexpressions of COX-2 and iNOS with increased PGE-2 and NO levels in the damaged muscle tissue were also exhibited. These abnormalities were suppressed markedly by XQAS treatment in a dose-dependent manner or by either CPS or IHS treatment, while the more significant suppression was found in the HXQAS-treated group compared to the CPS- or IHS-treated group, also suggesting a synergistic effect between both (Figures 2(c) and 2(d)).

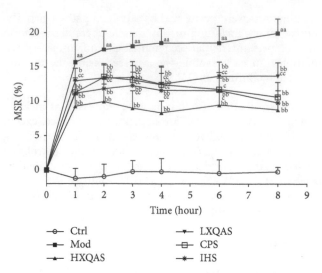

FIGURE 1: Effect of XQAS on muscle swelling rate (MSR) in the acute STI model induced by hitting hind leg muscle in rats. The rats were no modeling topically repeatedly treated with 150 μL/time vehicles in the control (Ctrl), or modeling topically repeatedly treated with 150 μL/time vehicles in the acute STI model (Mod), XQAS in the high-dose and low-dose XQAS-treated group (HXQAS and LXQAS, containing 0.50 or 0.25 g/mL both *CP* and *IH*, resp.), CPS (containing 1.0 g/mL *CP*) (CPS), or IHS (containing 1.0 g/mL *IH*) (IHS) for 8 h. The data were shown as mean ± SD (*n* = 8 per group). aa: *P* < 0.01 versus Ctrl; b: *P* < 0.05, or bb: *P* < 0.01 versus Mod. c: *P* < 0.05, or cc: *P* < 0.01 versus HXQAS.

3.2.3. Effects of XQAS on Oxidative Stress in the Injured Muscle Tissue. Oxidative stress in the injured skeletal muscle is produced, which is known to accelerate progression of muscle pathologies [20] and is able to be marked by increased MPO activity and MDA level with decreased SOD activity [21–23], which were detected in the damaged muscle tissue in this study. XQAS, CPS, and HIS treatment obviously inhibited these changes and XQAS effects showed a dose-dependent manner. With an equal-dose treatment, the XQAS showed more effective effects than CPS or HIS on suppressing production of oxidative stress in the injured muscle, indicating a synergistic effect between both (Figure 2(e)).

3.3. Evaluation of XQAS on Inhibition of Inflammation Signaling Pathway Activated by Acute STI

3.3.1. Effects of XQAS on Degradation of IκBα, Expression of NF-κB p65 mRNA, and Expressions of NF-κB p65 in the Nucleus and Cytosol in the Injured Muscle. NF-κB is thought of as a genetic switch to control the inflammation-related target genes and proteins expression [14]. In this acute STI model, an activated inflammatory signaling pathway was exhibited with downregulated IκBα expression in the cytosol, indicating that IκBα was degraded in the cytosol, upregulated expression of NF-κB p65 mRNA, and downregulated in the cytosol and upregulated in the nuclei NF-κB p65 expression, indicating that NF-κB p65 synthesis was enhanced and that more NF-κB p65 was translocated to the nucleus.

XQAS treatment dose-dependently inhibited hypoexpression of IκBα in the cytosol, hyperexpression of NF-κB p65 mRNA, and hypoexpression in the cytosol with hyperexpression in the nuclei of NF-κB p65 in the injured muscle, suggesting that XQAS can inhibit acute STI-induced IκBα degradation, overexpression of NF-κB p65 gene, and NF-κB p65 translocation into nuclei from cytosol, all of which results in an inhibition in activated inflammatory signaling pathway. Treatment with CPS or IHS alone, as an equal dose with XQAS, also showed similar effects with XQAS but inferior significantly to XQAS, indicating a synergistic effect between *CP* and *IH* on inhibiting acute STI-induced activation of inflammatory signaling pathway (Figures 3(a)–3(c)).

3.3.2. Effects of XQAS on Activation of AKT, p38, and JNK in the Injured Muscle. Activation of MAPK (p-38, JNK, etc.) and AKT signaling cascadedly activate their downstream NF-κB by promoting IκBα degradation and NF-κB gene expression [14]. In the present study, the levels of NF-κB gene expression significantly increased, followed by NF-κB expressions increased both in endochylema and in nucleus, while XQAS, CPS, and IHS treatment can inhibit NF-κB expressions abnormal increase in different degrees. The levels of total AKT (t-AKT), total p38 (t-p38), and total JNK (t-JNK) expression were not changed markedly in the injured muscle, while the levels of phosphorylation of AKT (p-AKT), phosphorylation of p38 (p-p38), and phosphorylation of JNK (p-JNK) expression were significantly increased, suggesting AKT, p38, and JNK were activated. XQAS treatment dose-dependently inhibited the activations of both p-AKT and p-p38 in the acute STI model. Notably, CPS treatment masterly suppressed p38 activated but almost did not change AKT activated with only a decreased tendency in phosphorylated AKT expression. However, IHS treatment, showing a contrary action with CPS, masterly suppressed AKT activated but almost did not change p38 activated with very little decrease in phosphorylated p38 expression. In addition, comparing the effects of XQAS, CPS, and IHS with an equal-dose treatment on suppressing both AKT and p38 activated, the XQAS effect was less than the CPS on suppressing p38 activated and was also less than the IHS on suppressing AKT activated. Treatment with XQAS, CPS, or IHS did not improve p-JNK activated in the injured muscle (Figure 3(d)).

3.4. Histopathologic Evaluation of Acute Injured Muscle Tissue with or without XQAS, CPS, and IHS Treatment. In the Ctrl group, no marked injury was exhibited in the muscle tissue, while in the model group, severe muscle tissue injury was exhibited with large areas of muscle fibers disruption, muscle cells necrosis and significant vascular damage leading to red blood cell accumulation in the interstitial space, and considerable inflammatory cells infiltration in the interstitial space. In the HXQAS group, injured muscle was significantly improved with greater reduced muscle fibers disruption and necrosis and significantly decreased interstitial ecchymosed following a few inflammatory cells infiltration. In the LXQAS group, the muscle-injured improvement was less than that in the HXQAS group, with a marked interstitial ecchymosis, muscle cell necrosis, and inflammatory cells infiltration.

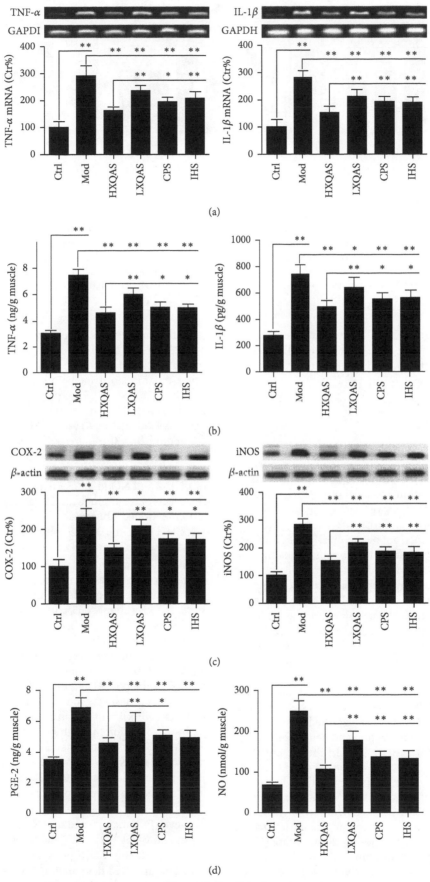

(a)

(b)

(c)

(d)

FIGURE 2: Continued.

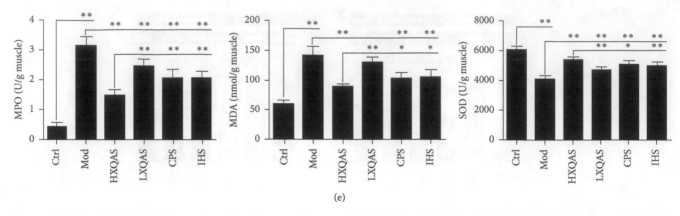

(e)

FIGURE 2: Effects of XQAS on inflammation-related agents with expressions of TNF-α ((a), left) and IL-1β ((a), right), mRNA and their levels (b), expressions of COX-2 ((c), left) and iNOS ((c), right), and levels of PGE-2 ((d), left) and NO ((d), right) and on oxidative stress-related agents with MPO activity ((e), left), MDA levels ((e), middle), and SOD activity ((e), right) in the control (Ctrl), acute STI model (Mod), high-dose XQAS-treated (HXQAS), low-dose XQAS-treated (LXQAS), CPS-treated (CPS), and IHS-treated (IHS) group after modeling with or without repeated drug treatment for 8 h. The data of mRNA or protein expression were shown as mean ± SD (n = 6 per group), while the data of biochemical indicators were shown as mean ± SD (n = 8 per group). $^{*}P < 0.05$; $^{**}P < 0.01$.

In the CPS or IHS group, the injured muscle was also improved significantly but less than that in the HXQAS group. Representative histopathological findings in each group are shown in Figure 4.

4. Discussion

The early recovery phase of STI is characterized by the overlapping processes of inflammation and following occurrence of secondary damage [4]. Within the injured muscle tissue there is leukocyte infiltration and local production of various pro- and anti-inflammatory cytokines, which are crucial for initiating the breakdown and the subsequent removal of damaged muscle fragments, but overexpression of proinflammatory cytokines can be infaust to subsequent healing [24]. In our present study, it was found that the proinflammatory cytokines and their gene overexpressions in the acute STI muscle tissue were notably suppressed by XQAS treatment, which demonstrates that XQAS has an efficacy to inhibiting inflammatory injuries in the acute closed STI. XQAS had quick treatment effects on acute STI, and the active components contained in the *CP* and *IH*, which compose XQAS formulation, have a synergistic effect on treating acute STI.

Free radical generation is known to accelerate progression of muscle pathologies [20]. Oxidative stress in skeletal muscle is increased during acute STI and is ascribed to increases in enzyme-initiated oxidant production and neutrophil-derived myeloperoxidase (MPO) activity [21]. In the present study, XQAS displayed a strong effect on reduction of MPO activity as well as attenuation of inflammatory cell infiltration in the interstitial space of injured muscle. Meanwhile, increased MDA level and decreased SOD activity, both of which are markers of oxidative stress [22], were significantly reversed by XQAS in a dose-dependent manner. Cyclooxygenase (COX), an enzyme that converts arachidonic acid to PGs, has been found to have two isoforms, namely, COX-1 and COX-2. COX-2 is responsible for production of large amounts of

proinflammatory PGs, especially PGE-2, at the inflammatory site [25]. PGE-2 has an effect on dilating blood vessels, resulting in fever and pain. It can also work synergistically with other inflammatory mediators to exacerbate inflammatory response [26]. NO, which is produced by iNOS activation, can regulate contractile function of skeletal muscle [27] and also lead to vasodilatation to increase perfusion, which is essential for remodeling the damaged muscle but results in tissue edema [28]. XQAS can also suppress STI-caused upregulations of COX-2 and iNOS expression with overproductions of PGE-2 and NO in a dose-dependent manner. In addition, the effects of treatment with CPS and IHS alone on improving aforementioned abnormality in the injured muscle tissue were less than the XQAS effects and there is a synergistic effect between *CP* and *IH* components in the XQAS.

NF-κB is a pivotal factor that transfers inflammatory signals from cytoplasm into the nucleus and induces a series of inflammatory responses in the cell [29]. During inactive state, NF-κB subunit p65/p50 is combined with its multiple inhibitors, IκBs such as IκBα, in the cytoplasm. IκBs can be phosphorylated by IκB kinase (IKKα and IKKβ) resulting in separation between IκB and NF-κB and IκB degradation via ubiquitination; the nuclear localization signal of NF-κB located in the p65 is then unmasked. Next, the NF-κB complex would translocate into the nucleus after separation with IκBs [14]. NF-κB activity can be regulated by MAPK and AKT pathway activation through promoting degradation of IκBα. The MAPK family consists of extracellular signal-regulated kinases 1/2 (ERK1/2), c-Jun N-terminal kinase (JNK), and p38 [30]. p38 not only leads to IκBα phosphorylation but also leads to nuclear p65 phosphorylation at Ser[276] via activating mitogen- and stress-activated protein kinase-1 (MSK-1) [31]. However, JNK mainly mediates NF-κB signaling via effects on c-Jun and c-Fos [32]. AKT mediates NF-κB activity mainly through inducing IKKβ phosphorylation and then leads to IκBs ubiquitinated degradation [33]. An important aspect of the significance of NF-kB p65/p50 in inflammatory reaction

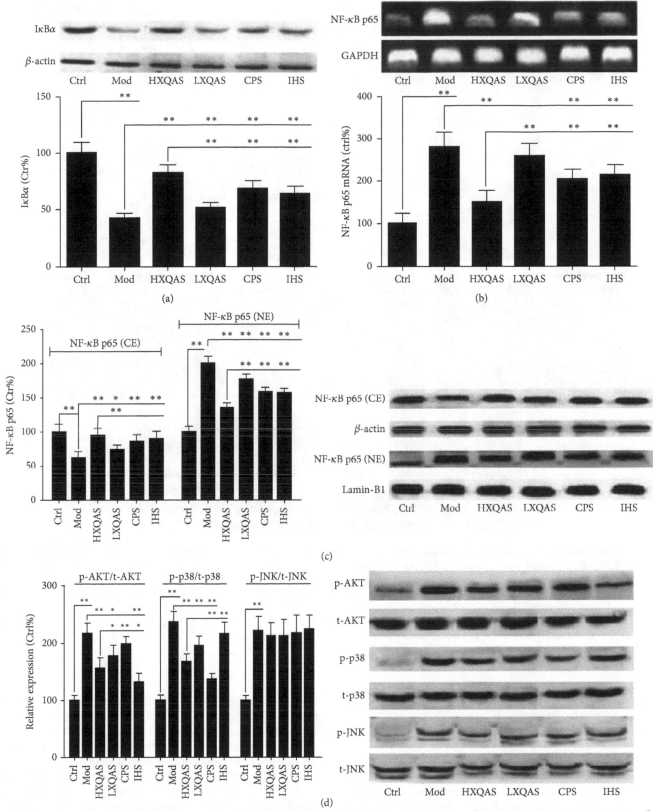

FIGURE 3: Effects of XQAS on inflammation-related signaling pathway with IκBα expression in cytosol (a), NF-κB p65 mRNA expression (b), NF-κB p65 expression in cytosol extraction (CE) and nuclei extraction (NE) (c), and expressions of total AKT (t-AKT), Ser^{473} phosphorylation of AKT (p-AKT), total p38 (t-p38), Thr^{180}/Tyr^{182} phosphorylation of p38 (p-p38), total JNK (t-JNK), and Thr^{183}/Tyr^{185} phosphorylation of JNK (p-JNK) in the control (Ctrl), acute STI model (Mod), high-dose XQAS-treated (HXQAS), low-dose XQAS-treated (LXQAS), CPS-treated (CPS), and IHS-treated (IHS) group after modeling with or without repeated drug treatment for 8 h. The data were shown as mean ± SD ($n = 6$ per group). $^*P < 0.05$; $^{**}P < 0.01$.

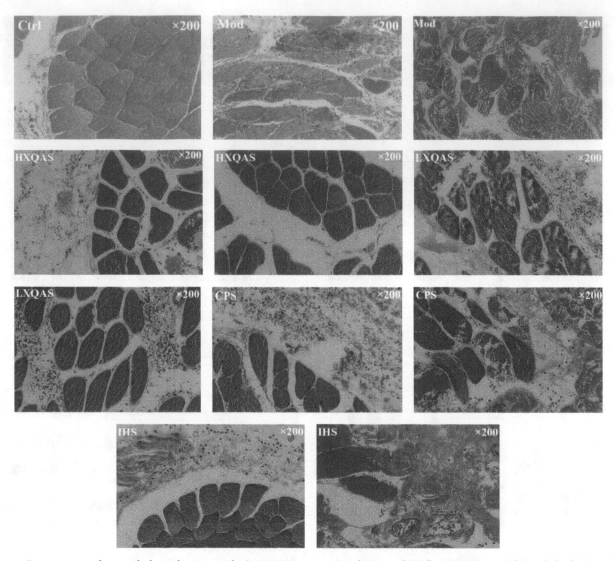

FIGURE 4: Representative histopathological micrographs (×200, HE staining) in the control (Ctrl), acute STI model (Mod), high-dose XQAS-treated (HXQAS), low-dose XQAS-treated (LXQAS), CPS-treated (CPS), and IHS-treated (IHS) group after modeling with or without repeated drug treatment for 8 h. Normal muscle tissue in Ctrl; severe muscle fibers disruption and necrosis, significant red blood cell accumulation in the interstitial space, and inflammatory cells infiltration in the Mod; very significant pathological improvement in injured muscle with markedly reduced area of the disruption and necrosis, decreased interstitial ecchymosed and inflammatory cells infiltration in the HXQAS group, and still marked muscle tissue injury but improved with marked muscle fibers disruption and necrosis, red blood cell accumulation in the interstitial space, and inflammatory cells infiltration in the LXQAS, CPS, and IHS group were shown.

stems from it both being activated by and inducing the expression of inflammatory cytokines [14].

A recent study has indicated that blockade of MAPK-NF-κB pathway activation protects mice from tissue injury by reducing the production of proinflammatory cytokines [34]. Suppression of AKT activation has also been shown to reduce LPS-induced inflammatory responses in the human endothelial cells [35]. From our results, we found that XQAS by suppressing activations of both AKT and p38 pathway quickly abolished activation of NF-κB p65. NF-κB gene expression and its translocation from cytosol to nucleus were enhanced owing to IκBα degraded in the acute injured muscle, while XQAS treatment led to a strong suppression on inflammatory

cascade to acute STI. XQAS combining characteristics of CPS and IHS, where CPS merely suppressed p38 activation while IHS suppressed AKT activation majorly, achieved a super effectiveness on preventing IκB degraded and NF-κB translocation into nucleus activated by STI. There is a synergistic effect between CPS and IHS active components in the XQAS. The critical super effectiveness of XQAS on injured muscle may be effective suppression on IκBα degradation to lead to abolishment of NF-κB translocation from cytosol to nucleus, resulting in a strong suppression on transcriptional activation of NF-κB itself and target with inflammation-related genes and on subsequent muscle necrosis, blood stasis in the interstitial space, inflammatory cells infiltration,

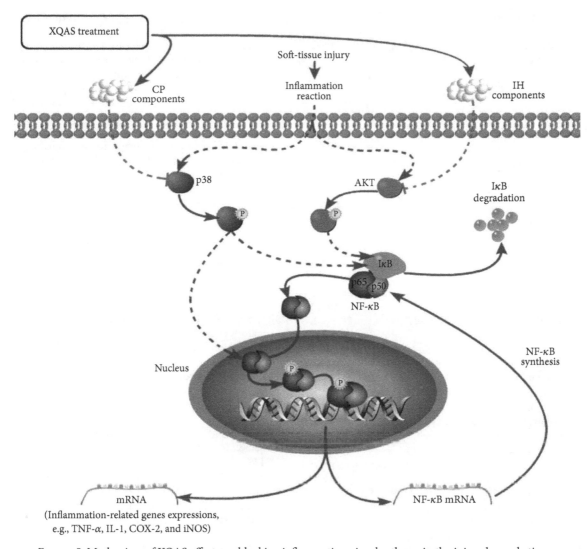

FIGURE 5: Mechanism of XQAS effects on blocking inflammation-signal pathway in the injured muscle tissue.

oxidative stress, and acute traumatic swelling. In addition, though JNK was also activated in the injured muscle tissue, XQAS, CPS, and IHS all did not alter the state of JNK activation.

Although inflammation is generally considered as a normal and necessary prerequisite to injury recovery [36, 37], it is indeed detrimental when inflammation cascade gets out of control, such as restricting the blood flow due to increased local hydrostatic pressure in the oedema site, pain, and reducing local oxygen levels, during acute STI [38]. Both our present study and previous study [16] indicated that instant suppression to acute STI-induced excess inflammation in the initiation of acute STI is very beneficial for prevention from secondary damage to normal muscle cells and muscle necrosis with subsequent degenerative processes to lead to muscle tissue replacement by excess fibrin deposits. The impressive effects of XQAS on treating STI probably owe to its very effective suppression to inflammatory cascade in the initiation of STI.

5. Conclusion

XQAS is a quite reasonable formulation with a combination of active components of *Cynanchum paniculatum* (*CP*) and *Illicium henryi* (*IH*) in treating acute STI. The mechanism of impressive effects of XQAS, at least majorly, is due to its anti-inflammatory and antioxidative activities with a synergistic effect between active components of *CP* and *IH*, in which the *CP* components suppress STI-induced p38 phosphorylated activation with intranuclear NF-κB p65 phosphorylation, while the *IH* components suppress STI-induced AKT phosphorylated activation; subsequently, IκB degradation in the cytoplasm, which is promoted by both p38 and AKT pathways activation, is blocked to lead to decrease in NF-κB p65/p50 translocated into the nucleus after separation with IκB; ultimately, NF-κB p65/p50 actions on transcriptional activation of NF-κB itself and target with inflammation-related genes, all of which are enhanced by both p38 and AKT pathways activation, are abolished. The mechanism process was shown in Figure 5.

Competing Interests

The authors declare that they have no competing interests regarding this paper.

Authors' Contributions

Shudong Wang, Tao Li, and Wei Qu equally contributed to this work.

Acknowledgments

The authors are grateful to Professor Wenxia Bai, an Associate Researcher at Jiangsu Center for Safety Evaluation of Drugs, China, for her contribution to the histopathological examination.

References

[1] D. Mantle, M. A. Gok, and T. W. J. Lennard, "Adverse and beneficial effects of plant extracts on skin and skin disorders," *Adverse Drug Reactions and Toxicological Reviews*, vol. 20, no. 2, pp. 89–103, 2001.

[2] D. De-Quan, N. Xing-Yan, and L. Fang, "Henry Anise spray combined with diode laser in the treatment of herpes zoster-induced neuralgia and postherpetic neuralgia," *Journal of Medical Postgraduates*, vol. 26, no. 10, pp. 1061–1063, 2013.

[3] W. Shu-Dong, L. Wen-Ya, and W. Zheng, "Analgesic effects of illicium henrys combined with cyuanchum panicalatum in different proportions," *Journal of Medical Postgraduates*, vol. 26, no. 2, pp. 134–136, 2013.

[4] C. Deng, N. Yao, B. Wang, and X. Zhang, "Development of microwave-assisted extraction followed by headspace single-drop microextraction for fast determination of paeonol in traditional Chinese medicines," *Journal of Chromatography A*, vol. 1103, no. 1, pp. 15–21, 2006.

[5] J. S. Liu and Q. R. Zhou, "The toxic principle of Illicium henryi Diels and structure of 6-deoxypseudoanisatin," *Acta Pharmaceutica Sinica*, vol. 23, no. 3, pp. 221–223, 1988.

[6] A. Hirai, T. Terano, T. Hamazaki et al., "Studies on the mechanism of antiaggregatory effect of moutan cortex," *Thrombosis Research*, vol. 31, no. 1, pp. 29–40, 1983.

[7] J. Robak and R. J. Gryglewski, "Flavonoids are scavengers of superoxide anions," *Biochemical Pharmacology*, vol. 37, no. 5, pp. 837–841, 1988.

[8] K. Murota and J. Terao, "Antioxidative flavonoid quercetin: implication of its intestinal absorption and metabolism," *Archives of Biochemistry and Biophysics*, vol. 417, no. 1, pp. 12–17, 2003.

[9] M. L. Urso, "Anti-inflammatory interventions and skeletal muscle injury: benefit or detriment?" *Journal of Applied Physiology*, vol. 115, no. 6, pp. 920–928, 2013.

[10] G. J. van der Vusse, M. van Bilsen, and R. S. Reneman, "Ischemia and reperfusion induced alterations in membrane phospholipids: an overview," *Annals of the New York Academy of Sciences*, vol. 723, pp. 1–14, 1994.

[11] D. K. Das, "Cellular, biochemical, and molecular aspects of reperfusion injury. Introduction," *Annals of the New York Academy of Sciences*, vol. 723, pp. 13–16, 1994.

[12] K.-D. Schaser, B. Vollmar, M. D. Menger et al., "In vivo analysis of microcirculation following closed soft-tissue injury," *Journal of Orthopaedic Research*, vol. 17, no. 5, pp. 678–685, 1999.

[13] J. R. Bunn, J. Canning, G. Burke, M. Mushipe, D. R. Marsh, and G. Li, "Production of consistent crush lesions in murine quadriceps muscle—a biomechanical, histomorphological and immunohistochemical study," *Journal of Orthopaedic Research*, vol. 22, no. 6, pp. 1336–1344, 2004.

[14] N. D. Perkins, "The Rel/NF-κB family: friend and foe," *Trends in Biochemical Sciences*, vol. 25, no. 9, pp. 434–440, 2000.

[15] R. Craig, A. Larkin, A. M. Mingo et al., "p38 MAPK and NF-κB collaborate to induce interleukin-6 gene expression and release. Evidence for a cytoprotective autocrine signaling pathway in a cardiac myocyte model system," *The Journal of Biological Chemistry*, vol. 275, no. 31, pp. 23814–23824, 2000.

[16] S. Wang, W. Qu, T. Li et al., "Xiangqing anodyne spray (XQAS): a combination of ethanol extracts of *Cynanchum paniculatum* and *Illicium henryi* for treating soft-tissue injury," *International Journal of Clinical and Experimental Medicine*, vol. 8, no. 8, pp. 12716–12725, 2015.

[17] S. A. Stratton, R. Heckmann, and R. S. Francis, "Therapeutic ultrasound: its effects on the Integrity of a nonpenetrating wound," *The Journal of Orthopaedic and Sports Physical Therapy*, vol. 5, no. 5, pp. 278–281, 1984.

[18] H. Süleyman, L. Ö. Demirezer, A. Kuruüzüm et al., "Antiinflammatory effect of the aqueous extract from *Rumex patientia* L. roots," *Journal of Ethnopharmacology*, vol. 65, no. 2, pp. 141–148, 1999.

[19] C. Gates and J. Huard, "Management of skeletal muscle injuries in military personnel," *Operative Techniques in Sports Medicine*, vol. 13, no. 4, pp. 247–256, 2005.

[20] L. L. Ji, M.-C. Gomez-Cabrera, and J. Vina, "Role of free radicals and antioxidant signaling in skeletal muscle health and pathology," *Infectious Disorders—Drug Targets*, vol. 9, no. 4, pp. 428–444, 2009.

[21] A. R. Judge and S. L. Dodd, "Xanthine oxidase and activated neutrophils cause oxidative damage to skeletal muscle after contractile claudication," *American Journal of Physiology—Heart and Circulatory Physiology*, vol. 286, no. 1, pp. H252–H256, 2004.

[22] V. Hernández, M. Miranda, I. Pascual et al., "Malondialdehyde in early phase of acute pancreatitis," *Revista Española de Enfermedades Digestivas*, vol. 103, no. 11, pp. 563–569, 2011.

[23] M. Assady, A. Farahnak, A. Golestani, and M. R. Esharghian, "Superoxide dismutase (SOD) enzyme activity assay in *Fasciola* spp. parasites and liver tissue extract," *Iranian Journal of Parasitology*, vol. 6, no. 4, pp. 17–22, 2011.

[24] J. G. Tidball, "Inflammatory processes in muscle injury and repair," *The American Journal of Physiology—Regulatory Integrative and Comparative Physiology*, vol. 288, no. 2, pp. R345–R353, 2005.

[25] S. H. Lee, E. Soyoola, P. Chanmugam et al., "Selective expression of mitogen-inducible cyclooxygenase in macrophages stimulated with lipopolysaccharide," *The Journal of Biological Chemistry*, vol. 267, no. 36, pp. 25934–25938, 1992.

[26] J.-H. Choi, B.-H. Jung, O.-H. Kang et al., "The anti-inflammatory and anti-nociceptive effects of ethyl acetate fraction of cynanchi paniculati radix," *Biological & Pharmaceutical Bulletin*, vol. 29, no. 5, pp. 971–975, 2006.

[27] L. Kobzik, M. B. Reid, D. S. Bredt, and J. S. Stamler, "Nitric oxide in skeletal muscle," *Nature*, vol. 372, no. 6506, pp. 546–548, 1994.

[28] I. Rubinstein, Z. Abassi, R. Coleman, F. Milman, J. Winaver, and O. S. Better, "Involvement of nitric oxide system in experimental muscle crush injury," *The Journal of Clinical Investigation*, vol. 101, no. 6, pp. 1325–1333, 1998.

[29] L. Zhao, S.-L. Zhang, J.-Y. Tao et al., "Anti-inflammatory mechanism of a folk herbal medicine, *Duchesnea indica* (Andr) Focke at RAW264.7 cell line," *Immunological Investigations*, vol. 37, no. 4, pp. 339–357, 2008.

[30] M. Cargnello and P. P. Roux, "Activation and function of the MAPKs and their substrates, the MAPK-activated protein kinases," *Microbiology and Molecular Biology Reviews*, vol. 76, no. 2, p. 496, 2012.

[31] L. Vermeulen, G. De Wilde, P. Van Damme, W. V. Berghe, and G. Haegeman, "Transcriptional activation of the NF-κB p65 subunit by mitogen- and stress-activated protein kinase-1 (MSK1)," *The EMBO Journal*, vol. 22, no. 6, pp. 1313–1324, 2003.

[32] S. Papa, F. Zazzeroni, C. Bubici et al., "Gadd45β mediates the NF-κB suppression of JNK signalling by targeting MKK7/JNKK2," *Nature Cell Biology*, vol. 6, no. 2, pp. 146–153, 2004.

[33] H. C. Dan, M. J. Cooper, P. C. Cogswell, J. A. Duncan, J. P.-Y. Ting, and A. S. Baldwin, "Akt-dependent regulation of NF-κB is controlled by mTOR and Raptor in association with IKK," *Genes & Development*, vol. 22, no. 11, pp. 1490–1500, 2008.

[34] C.-C. Hsu, J.-C. Lien, C.-W. Chang, C.-H. Chang, S.-C. Kuo, and T.-F. Huang, "Yuwen02f1 suppresses LPS-induced endotoxemia and adjuvant-induced arthritis primarily through blockade of ROS formation, NFkB and MAPK activation," *Biochemical Pharmacology*, vol. 85, no. 3, pp. 385–395, 2013.

[35] S.-J. Jiang, S.-Y. Hsu, C.-R. Deng et al., "Dextromethorphan attenuates LPS-induced adhesion molecule expression in human endothelial cells," *Microcirculation*, vol. 20, no. 2, pp. 190–201, 2013.

[36] S. G. Dakin, J. Dudhia, and R. K. W. Smith, "Resolving an inflammatory concept: the importance of inflammation and resolution in tendinopathy," *Veterinary Immunology and Immunopathology*, vol. 158, no. 3-4, pp. 121–127, 2014.

[37] J. D. Rees, M. Stride, and A. Scott, "Tendons—time to revisit inflammation," *British Journal of Sports Medicine*, vol. 48, no. 21, pp. 1553–1557, 2014.

[38] L. Poltawski and T. Watson, "Bioelectricity and microcurrent therapy for tissue healing—a narrative review," *Physical Therapy Reviews*, vol. 14, no. 2, pp. 104–114, 2009.

9

Influence of the *Melissa officinalis* Leaf Extract on Long-Term Memory in Scopolamine Animal Model with Assessment of Mechanism of Action

Marcin Ozarowski,[1,2] **Przemyslaw L. Mikolajczak,**[2,3] **Anna Piasecka,**[4] **Piotr Kachlicki,**[4] **Radoslaw Kujawski,**[2] **Anna Bogacz,**[5,6] **Joanna Bartkowiak-Wieczorek,**[5] **Michal Szulc,**[3] **Ewa Kaminska,**[3] **Malgorzata Kujawska,**[7] **Jadwiga Jodynis-Liebert,**[7] **Agnieszka Gryszczynska,**[2] **Bogna Opala,**[2] **Zdzislaw Lowicki,**[2] **Agnieszka Seremak-Mrozikiewicz,**[2,8,9] **and Boguslaw Czerny**[6,10]

[1] *Department of Pharmaceutical Botany and Plant Biotechnology, Poznan University of Medical Sciences, Sw. Marii Magdaleny 14, 61-861 Poznan, Poland*
[2] *Department of Pharmacology and Phytochemistry, Institute of Natural Fibres and Medicinal Plants, Wojska Polskiego 71b, 60-630 Poznan, Poland*
[3] *Department of Pharmacology, University of Medical Sciences, Rokietnicka 5a, 60-806 Poznan, Poland*
[4] *Department of Pathogen Genetics and Plant Resistance, Metabolomics Team, Institute of Plant Genetics of the Polish Academy of Science, Strzeszynska 34, 60-479 Poznan, Poland*
[5] *Laboratory of Experimental Pharmacogenetics, Department of Clinical Pharmacy and Biopharmacy, University of Medical Sciences, 14 Sw. Marii Magdaleny, 61-861 Poznan, Poland*
[6] *Department of Stem Cells and Regenerative Medicine, Institute of Natural Fibres and Medicinal Plants, Wojska Polskiego 71b, 60-630 Poznan, Poland*
[7] *Department of Toxicology, Poznan University of Medical Sciences, Dojazd 30, 60-631 Poznan, Poland*
[8] *Division of Perinatology and Women's Diseases, Poznan University of Medical Sciences, Polna 33, 60-535 Poznan, Poland*
[9] *Laboratory of Molecular Biology, Poznan University of Medical Sciences, Polna 33, 60-535 Poznan, Poland*
[10] *Department of General Pharmacology and Pharmacoeconomics, Pomeranian Medical University, Zolnierska 48, 70-204 Szczecin, Poland*

Correspondence should be addressed to Marcin Ozarowski; mozarow@ump.edu.pl

Academic Editor: Helmut Hugel

Melissa officinalis (MO, English: lemon balm, Lamiaceae), one of the oldest and still most popular aromatic medicinal plants, is used in phytomedicine for the prevention and treatment of nervous disturbances. The aim of our study was to assess the effect of subchronic (28-fold) administration of a 50% ethanol extract of MO leaves (200 mg/kg, p.o.) compared with rosmarinic acid (RA, 10 mg/kg, p.o.) and huperzine A (HU, 0.5 mg/kg, p.o.) on behavioral and cognitive responses in scopolamine-induced rats. The results were linked with acetylcholinesterase (AChE), butyrylcholinesterase (BuChE), and beta-secretase (BACE-1) mRNA levels and AChE and BuChE activities in the hippocampus and frontal cortex of rats. In our study, MO and HU, but not RA, showed an improvement in long-term memory. The results were in line with mRNA levels, since MO produced a decrease of AChE mRNA level by 52% in the cortex and caused a strong significant inhibition of BACE1 mRNA transcription (64% in the frontal cortex; 50% in the hippocampus). However, the extract produced only an insignificant inhibition of AChE activity in the frontal cortex. The mechanisms of MO action are probably more complicated, since its role as a modulator of beta-secretase activity should be taken into consideration.

1. Introduction

Neurodegenerative disorders including Alzheimer's disease, characterized by loss of memory and learning ability, are the increasing public health problem worldwide [1, 2]. Plants with neurobiological activity may be potential targets for drug discovery [3]. Searching for new drugs and explaining their mechanisms of action are one of the most intensively developing areas of scientific platform. Moreover plant origin substances can be a valuable alternative way in the prevention and treatment of dementias as component of healthy diet.

Melissa officinalis (*MO*, English: lemon balm, Lamiaceae), one of the oldest and still most popular aromatic medicinal plants, is used in phytotherapy for the prevention and treatment of nervous disturbances of sleep and gastrointestinal disorders as sedative and antispasmodic medicine [4]. New neuropharmacological investigations showed that ethanol extracts of *MO* exerted also neuroprotective [5, 6], antioxidant, cyclooxygenase-2 inhibitory [7], and antinociceptive activities [6, 8]. Moreover, it is known that *MO* is used for memory-enhancing effects in European folk medicine [9–12]. Indeed, Akhondzadeh et al. [13] carried out the clinical trial in which *MO* extract produced a significantly better outcome on cognitive function than placebo in patients with mild to moderate Alzheimer's disease. In other clinical studies, Kennedy et al. [14–16] observed that a treatment combining both calming effects and beneficial cholinergic modulation may well prove to be a novel treatment for Alzheimer's disease. Studies of molecular mechanisms showed that *MO* extracts exhibited cholinergic (nicotinic and muscarinic) receptor-binding properties in human cerebral cortex tissue [15]. Moreover, it was observed that both fractions and crude ethanol extract of *MO* inhibited acetylcholinesterase (AChE) of rats brain [17, 18] and also *in vitro* [9, 19, 20], but only two studies analyzed behavioral mechanism of action of *MO* extracts on scopolamine-induced memory impairment in rats [12, 18]. One study showed that *MO* extract (after intraperitoneal injection) significantly enhanced learning and memory of rats and significantly ameliorated scopolamine-induced learning deficit [18]; however in another study, it was observed that *MO* extract was completely inactive [12]. Moreover, in these studies, attention has not been paid to the influence of the *MO* extract on the expression of genes participating in the conditioning of the synaptic cholinergic equilibrium, AChE and bytyrylcholinesterase (BuChE) or even the beta-secretase (BACE1), in rats brain, being responsible for beta-amyloid deposition in Alzheimer's disease [1].

On the other hand, it is well known that essential oil in leaf of *MO* is considered to be the therapeutic principle mainly responsible for most of the abovementioned activities, but also plant phenolics are considered as an important factor in *MO* therapeutic effects [6, 21]. It was shown that ethanol extract contains rosmarinic acid (RA) as the major compound [7]; however there is no detailed information about full phenolic profile of extract from *MO* leaves being probably responsible for pharmacological effects as well. This becomes especially important given the results of previous studies showing that RA did not affect short- and long-term memory [22] or marginally improved long-term memory in rats model [23], although it was observed that RA had an ability to inhibit AChE in the frontal cortex and in the hippocampus of rats [23]. On the other hand, polyphenols still constitute a promising source of new drugs and there is a high interest in understanding their mechanisms in prevention and treatment of Alzheimer's disease [16, 23, 24].

2. Objectives

The aim of this study was to evaluate the influence of subchronic (28-fold) intragastrical administration of ethanol extract of *MO* leaves and rosmarinic acid on scopolamine (SC) impaired memory in animal model. Furthermore, acetylcholinesterase (AChE) and butyrylcholinesterase (BuChE) activities assessment in hippocampus and frontal cortex were studied. Moreover, gene expression levels for AChE, BuChE, and BACE-1 in the hippocampus and frontal cortex were investigated. The *MO* ethanolic extract was phytochemically investigated (HPLC-ESI-MS^n, UPLC-PDA) in order to identify phytochemicals present in plant extract.

3. Materials and Methods

3.1. Plant Material. The leaves of *Melissa officinalis* L. (Lamiaceae) were obtained from an herbal company "Kawon-Hurt" (Gostyn Wlkp., Poland). The plant material was identified in the Department of Pharmaceutical Botany and Plant Biotechnology, Faculty of Pharmacy, Poznan University of Medical Sciences. The voucher specimen has been deposited in the Herbarium of the Institute of Natural Fibres and Medicinal Plants in Poznan (Plewiska), Poland.

3.2. Chemical and Drugs. All reagents for HPLC analysis, scopolamine hydrobromide trihydrate (SC), and rosmarinic acid (RA) and reagents for biochemical analyses were purchased from Sigma-Aldrich (Poland). Huperzine A (HU) was obtained from Enzo Life Sciences AG (Alexis Corporation, Biomibo Distribution, Poland). Chemicals for gene expression analysis were obtained from Roche Diagnostic and ALAB (Poland). All chemicals and drugs were *ex tempore* prepared on the day of the experiment.

3.3. Preparation of the Extract. 1000 g of raw plant material was extracted with 50% ethanol by percolation (24 h) at room temperature (22 ± 1°C). After filtration, the extract was concentrated under vacuum to eliminate the ethanol content. The concentrated extract was frozen and freeze-dried. The final product yielded 248.21 g of solid extract.

3.4. Metabolites Identification with LC-MS. Metabolomic analyses were performed using two complementary LC-MS systems. The first one, HPLC-DAD-MS^n, consisted of an Agilent 1100 HPLC instrument with a diode-array detector (DAD) (Agilent, Palo Alto, CA, USA) and an Esquire 3000 ion trap mass spectrometer (Bruker Daltonics, Bremen, Germany). Chromatographic separations by HPLC were carried out on an XBridge C18 column (150 × 2,1 mm, 3,5 μm particle size) using water acidified with 0.1% formic acid (solvent A) and acetonitrile (solvent B) with the mobile phase flow of 0.2 mL/min in the following gradient: 0–25 min from 10% to 30% B, 25–46 min to 98% B, and being maintained at these conditions until 51 min. Up to 52 min system returned to the starting conditions and was reequilibrated for 5 min. The most important MS parameters were as follows: the ion source ESI voltage −4 kV or 4 kV, nebulization of nitrogen at a pressure of 30 psi at a gas flow rate 9 L/min, ion source temperature at 310°C, and skimmer 1: −10 V. The spectra were scanned in the range of 50–3000 m/z. The second system consisted of UPLC (the Acquity system, Waters, Milford, USA) hyphenated to QExactive hybrid MS/MS quadrupole-Orbitrap mass spectrometer. Chromatographic separations in this system were carried out using water acidified with 0.1% formic acid (solvent A) and acetonitrile (solvent B) with the mobile phase flow of 0.4 mL/min in the following gradient: 0–5 min from 10% to 25% B, 5–13 min to 98% B, and being maintained at these conditions until 14.5 min. Up to 15 min system returned to the starting conditions and was reequilibrated for 3 min. QExactive MS operated upon the following settings: the HESI ion source voltage −3 kV or 3 kV. The sheath gas flow was 48 L/min, auxiliary gas flow 13 L/min, ion source capillary temperature 250°C, and auxiliary gas heater temperature 380°C. The CID MS/MS experiments were performed using collision energy of 15 eV. The MS^n (up to the MS5) and MS/MS spectra were recorded in the negative and positive ion modes using the previously published approach [23, 25, 26]. The individual compounds were identified via comparison of the exact molecular masses (measured in most cases with Δ below 1 ppm), mass spectra, and retention times to those of the standard compounds, as well as the databases available online (PubChem, ChEBI, Metlin, and KNApSAck) and literature data.

3.5. Quantitative HPLC Analysis.

Sample was extracted by 70% ethanol. After sonification, solution was cooled down and filtered through membrane filter. HPLC method was used to determine RA in a dry ethanolic extract. The Lichrospher 100 RP-18e (125 mm; 4,0 mm; 5 um, Merck) was applied for identification of this active compound. Temperature of column was 35°C, detection of RA was at 205 nm, and flow rate was 1,5 mL/min. Mobile phase A was $H_3PO_4 : H_2O$ (1 : 999); mobile phase B was acetonitrile. Time was as follows: 0 min, 10% B; 13 min, 22% B; 14 min, 40% B; 25 min, 40% B.

Moreover, for identification of other chemical compounds, a Zorbax Poroshell 120 SB-C18 column, 2.7 mm 3.0 mm × 100 mm (Agilent), was used. The lithospermic acid and salvianolic acid B were detected at 250 nm; salvianolic acid A was detected at 280 nm. The gradient mixtures of phase A—water : H_3PO_4 (100 : 0.02, V/V)—and of phase B—acetonitrile : tetrahydrofurane (100 : 2, V/V)—were used as eluents. Peaks were identified by addition of standard solutions and by UV-Vis spectra. The quantification of these compounds was achieved using calibration curves prepared with pure compounds. The flow rate was 0.7 mL/min, column temperature 27°C, and sample injection 5 mL. The gradient

mixtures program was as follows: 0 min: 5% B; 3 min: 10% B; 5 min: 12% B; 11 min: 21.7% B; 15 min: 39% B; 39 min: 39% B; 70 min: 70% B; and detection of compounds took place at 250 nm, 280 nm, and 330 nm [27].

3.6. Determination of Total Phenolic Compounds in the Extract.

The calculation of polyphenols to gallic acid was done using the Folin-Ciocalteu reagent with the spectrophotometric modified method described by Slinkart and Singleton [28].

3.7. Determination of Total Hydroxycinnamic Acid Derivatives.

Determination of total hydroxycinnamic acid derivatives calculated on rosmarinic acid was performed according to the procedure described in EurPh. 5.0.

3.8. Distillation of Essential Oil.

The essential oil contents were determined by way of stream distillation in Deryng's apparatus according to EurPh. 5.0. 100.0 g of the dry hydroethanolic MO leaf extract (separate sample) was placed in a round-bottom flask. Then, 500.0 mL distilled water and 0.3 mL xylen were added and boiled in Deryng's apparatus for 3 h.

3.9. Gas Chromatography Analysis.

Gas chromatography (GC) analyses were carried out using a Perkin-Elmer Clarus 500 gas chromatograph with a data processing system and an FID (GC-FID). Separation was achieved by using an Elite FFAP fused-silica capillary column (30 m long, 0.32 mm in internal diameter, and 0.25 μm of film thickness). The injector and detector temperatures were 220°C. Helium was used as a carrier gas with a flow of 1.5 mL min^{-1}. A sample of 1.0 μL was injected, using slit mode (split ratio 1 : 100). The results were reported as the relative percentage of the total peak area.

3.10. Animals.

Experiments with rats were performed in accordance with Polish governmental regulations (Dz. U. 05.33.289). The study was conducted in accordance with ethical guidelines for investigations in conscious animals and the study protocol was approved by the Local Ethics Committee of the Use of Laboratory Animals in Poznan, Poland (64/2008). The experiments were performed on male six-week-old Wistar rats housed in controlled room temperature (20 ± 0.2 C) and humidity (65–75%) under a 12 h : 12 h light-dark cycle (lights on at 7 a.m.). Animals were kept in groups in amounts of 8–10 in light plastic cages (60 × 40 × 40 cm) and had a free access to standard laboratory diet (pellets-Labofeed B) and to tap water in their cages.

3.11. Treatments.

The rats were treated with hydroethanolic extract of Melissa officinalis leaf (MO) in a dose of 200 mg/kg b.w., intragastrically (p.o.) (groups MO + H_2O and MO + SC) for 28 (28x) consecutive days. For comparative purposes, huperzine A (HU) was administered chronically (28x) in a dose 0.5 mg/kg b.w. (p.o.) (groups HU + H_2O and HU + SC) as a known acetylcholinesterase inhibitor. Moreover, rosmarinic acid (Sigma-Aldrich) (RA) was applied (28x) in a dose of 10 mg/kg b.w. (p.o.) (groups RA + H_2O and RA + SC) as a comparative chemical compound. On the last day, 30 min after the last dose of *MO*, or *HU*, SC was given intraperitoneally (i.p.) in a dose of 0.5 mg/kg b.w. Control groups were treated with 0.5% methylcellulose (MC), whereas water for injection (H_2O) was used as a vehicle for SC (groups MC + H_2O and MC + SC). *MO* was prepared ex tempore before administration and suspended in MC in concentrations of 20 mg/mL. On day 28 of the experiment, 1 h after the last dose, the animals were killed by decapitation and hippocampus and part of frontal cortex were collected from brain of rats. The tissue samples were then stored at −80°C until measurement of acetylcholinesterase (AChE) and butyrylcholinesterase (BuChE) activities or mRNA level changes.

3.12. Cognitive and Behavioral Tests. Cognitive and behavioral tests were used in the present study similarly as in our previous report [23]: (1) sedative activity was assessed using a locomotor activity test, (2) motor coordination assessment was done using a "chimney" test, (3) the passive avoidance test was performed as an animal model for the assessment of long-term memory, and (4) the object recognition test was used as an animal model for the assessment of short-term memory.

3.12.1. Measurement of Locomotor Activity. Locomotor activity assessment was performed with licensed activity meter (Activity Cage, Ugo Basile, Italy) by placing the animals in the centre of the apparatus and recording their horizontal activity [23]. The data obtained were expressed as signals corresponding to animal movements for 5 minutes. The locomotor activity was measured 30 minutes after the administration of a single dose of SC H_2O. Any distracting factors were reduced to the minimum (noise, presence of people, and presence of other rats).

3.12.2. Measurement of Motor Coordination. Motor coordination was evaluated using "chimney" test described originally for mice [29]. Thirty minutes after SC or vehicle injection, rat was allowed to enter a glass laboratory cylinder that is 500 mm long and 80 mm in diameter laid on its side. Upon reaching its bottom by the animal, position of the cylinder was rapidly changed from horizontal to vertical and a timer started. The animal immediately began to move backwards. The timer was stopped after the rat left the cylinder and assumed a sitting posture on the top of the vessel. The time of exit from the cylinder was accepted as a measure of motor coordination. Motor impairment was assessed as the inability of rats to climb backwards up the tube within 60 s.

3.12.3. Passive Avoidance Test. Passive avoidance test was used as an animal model for the assessment of long-term memory (effects on retrieval and memory consolidation) [30]. The test relies on the natural preference of rats for darkness. After 2 minutes of habituation to a dark compartment, a rat was placed on the illuminated platform and allowed to enter the dark compartment using licensed apparatus (Passive Avoidance System, step through, Ugo Basile, Italy). Two more approach trials were allowed on the following day with a two-minute interval between them. At the end of

the second trial, an unavoidable scrambled electric footshock (500 μA, AC, 3 s) was delivered through the grid floor of the dark compartment (learning trial). Retention of the passive avoidance response (latency) was tested 24 h later by placing the animal on the platform and measuring the latency in reentering the dark compartment against the arbitrary maximum time of 180 s. The test was performed after 30 minutes after the administration of a single dose of SC or the vehicle.

3.12.4. Object Recognition Test. Object recognition test was used as an animal model for the assessment of short-term memory [31]. The object recognition task took place in a 40 × 60 cm open box surrounded by 40 cm high walls made of plywood with a frontal glass wall. All animals were submitted to a habituation session where they were allowed to freely explore the open field for 5 min. No objects were placed in the box during the habituation trial. On the day of testing, the animals were given an additional 3 min rehabituation period prior to commencing the test. The test was divided into three phases with two trials, the acquisition trial, the retention trial, and an intertrial interval of varying times.

(i) Acquisition trial: in this first trial, the animals explored two identical objects (*A*1 and *A*2) for a period of 3 min positioned in two adjacent corners, 10 cm from the walls.

(ii) Intertrial interval (ITI): the animals were returned to the home cage for 30 min.

(iii) Retention trial: in this second trial, the animals explored a familiar object (*A**) that is a duplicate of those objects from the acquisition trial (to minimize olfactory cues) and a novel object (*B*) for a further 3 min.

They were made of a biologically inert substance (plastic) and were chosen to enable ease of cleaning (10% alcohol) between subjects in an attempt to remove olfactory cues. Object exploration is defined by animals licking, sniffing, or touching the object whilst sniffing but not leaning against, turning round, or standing or sitting on the object. Objects were of sufficient weight and were secured to the floor of the arena to ensure that they could not be knocked over or moved around by the animal. The exploration time (s) of all objects was recorded via stopwatch for subsequent statistical analysis. The time measured as an exploration behavior was used to calculate a memory discrimination index (OR) as reported by Blalock et al. [31]: $OR = (B-A^*)/(B+A)$, where B was the time spent exploring the new object and A^* was the time spent exploring the familiar object. Higher OR was considered to reflect greater memory ability [31]. The test was performed after 30 minutes after the administration of a single dose of SC or the vehicle.

3.13. Acetylcholinesterase and Butyrylcholinesterase Activities Assay in Brain of Rats. Acetylcholinesterase (AChE) and butyrylcholinesterase (BuChE) activities were performed by modifying spectrophotometric Ellman's method according to Isomae et al. [32]. The activities of AChE and BuChE

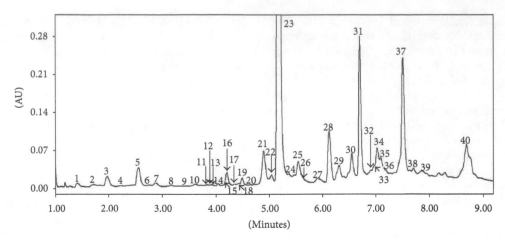

FIGURE 1: Chromatogram UV of *Melissa officinalis* leaf extract obtained at 270 nm with peaks identified by HPLC-UV-MS.

were determined by measuring the formation of the yellow anion obtained from the reaction between Ellman's reagent and the thiocholine generated by the enzymatic hydrolysis of acetylthiocholine iodide (ATCh) and butyrylthiocholine (BTCh), respectively (sample 0.1 mL, PBS 0.8 mL, DTNB 0.1 mL, ATCh 0.20 mL, and BTCh 0.20 mL). The biochemical assay of AChE and BuChE in homogenate of brain samples was expressed as μmol/min/mg protein by using spectrophotometric method (λ = 412 nm).

3.14. RNA Isolation and Reverse Transcription Reaction.

Total RNA isolation from the rats brain tissues homogenates (frontal cortex, hippocampus) was carried out using TriPure Isolation Reagent (Roche) according to manufacturer's protocol. The integrity of RNA was visually assessed by a conventional agarose gel electrophoresis and the concentration will be evaluated by measuring the absorbance at 260 and 280 nm in a spectrophotometer (BioPhotometer Eppendorf). RNA samples were stored at −80°C until use. The 1 μg of total RNA from all samples was used for the reverse transcription into cDNA using Transcriptor First Strand Synthesis Kit (Roche) according to manufacturer's protocol. Obtained cDNA samples was stored at −20°C or used directly for the quantitative real-time PCR (qRT-PCR).

3.15. Real-Time PCR mRNA Quantification.

The acetylcholinesterase (AChE), butyrylcholinesterase (BChE), and beta-secretase (BACE1) genes expression level was analyzed by two-step quantitative real-time PCR (qRT-PCR), in a volume of 10 μL reaction mixture, using relative quantification methodology with a LightCycler TM Instrument (Roche, Germany) and a LightCycler Fast Start DNA Master SYBR Green I kit (Roche Applied Science) according to the instructions of the manufacturer. All primers sequences were designed and custom-designed using the Oligo 6.0 software (National Biosciences) and were verified by assessment of a single PCR product on agarose gel and by a single temperature dissociation peak (melting curve analysis) of each cDNA amplification product. An GAPDH gene was used as a housekeeping gene (endogenous internal standard) for

normalization of qPCR. For each quantified gene, standard curves were prepared from dilution of cDNA and generated from a minimum of four data points. All quantitative PCR were repeated twice. The data were evaluated using LightCycler Run 4.5 software (Roche Applied Science). Each PCR run included a nontemplate control to detect potential contamination of reagents.

3.16. Statistical Analysis.

All values were expressed as means ± SEM. The statistical comparison of results was carried out using one-way analysis of variance (ANOVA) followed by Duncan's *post hoc* test for detailed data analysis. The values of $p < 0.05$ were considered as a statistical significant difference.

4. Results

4.1. Phytochemical Profile of Extract

4.1.1. Identification of Metabolites.

Forty phenolic metabolites were identified in hydroethanolic *Melissa officinalis* leaf extract (Table 1, Figure 1). The predominant identified compounds were bioactive caffeic acid esters and glycosides of flavones. The caffeic acid dimer, rosmarinic acid (metabolite **23**), and caffeate trimer (lithospermic acid, **31**) were the principal caffeic acid derivatives in the analyzed samples. Hydroxyjasmonic acid and its derivatives, teucrol as well as sagecoumarin, were identified for the first time in the genus *Melissa* while luteolin and apigenin glycoconjugates are well known phytochemicals in this species [33]. Multistep fragmentation with accurate mass measurement enabled confirming that the losses of fragment 79.9573 amu from the [M-H]$^-$ ions of compounds **4, 9, 27, 30,** and **32** referred to sulphate groups. The first-order fragmentation of **30** revealed the loss of 79.9573 and yielded the product ion at 719.1622 m/z. The following fragmentation of this ion corresponded to that of the sagerinic acid (dimer of rosmarinic acid) described by Barros et al. [34]. The exact placement of the sulphation position would require in-depth chemical analysis. Thus, **30** was tentatively assigned as sulphated sagerinic acid.

Table 1: Metabolites detected in *Melissa officinalis* leaf extract by UPLC-MS.

No	RT [min]	Metabolite identification	Chemical formula	Exact mass of [M-H]⁻ Measured	Calculated	Δppm	Fragmentation Negative ion mode (ESI−)	Fragmentation Positive ion mode (ESI+)	λmax [nm]	CID[a]	Identification level[b]	Reference
1	1.41	2-Hydroxy-3-(3,4-dihydroxyphenyl)-propanoic acid	$C_9H_9O_5$	197.045	197.0455	−4.1775	197, 179, 135	199, 163	283, 312	8143997	2	[34]
2	1.73	Dihydroxybenzoic acid hexoside	$C_{13}H_{15}O_9$	315.072	315.0722	0.8346	315, 153, 109	317, 155	282	54726828	3	[35]
3	1.98	Caftaric acid	$C_{13}H_{11}O_9$	311.041	311.0409	0.6141	311, 221, 179, 149		318	6440397	2	[35]
4	2.24	2-Hydroxy-3-(3,4-dihydroxyphenyl)-propanoic acid sulphated	$C_9H_9O_8S$	277.003	277.0024	0.3998	277, 197, 179, 135		312		3	[35]
5	2.56	Hydroxyjjasmonic acid hexoside	$C_{18}H_{27}O_9$	387.166	387.1661	0.9214	387, 207, 163		323	44237366	2	[17]
6	2.76	Caffeic acid	$C_9H_7O_4$	179.034	179.0451	−4.9075	179, 135	181, 163	275	689043	1	std
7	2.89	Salvianolic acid E	$C_{36}H_{29}O_{16}$	717.1450	717.1467	2.313	717, 519, 339, 321, 295, 277		275, 325	49770697	2	[35]
8	3.17	Salvianolic acid H/I (isomer)	$C_{27}H_{21}O_{12}$	537.104	537.1038	0.8562	537, 493, 359, 295		281, 325		2	[35]
9	3.45	Hydroxyjjasmonic acid sulphated	$C_{12}H_{17}O_7S$	305.07	305.07	1.117	305, 225, 194, 147		275, 330		3	[17]
10	3.62	Nepetoidin B	$C_{17}H_{13}O_6$	313.072	313.0718	1.1232	nd		282, 316	5316819	2	[73]
11	3.7	Yunnaneic acid F	$C_{26}H_{25}O_{14}$	597.1255	597.1244	1.8743	597, 509, 311, 197		Masked		2	[34]
12	3.83	Decarboxyrosmarinic acid (teucrol)	$C_{17}H_{15}O_6$	315.088	315.0874	0.9396	315, 179, 135		275, 330	637829	2	[74]
13	3.9	Caffeoylcaftaric acid	$C_{22}H_{17}O_{12}$	473.073	473.0725	0.7555	173, 311, 149		Masked	65018	3	[35]
14	3.97	Apigenin glucosylrhamnoside	$C_{27}H_{29}O_{14}$	577.157	577.1563	1.1136	577, 269	579, 433, 271	275, 340	92741003	3	[33]
15	4.04	Luteolin 7-O-glucoside 3'-O-glucuronide	$C_{27}H_{27}O_{17}$	623.126	623.1254	0.9696	623, 461, 447, 285, 255	625, 463, 287	273, 343		2	[33]
16	4.21	Rosmarinic acid hexoside	$C_{24}H_{25}O_{13}$	521.13	521.1301	0.3551	521, 359, 161	523, 361, 325, 163	329	25245848	2	[34]
17	4.3	Luteolin O-diglucoside	$C_{27}H_{29}O_{16}$	609.147	609.1461	0.7183	609, 285	611, 287	269, 349		3	[33]
18	4.41	Luteolin glucosylrhamnoside	$C_{27}H_{29}O_{15}$	593.152	593.1512	0.8077	593, 447, 285	595, 449, 287	271, 343		3	[33]
19	4.49	Luteolin 4'-O-glucoside	$C_{21}H_{19}O_{11}$	447.094	447.0933	0.9728	447, 285	449, 287	271, 343	5319116	3	[33]
20	4.5	Sagerinic acid 2-hydroxy-3-(3,4-dihydroxyphenyl)-propanoide	$C_{45}H_{39}O_{20}$	899.205	899.204	1.0448	899, 719, 591, 475, 295		Masked		3	[35]
21	4.9	Salvianolic acid B (lithospermic acid B)	$C_{36}H_{29}O_{16}$	717.146	717.1461	0.1846	717, 519, 359, 161		327	6441188	2	[34]
22	5.04	Sagerinic acid	$C_{36}H_{31}O_{16}$	719.163	719.1618	0.9979	719, 519, 359, 161		287, 330		2	[34]
23	5.14	Rosmarinic acid	$C_{18}H_{15}O_8$	359.077	359.0772	0.002	359, 161	361, 163	329	5281792	1	std

TABLE 1: Continued.

No	RT [min]	Metabolite identification	Chemical formula	Exact mass of $[M-H]^-$ Measured	Calculated	Δppm	Fragmentation in Negative ion mode (ESI−)	Fragmentation in Positive ion mode (ESI+)	λ_{max} [nm]	CID[a]	Identification level[b]	Reference
24	5.55	Salvianolic acid B 2-hydroxy-3-(3,4-dihydroxyphenyl)-propanoide	$C_{45}H_{37}O_{20}$	897.19	897.1884	1.6873	897, 717, 519, 359, 161		330		3	[35]
25	5.6	Sagerinic acid di-2-hydroxy-3-(3,4-dihydroxyphenyl)-propanoide	$C_{54}H_{47}O_{24}$	1079.2449	1079.2457	−0.7911	1079, 897, 719, 539, 359, 295		288, 330		3	[35]
26	5.92	Sagecoumarin di-2-hydroxy-3-(3,4-dihydroxyphenyl)-propanoide caffeide	$C_{54}H_{43}O_{24}$	1075.2156	1075.2150	0.559	1077, 897, 717, 537, 409, 359, 339, 277		322		3	[35]
27	5.98	Rosmarinic acid sulphated I isomer	$C_{18}H_{15}O_{11}S$	439.035	439.0341	2.0214	439, 359, 341, 163		Masked		2	[34]
28	6.13	Luteolin 3′-O-glucuronide	$C_{21}H_{17}O_{12}$	461.073	461.072	1.634	461, 285	463, 287	269, 340	170474237	2	[33]
29	6.32	Salvianolic acid A	$C_{26}H_{21}O_{10}$	493.115	493.114	1.1011	493, 359, 295, 179		298, 327	5281793	2	[34]
30	6.56	Sagerinic acid sulphated	$C_{36}H_{31}O_{19}S$	799.1196	799.1186	0.954	799, 719, 619, 519, 359, 161		325		3	[35]
31	6.71	Lithospermic acid	$C_{27}H_{21}O_{12}$	537.104	537.1048	0.9698	537, 493, 359, 161		292, 329	6441498	2	[35]
32	6.8	Rosmarinic acid sulphated II isomer	$C_{18}H_{15}O_{11}S$	439.034	439.0341	0.2837	439, 359, 341, 163		Masked		2	[34]
33	6.89	Sagecoumarin	$C_{27}H_{19}O_{12}$	535.088	535.0882	0.1204	535, 311, 267, 177		Masked		2	[36]
34	7.03	Salvianolic acid L I isomer	$C_{36}H_{29}O_{16}$	717.146	717.1461	0.2697	717, 519, 359		284, 329		2	[35]
35	7.1	Salvianolic acid L hydroxycaffeide	$C_{45}H_{35}O_{20}$	895.173	895.1727	0.6282	895, 519, 359, 161		Masked		3	[35]
36	7.4	Sagecoumarin caffaride	$C_{40}H_{29}O_{20}$	829.126	829.1258	0.6953	829, 667, 535, 355, 311		Masked		3	[36]
37	7.51	Sagecoumarin 2-hydroxy-3-(3,4-dihydroxyphenyl)-propanoide	$C_{36}H_{27}O_{16}$	715.131	715.1305	0.8176	715, 535, 311, 267		319		3	[34]
38	7.71	Unknown	$C_{36}H_{57}O_{14}S$	745.348	745.3475	0.4402			281, 326		4	[35]
39	7.85	Methyl rosmarinate	$C_{19}H_{17}O_{8}$	373.093	373.0929	0.1765	373, 359, 161		284, 323	6479915	2	[75]
40	8.69	Salvianolic acid C caffeoylhydroxycaffeide	$C_{44}H_{33}O_{18}$	849.168	849.1672	0.8615	849, 687, 491, 359, 327, 255		286, 318		3	[35]

[a]CID: identifier for a chemical structure in the PubChem Compound database.
[b]Metabolite identification level according to Metabolomics Standards Initiative recommendation [76].
std: identification on the basis of standard compound fragmentation.
nd: not detected.

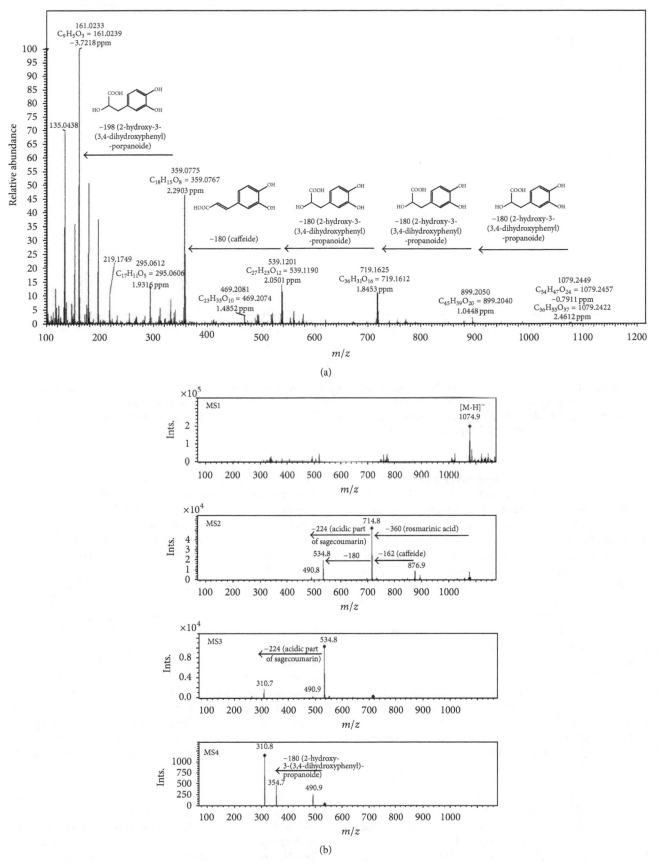

Figure 2: Continued.

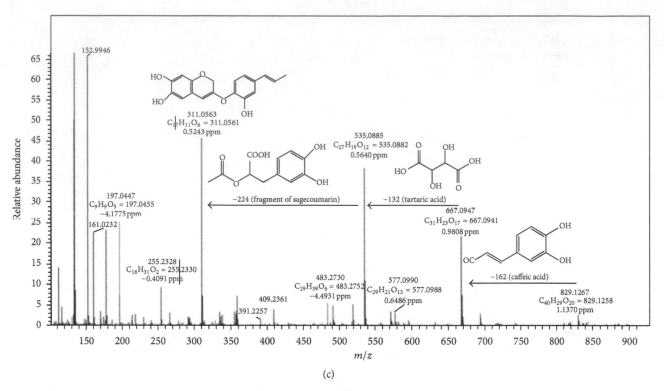

FIGURE 2: (a) Mass spectra in negative ionization mode and simplified fragmentation scheme of compound **25** (pentameric ester of caffeic acid). (b) Mass spectra in negative ionization mode and simplified fragmentation scheme of compound **26** (pentameric structure of sagecoumarin di-2-hydroxy-3-(3,4-dihydroxyphenyl)-propanoide caffeide). (c) Mass spectra in negative ionization mode and simplified fragmentation scheme of compound **36** (pentameric structure of sagecoumarin caftaride).

Tetrameric structures of hydroxycinnamic acids were identified in lemon balm recently [34, 35]. The measurement of accurate masses allowed the identification of compound **25**, which was tentatively identified as pentameric ester of caffeic acid (Figure 2(a)). In **25**, the double loss of 180.0421 amu corresponded to fragments with the molecular formula of $C_9H_8O_4$, adequate to dehydroxylated 2-hydroxy-3-(3,4-dihydroxyphenyl)-propanoic acid. The product ion at 719.1623 m/z and its further fragmentation are similar to those of metabolite **22** as described previously [34, 35]. Therefore, metabolite **25** was tentatively assigned as sagerinic acid di-2-hydroxy-3-(3,4-dihydroxyphenyl)-propanoide. Nevertheless, comprehensive studies by nuclear magnetic resonance are required to complete elucidation of substitution pattern for particular components of those pentamers.

Sagecoumarins were previously identified in *Salvia officinalis* as caffeic acid trimers [36]. Our MS analysis indicated the presence of such compounds and their derivatives also in *M. officinalis*. The pseudomolecular ion of compound **33** observed in the negative ionization mode had the accurate mass of 535.0880 m/z which corresponded to the chemical formula $C_{27}H_{19}O_{12}$ adequate for sagecoumarin (according to the Metlin and KNApSAck databases). Noteworthy, **26**, **33**, **36**, and **37** had the same fragmentation pattern of the product ion obtained in the MS/MS and MS^n in the negative ionization mode. The [M-H-180.0422]$^-$ ion corresponded to the detachment of 2-hydroxy-3-(3,4-dihydroxyphenyl)-propanoic acid; thus **37** was tentatively

assigned as tetrameric sagecoumarin 2-hydroxy-3-(3,4-dihydroxyphenyl)-propanoide. The [M-H-360.0846]$^-$ ion in **26** was indicated on rosmarinic acid substitution to **37**. Mass spectra of MS^n in negative ionization of the compound provided complementary information to HR-MS/MS mass spectra indicated on caffeic acid as internal component of the dimer. In addition, simultaneous loss of fragments 180 amu and 224 amu in MS3 and MS4 indicated that the two components cannot be linked (Figure 2(b)). However, detailed analysis of substitution pattern of **26** should be done. Therefore, **26** was tentatively assigned as pentameric structure of sagecoumarin di-2-hydroxy-3-(3,4-dihydroxyphenyl)-propanoide caffeide. Rupture of caffeic and tartaric acid moieties from the product ion at 535.0885 m/z was observed for compound **36** (Figure 2(c)). Detection of the accurate masses of these two detached fragments with Δ less than 1 ppm eliminated the possibility of hexose and pentose substitution which have the same nominal masses as caffeic and tartaric acid, respectively. Therefore, **36** was tentatively identified as another pentameric structure of sagecoumarin caftaride.

Metabolite **28** with the accurate masses of 461.073 m/z was tentatively identified as luteolin O-glucuronide. The [M-H-176.0324]$^-$ ion is indicated on loss of structure $C_6H_8O_6$ corresponding to glucuronide moiety. The product ion at 285.0405 m/z was indicated on flavone luteolin. The place of substitution of the carboxylic acid on flavone skeleton is problematic due to different isomers reported in lemon balm:

TABLE 2: Effect of *Melissa officinalis* leaf extract (200 mg/kg, p.o.) treatment on sedative activity, motor coordination, and memory in rats.

Group	n	Locomotor activity [number of impulses/5 min]	Motor coordination, exit time [s]	Short-term memory[e] OR	Long-term memory, latency [s]
MC + H$_2$O	18	390 ± 24	17 ± 3	0.40 ± 0.06	47 ± 14
MC + SC	18	526 ± 48*	32 ± 5*	0.32 ± 0.05	12 ± 3*
MO + H$_2$O	10	231 ± 48*	32 ± 7*	0.43 ± 0.07	169 ± 11*
MO + SC	9	436 ± 60	43 ± 7	0.09 ± 0.11*	23 ± 6
HU + H$_2$O	9	515 ± 32	15 ± 2	0.37 ± 0.09	158 ± 14*
HU + SC	8	639 ± 71*	56 ± 3	0.22 ± 0.06	49 ± 18#
RA + H$_2$O	8	406 ± 59	21 ± 5	0.45 ± 0.05	58 ± 28
RA + SC	8	605 ± 55	28 ± 7	0.45 ± 0.05	20 ± 7

Means ± SEM.
[n]Number of animals.
MC + H$_2$O: control rats.
SC: scopolamine (0.5 mg/kg b.w., i.p.).
HU: huperzine A (0.5 mg/kg b.w., p.o.).
RA: rosmarinic acid (10 mg/kg b.w., p.o.).
[e]Expressed as ratio OR = $(B − A^*)/(B + A)$; for details see Section 3.
*Versus MC + H$_2$O, $p < 0.05$.
#Versus MC + SC, $p < 0.05$.

luteolin 3'-O- and 7-O-glucuronide [33]. It is impossible to distinguish both structures by mass spectrometry. Only one chromatographic peak corresponding to the [M-H]$^-$ ion at 461.073 m/z was observed in our study. Since luteolin 3'-O-glucuronide was assigned as the most abundant flavonoid in lemon balm [33], we assumed that **28** corresponded to this structure.

4.1.2. Flavonoids and Polyphenolic Acids.

The major compound, from the 40 chemical compounds identified in hydroethanolic *MO* leaf extract established by HPLC, was RA (8.85 g/100 g) (Table 1, Figure 1).

Other chemical compounds with neuromodulatory activities such as lithospermic acid (0.042 g/100 g), salvianolic acid A (0.040 g/100 g), salvianolic acid B (0.023 g/100 g), and caffeic acid (0.087 g/100 g) were also documented in literature. Moreover, the total polyphenolic compounds content of *MO*, determined with the use of Folin–Ciocalteu assay, was 33.97%, calculated as gallic acid. The total hydroxycinnamic derivatives content expressed spectrophotometrically as rosmarinic acid was 21.15 g/100 g.

4.1.3. Essential Oil Composition.

Hydroethanolic *MO* leaf extract contained 0.08% of total essential oil. The GC/FID analysis showed that the extract comprised camphene (0.04%), alfa-pinene (0.07%), beta-pinene (16.47%), and myrcene (19.51%). Moreover, according to retention time, 16 compounds were identified as follows: alfa-bisabolol, borneol, carvone, chamazulene, cineole, eugenol, gamma-terpineol, guaiazulene, isopulegol, linalool, limonene, menthol, menthyl acetate, pulegone, terpine, and thymol. These compounds are present in the essential oil in trace amounts which do not allow the quantitative interpretation.

4.2. Cognitive and Behavioral Experiments

4.2.1. Locomotor Activity.

A one-way ANOVA analysis revealed significant differences in the locomotor activity of rats expressed as their horizontal spontaneous activity after *MO* administration (ANOVA, $F(7, 80) = 6.46$, $p < 0.05$) (Table 2). Detailed *post hoc* analysis showed that *MO* + H$_2$O decreased the locomotor activity of rats by 40.31%, but HU + H$_2$O did not affect this activity when compared with control group (MC + H$_2$O). We observed also that RA + H$_2$O did not change the locomotor activity of rats. Stimulating effects in the locomotor activity of rats were observed after an acute SC injection (MC + SC versus MC + H$_2$O, $p < 0.05$) and this effect was observed in all SC-treated rats when compared with the proper non-SC-treated animals. On the contrary, these SC-treated animals did not differ in comparison to animals that received SC only (*MO* + SC versus MC + SC, $p > 0.05$; HU + SC versus MC + SC, $p > 0.05$; RA + SC versus MC + SC, $p > 0.05$).

4.2.2. Motor Coordination.

A one-way ANOVA analysis revealed significant differences in motor coordination of rats expressed as their exit time from the cylinder ($F(5, 73) = 2.84$, $p < 0.05$) (Table 2). Detailed analysis showed that the multiple administration of RA + H$_2$O and HU + H$_2$O did not affect significantly this paradigm when compared with control rats ($p > 0.05$), whereas *MO* treatment led to prolonged exit time (*MO* + H$_2$O versus MC + H$_2$O, $p < 0.05$). Moreover, generally SC-treated animals showed produced prolongation of exit time and the effects were statistically significant not only in control groups (MC + SC versus MC + H$_2$O, $p < 0.05$), but also in RA-treated rats (RA + SC versus MC + SC, $p < 0.05$). However, the rest of the SC-treated animals did not differ in comparison to animals receiving SC only (*MO* + SC versus MC + SC, $p > 0.05$; HU + SC versus MC + SC, $p > 0.05$).

4.2.3. Long-Term Memory.

A one-way ANOVA analysis revealed significant differences in long-term memory after using a passive avoidance test ($F(7, 77) = 20.1$; $p < 0.05$, Table 2). It was shown that the strongest effect leading to

TABLE 3: The effect of *Melissa officinalis* leaf extract on acetylcholinesterase (AChE) and butyrylcholinesterase (BuChE) activities and AChE, BuAChE, or beta-secretase (BACE1) mRNA expression levels in frontal cortex (FC) or hippocampus (Hipp) of rats.

| Group[n] | Enzyme activity [nmol/min/mg protein] | | | | mRNA expression[#] [%] | | | | | |
| | AChE | | BuChE | | ACHE | | BuChE | | BACE1 | |
	FC	Hipp	FC	Hipp	FC	Hipp	FC	Hipp	FC	Hipp
MC + H_2O	363 ± 49	439 ± 73	65 ± 11	53 ± 8	100 ± 12	100 ± 11	100 ± 18	100 ± 11	100 ± 16	100 ± 8
MO + H_2O	276 ± 34	409 ± 28	69 ± 6	62 ± 4	$48 \pm 4^*$	$31 \pm 7^*$	$16 \pm 2^*$	$64 \pm 21^{\&}$	$36 \pm 3^*$	$50 \pm 8^*$
HU + H_2O	$189 \pm 15^*$	$239 \pm 15^*$	58 ± 6	51 ± 4	$53 \pm 13^*$	85 ± 5	$42 \pm 9^*$	102 ± 11	$62 \pm 6^*$	98 ± 4
RA + H_2O	$224 \pm 16^*$	$251 \pm 12^*$	77 ± 7	$99 \pm 7^*$	101 ± 12	103 ± 5	$184 \pm 31^*$	$56 \pm 7^*$	$126 \pm 13^{\&}$	98 ± 3

Means ± SEM.
[n]Number of animals: 7–10.
[#]Values expressed as a ratio: the gene/GAPDH.
MC + H_2O: control group.
HU: huperzine A (0.5 mg/kg b.w., p.o.).
RA: rosmarinic acid (10 mg/kg b.w., p.o.).
[*,&]Versus MC + H_2O, $p < 0.05$ or $p < 0.07$, respectively.

an improvement of this paradigm was produced by extract of *MO* and HU, but not RA, when compared with control animals (*MO* + H_2O versus MC + H_2O, $p < 0.05$; HU + H_2O versus MC + H_2O, $p < 0.05$; RA + H_2O versus MC + H_2O, $p > 0.05$), However, the administration of SC to rats significantly decreased the latency time of passive avoidance task (MC + SC versus MC + H_2O, $p < 0.05$). After *MO* or RA combined treatment with SC, no improvement of long-term memory was observed, but HU given with SC showed enhancement of this paradigm in rats (HU + SC versus MC + SC, $p < 0.05$). Therefore, it can be concluded that administration of HU overcomes the effect shown by SC only (Table 1).

4.2.4. Short-Term Memory. The results of the object recognition test showed that an administration of the compounds or extract did affect the rats' short-term memory (ANOVA $F_{(7, 78)} = 2.73$, $p < 0.05$) (Table 2).

Detailed *post hoc* analysis showed that only SC significantly decreased the short-term memory in *MO*-treated rats (*MO* + SC versus *MO* + H_2O, $p < 0.05$; *MO* + SC versus MC + SC, $p < 0.05$), whereas the differences between rest of the animals did not reach statistical significance ($p > 0.05$).

4.3. AChE and BuChE Activities in Rat Brain. A one-way ANOVA revealed significant differences between groups in the activity of AChE in both the cortex and the hippocampus (frontal cortex: $F_{(3, 27)} = 5.65$, $p < 0.05$; hippocampus: ANOVA $F_{(3, 29)} = 7.96$, $p < 0.05$). It was found out that *MO* showed an insignificant inhibition of AChE activity in the frontal cortex by 24% when compared with control rats (MC + H_2O, $p < 0.06$) and in the hippocampus by 7% (Table 3), whereas HU produced a distinct significant inhibition of AChE activity in comparison to control group by 48% ($p < 0.05$) and 47% ($p < 0.05$) in the cortex and the hippocampus, respectively. Also, RA lowered significantly AChE activity both in the cortex (38%) and in the hippocampus (43%). Moreover, there were not significant differences between the values of BuChE activities for *MO* and HU when compared

with control group in the frontal cortex (ANOVA $F_{(3, 30)} = 1.01$, $p > 0.05$), whereas in the hippocampus the differences reached statistical significance (ANOVA $F_{(3, 27)} = 14.1$, $p < 0.05$). Detailed analysis showed that only RA effect was significant and increased BuChE activity in the hippocampus when compared with the control rats ($p < 0.05$).

4.4. AChE, BuChE, and BACE1 mRNA Level Changes in Rat Brain. A one-way ANOVA analysis revealed significant differences of AChE mRNA transcription profile in the cortex (ANOVA $F_{(3, 27)} = 8.57$, $p < 0.05$). As shown in Table 3, the multiple treatment of *MO* produced in the cortex a statistically significant decrease of AChE mRNA level by 52%; the administration of HU caused decrease of its level by 44% ($p < 0.05$), whereas RA did not affect this parameter when compared to the control.

There were significant differences between the relative values of BuChE mRNA levels in this region of brain in rats (frontal cortex: ANOVA $F_{(3, 25)} = 16.2$, $p < 0.05$). The *MO* treatment led to a decrease in the BuChE mRNA level by 84% (versus MC + H_2O, $p < 0.05$), the prolonged HU administration resulted in a decrease of the transcript level in the cortex by 58% (versus MC + H_2O, $p < 0.05$), but RA increased this parameter in the cortex by 84% (versus MC + H_2O, $p < 0.05$).

The significant differences of mRNA transcription level of AChE mRNA level in the hippocampus (ANOVA $F_{(3, 31)} = 21.2$, $p < 0.05$) have been observed. The detailed analysis shown that, in the case of AChE after *MO* treatment, mRNA level significantly decreased by 69% (versus MC + H_2O, $p < 0.05$), while the administration of HU resulted in a statistically insignificant decrease of AChE mRNA level by 18%, when compared with control group. Also RA did not change the level of transcript.

In the case of BuChE mRNA expression in the hippocampus, there were statistically significant differences between groups (ANOVA $F_{(3, 27)} = 3.10$; $p < 0.05$). Detailed analysis showed that, in the *MO* + H_2O treated group, the expression lowered by 36%, but the difference did not reach strong significance when compared with the control values ($p < 0.07$) and no change in the expression level of this enzyme was shown after the administration of HU. On the contrary, RA produced an increase of BuChE mRNA expression in the hippocampus by 44% (versus MC + H_2O, $p < 0.05$).

Further analysis showed the significant differences in BACE1 mRNA expression in both brain regions of rats (in the cortex and the hippocampus) (frontal cortex: ANOVA $F(3, 27) = 16.3$, $p < 0.05$; hippocampus: ANOVA $F(3, 27) = 13.3$, $p > 0.05$). It was observed that MO produced a statistically significant decrease of the BACE1 expression level by 64% in the cortex (versus MC + H_2O, $p < 0.05$) and by 50% in the hippocampus (versus MC + H_2O, $p < 0.05$). For comparison, HU treatment led to a decrease in the mRNA expression level by 38% in the cortex (versus MC + H_2O, $p < 0.05$), but not in the hippocampus. On the contrary, RA produced an increase of this transcript in the cortex by 26%, but the effect did not reach a strong statistical significance (versus MC + H_2O, $p < 0.07$), whereas in the hippocampus there was no difference between RA and control group.

5. Discussion

Cognitive and Behavioral Experiments. The present study investigated the influence of subchronic (28-fold) administration of standardized 50% EtOH extract of *Melisa officinalis* leaf extract (MO) (200 mg/kg, p.o., containing 17.7 mg/kg of RA) on SC-induced impairment of short-term and long-term memory in rats. The results were compared with the activity of cholinesterases (AChE and BuChE) as well as with AChE, BuChE, and BACE1 gene expression levels in the cortex and hippocampus of the rat brain. So far, little evidence is yet available as regards mechanisms of MO leaf extract action that are potentially relevant to cognitive function of rats after *per os* administration. MO is traditionally used in treating neurological disorders through its anti-AChE [18] and antiagitation properties [37]. Moreover, Wake et al. [38] and Kennedy et al. [15] showed that MO extract has nicotinic receptor activity and that it can displace [3H]-(N)-nicotine from nicotinic receptors in homogenates of human cerebral cortex tissue and they suggested that these mechanisms can explain activity of MO extract in amnesia model. Recently, Soodi et al. [18] observed that intraperitoneal injections of MO extract (200 mg/kg) in rats could significantly enhance learning and memory processes in animals since the extract significantly ameliorates SC-induced learning deficit in Morris water maze test. On the contrary, in higher dose, it can be observed that MO extract (400 mg/kg) could not reverse SC-induced memory impairment [18]. In our study, administration of MO extract at a dose of 200 mg/kg (p.o.) showed the effect leading to improvement of long-term memory in a passive avoidance test in rats. However, after MO combined treatment with SC, MO did not overcome the impairment shown by SC (Table 2). It should be emphasized that it is not clear whether the effect shown in our study by MO in non-SC-treated rats is specific, since the MO treatment produced significant lowering of locomotor activity of rats; therefore the sedative profile of MO cannot be excluded.

On the other hand, Ryu et al. [39] observed that agitation and aggression are highly prevalent in patients with dementia. According to Gitlin et al. [40], nonpharmacological interventions are recommended as first-line therapy. Although antipsychotics have shown benefit for Alzheimer's disease-related psychosis, their use is associated with several serious adverse effects [40]. Thus, it seems that the use of MO extract can provide dual benefits, both in aspect of inhibition of agitation and in improving the memory of patients with Alzheimer's disease.

Furthermore, in our study, RA in the dose of 10 mg/kg b.w. (p.o.) did not affect either short- or long-term memory, although RA lowered significantly AChE activity both in the cortex and in the hippocampus. Moreover, we observed that the repeated administration of RA in non-scopolamine-treated rats did not produce any changes of locomotor activity, similarly to our previous study [23].

It is possible that other chemical compounds can influence the memory in rats by synergic interactions in plant extract. According to our calculations, caffeic acid (0.174 mg in a single dose of extract administered to animals per kg b.w.), lithospermic acid (0.084 mg/kg), salvianolic acid A (0.08 mg/kg), and salvianolic acid B (0.046 mg/kg) may be responsible for observed pharmacological effects. On the other hand, results from few studies showed that salvianolic acids do not cross the blood brain barrier (BBB) [41, 42] and also lithospermic acid does not efficiently cross the BBB [43]. For this reason, the interpretation of our results is more complicated.

Firstly, Xu et al. [44] demonstrated that Sal A is a metabolically unstable compound that would undergo rapid methylation metabolism catalyzed by catechol O-methyltransferase *in vivo* into four major methylated metabolites of Sal A (3-O-methyl, 3′-O-methyl, 3,3″-O-dimethyl, and 3′,3″-O-dimethyl salvianolic acid A). These generated O-methylated metabolites may be largely responsible for its *in vivo* pharmacological effects. Although there are no available recent studies on the ability of these compounds to pass the BBB, such possibility should not be excluded.

Secondly, several studies showed central pharmacological effects in animals after *per os* administration of Sal B [45, 46], Sal A [47], and caffeic acid [48]. It was proved, for example, that salvianolic acid B (10 mg/kg, p.o.) significantly rescued the $A\beta25-35$ peptide-induced decrease of choline acetyltransferase and brain-derived neurotrophic factor protein levels in an amyloid β ($A\beta$) peptide-induced Alzheimer's disease mouse model [49]. It also significantly reversed (10 mg/kg, p.o.) the cognitive impairments induced by scopolamine (1 mg/kg, i.p.) or $A\beta$ (25–35) (10 nmol/5 μL, i.c.v.) injection in mice [45]. Previous studies [46, 47] showed also that both Sal A and Sal B are able to improve the impaired memory function induced by cerebral ischemia-reperfusion in mice. The stimulation of neurogenesis process in both subgranular zone (SGZ) and subventricular zone (SVZ) after brain ischemia and also alleviation neural cells loss and improved motor function recovery after brain ischemia in rats after the Sal B administration were also observed by Zhong et al. [50]. Moreover, the exposure to Sal B can maintain the proliferation of neural stem/progenitor cells (NSPCs) after cerebral ischemia and improve cognitive postischemic impairment after stroke in rats using Morris water maze test; therefore authors concluded that Sal B may act as a potential drug in treatment of brain injury or neurodegenerative disease [51]. Additionally, the improvement of motor function after cerebral ischemia in rats after salvianolic acid B administration was also demonstrated [52]. The clue to pass through the BBB Sal B provided also results of Li et al. indicating its protective effect on BBB in rats after cerebral ischemia-reperfusion by inhibiting the MAPK pathway [53]. In addition to this, it was shown that lithospermic acid and salvianolic acids exerted neuroprotective activity in various experimental models. Lithospermic acid significantly attenuates neurotoxicity *in vitro* and *in vivo* induced by 1-methyl-4-phenylpyridin (MPP(+)) by blocking neuronal apoptotic and neuroinflammatory pathways [54]. Salvianolic acid B inhibited amyloid beta-protein aggregation and fibril formation, as well as directly inhibiting the cellular toxicity of amyloid beta-protein in PC12 cells [55], and significantly reduced its cytotoxic effects on human neuroblastoma SH-SY5Y cells [56].

For an explanation of our results, observations of Pinheiro Fernandes et al. [57] may be very helpful, which showed that caffeic acid, nonflavanoid catecholic compound, whose derivatives are occurring in *MO* extract, improved the working, spatial, and long-term aversive memory deficits induced by focal cerebral ischemia in mice. Anwar et al. [48] showed also that caffeic acid (100 mg/kg) improved the step-down latencies in the inhibitory avoidance in rats. Tsai et al. [58] showed that caffeic acid is a potent neuroprotective agent in brain of 1-methyl-4-phenyl-1,2,3,6-tetrahydropyridine (MPTP) treated mice. Moreover, caffeic acid improves Aβ25–35-induced memory deficits and cognitive impairment in mice [59]. In another study, it was also shown that this compound has a significant protective effect on global cerebral ischemia-reperfusion injury in rats [60]. For instance, 12.4 ± 1.8 mg/100 g of caffeic acid was detected in the brain of mice with a diet containing 2% caffeic acid for 4 weeks [58]. Thus, there is progressive evidence that this compound passes through the BBB and has a central pharmacological activity.

Also results by Yoo et al. are also worth noting [61] which showed, also in a rat model of scopolamine-induced amnesia, that administration of luteolin (a common flavonoid from many plants including *M. officinalis*) at dose of 10 mg/kg caused the increase in the brain-derived neurotrophic factor (BDNF), acetylcholine, and the decrease in lipid peroxidation. Liu et al. [62] observed that chronic treatment with luteolin (50 and 100 mg/kg) improved neuronal injury and cognitive performance by attenuating oxidative stress and cholinesterase activity in streptozotocin-induced diabetes in rats. In our study, ethanolic extract of *MO* administered to rats significantly improved long-term memory after using a passive avoidance test, but after *MO* combined treatment with SC no improvement of this paradigm was observed (Table 2).

Thirdly, available pharmacokinetic studies were carried out for the pure compounds (Sal A and B) and the extract of the roots of *Salvia miltiorrhiza* [42, 63], but there are not available studies of bioavailability of these compounds after administration of *Melissa officinalis* leaf extract, containing other compounds as compared with the extract of *Salvia miltiorrhiza*. Moreover, there is a lack of data about how scopolamine may influence the penetration of the salvianolic acids (and other compounds) across the BBB. Hence, there is a need to study the pharmacokinetic parameters of these compounds in the group of animals treated with scopolamine in comparison with control group.

AChE and BuChE Activities in Rat Brain. To date, several studies have focused on explaining the mechanism of action of the MS extract and its active compounds. Soodi et al. [18] showed that treatment of animals with *MO* extract (400 mg/kg) prior to scopolamine injection could ameliorate scopolamine-induced enhancement in AChE activity. This dose of *MO* extract inhibited the AChE activity in the hippocampus of rats (51.9% versus 100.4% in normal saline group, $p < 0.05$; 91.4% in group treated with scopolamine + *MO* versus 128.1% in scopolamine group, $p < 0.05$). In another study, Anwar et al. [48] showed that 50 and 100 mg/kg of caffeic acid decreased *in vivo* the AChE activity in the cerebral cortex and striatum and increased the activity of this enzyme in the cerebellum, hippocampus, hypothalamus, pons, lymphocytes, and muscles when compared to the control group ($p < 0.05$). Our study showed that ethanolic extract of *MO* produced an insignificant and slight inhibition of AChE and BuChE activity in the frontal cortex and in the hippocampus (especially). However, it was observed previously [23] that RA inhibited the AChE activity in the rats frontal cortex and hippocampus. Moreover, we showed that RA possess a strong stimulatory effect on BuChE in the hippocampus.

AChE, BuChE, and BACE1 mRNA Level Changes in Rat Brain. So far, no results have been published of studies concerning the *in vivo* assessment of changes in AChE, BuChE, and BACE1 gene expression profile in different brain regions under the influence of *MO* extracts or their key bioactive metabolites. Such studies focused overwhelmingly on the analysis of their *in vitro* activities, to a lesser extent in animal experiments.

In our study, in the frontal cortex, we have observed the strongest inhibition of both AChE and BuCHE mRNA transcription under the influence of *M. officinalis* extract and huperzine A (Table 3). However, a more significant difference in the level of transcript was seen in the frontal cortex, in particular in the case of BuCHE mRNA of experimental rats (a decrease by 51.6% and 44% for *MO* and HU versus control, resp.). The strong inhibition of transcription of AChE mRNA was also observed in the hippocampus of *MO*-treated rats (a decrease by 69%). The BuChE mRNA transcription in animals receiving *MO* was lowered in a moderate way (decrease by 36%). Huperzine A alone has not caused changes that were observed in the group of *MO* (Table 2). Our findings mostly correlate with the observed changes in activities of AChE and BuChE in different groups of animals. In the case of BuChE, slightly different results between its activity and expression profile were especially seen in the frontal cortex and hippocampus of animals receiving *MO* (Table 3).

To date, there is a lack of published results of studies making an attempt to clarify the potential differences in the transcriptional profile and activity of AChE and BuChE under the influence of *MO* and its bioactive metabolites. It cannot be excluded that the key for the observed differences in the level of AChE activities and mRNA level can be caused by changes in the activity of AChE in other regions of the brain, not analyzed in this study, such as substantia nigra, cerebellum, globus pallidus, and hypothalamus, where it exerts nonenzymatic neuromodulatory functions affecting neurite outgrowth and synaptogenesis, modulating the activity of other proteins regional cerebral blood flow, and other functions [64]. But it is difficult to clearly explain why diminishing of AChE and BuChE mRNAs did not always correlate with the lowering of activity of these enzymes, although it has been recently noted that AChE activity was not paralleled by an increase in mRNA levels [65]. The authors explained this fact by stating that AChE levels are regulated at transcriptional, posttranscriptional, and posttranslational levels leading to complex expression patterns which can be modulated by physiological and pathological conditions. However, these mechanisms are not fully understood and further studies are needed in this field.

The cause of observed different degree of inhibition of activity and transcription status of studied genes, especially of BuChE (and AChE), may lie in a so-called "negative feedback" consisting of a complicated transcription/translation regulation, protein-protein interactions/modifications, and a metabolic network, together forming a system that allows the cell to respond sensibly to the multiple signal molecules that exist in its environment [66].

Because of that, we propose that the reason for differences between AChE and BuChE activities in the cortex and hippocampus under the *MO* may be due to the fact of insufficiency of applied dose and the duration of the experiment, affecting the transcriptional, tissue-specific, cellular machinery regulating BuChE transcription without affecting its activity. Moreover, the administration of higher doses of *MO* and extended period of time could lead to sufficient inhibition of its activity.

There is a need to conduct further studies to determine the molecular degree of dependence between changes in AChE and BuChE activities and activities of potential key factors regulating expression of these genes in the frontal cortex and hippocampus under the influence of extracts of *MO* and active metabolites. Another study determining the effectiveness of their actions on the cholinergic system in experimental animal models of memory impairment, with particular emphasis on scopolamine, including the determination of changes at the molecular level should be therefore carried out.

Alterations in BACE1 protein level have been proved in postmortem brain tissue from individuals with AD, with increases, decreases, and also no change reported [1, 67, 68]. An example of confirmation of these findings at the mRNA level is results of study by Coulson et al. [69]. Based on conducted studies, some authors suggested that increased BACE1 mRNA transcription in remaining neuronal cells may contribute to the increased BACE1 protein levels and activity found in brain regions affected by AD [70].

Results of many studies concerning the elevated level of BACE1 mRNA and protein in Alzheimer's disease provide direct and compelling reasons to develop therapies directed at BACE1 inhibition, thus reducing β-amyloid and its associated toxicities [67, 68].

In our study, we have observed that BACE mRNA expression statistically significantly decreased after *MO* administration in frontal cortex and hippocampus. These results suggest that the *MO* extract may act to inhibit BACE1 mRNA level, given the fact that the percentage of inhibition of the expression (64% in the frontal cortex, 50% in the hippocampus) is higher than that in the case of HU (38% in the cortex and the lack of changes in the hippocampus). A careful analysis of the literature data shows that there are no studies which analyzed the impact of *MO* extract on the expression level of BACE1 in Alzheimer's disease.

Furthermore, a literature analysis does not indicate already published results conducted by other teams attempting to assess the impact of RA on the transcriptional activity of AChE, BuChE, and BACE1. Although several studies (already mentioned and others [70, 71]) highlighted the RA and other caffeic acid derivatives capability of acetylcholinesterases inhibition, none of these studies does not touch the question of the molecular basis of their impact on the transcriptional machinery that regulates *in vivo* the expression of studied genes. Hence, in our opinion, obtained by our team results, they are one of the first of this type and, in general, correlate with the results of our previous study [23]. In this case, there is no clear evidence explaining different responses at the transcriptional level under the influence of RA, especially in the case of BuChE encoding gene in the hippocampus (Table 2). It is possible that the observed differentiation of BuChE transcriptional activity between the frontal cortex and the hippocampus may be due to the differences of butyrylcholinesterase localization and substrate affinity [72]. Since in our experiment we have carried out a quantitative analysis of AChE, BuChE, and BACE1 transcripts in brain homogenates of tested animals, rather than in individual, isolated cell fractions, therefore the obtained results constitute an overall "picture" of both studied genes transcriptional changes occurring in the brain areas of studied animals under the influence of the RA and the whole plant extract as well.

6. Conclusion

The subchronic administration of *MO* led to an improvement of long-term memory of rats; however the mechanisms of *MO* action are probably more complicated, since its role as a modulator of beta-secretase activity (due to inhibition of BACE1 mRNA expression in frontal cortex) should be taken into consideration.

It should be noted that we have studied a crude extract from leaf of *Melissa officinalis*, not a single pure chemical compound. This plant extract is a complex mixture, and its action may be a result of the summation of activities of several components (synergism/additive action of caffeic acid with salvianolic acids, rosmarinic acid, and others). In the case of extract from leaves of *Melissa officinalis*, it is possible that interactions occur between the 40 chemical compounds identified by HPLC system.

Taken together, it seems that the *MO* activity represents a possible option as complementary interventions to relieve the symptoms of mild dementia.

Competing Interests

The authors declare that they have no competing interests.

Acknowledgments

This work was supported by the Ministry of Science and Higher Education, Warsaw, Poland, from educational sources (2008–2011, Grant no. N 405417836).

References

[1] S. L. Cole and R. Vassar, "The Alzheimer's disease β-secretase enzyme, BACE1," *Molecular Neurodegeneration*, vol. 2, no. 1, article 22, 2007.

[2] L. A. Craig, N. S. Hong, and R. J. McDonald, "Revisiting the cholinergic hypothesis in the development of Alzheimer's disease," *Neuroscience & Biobehavioral Reviews*, vol. 35, no. 6, pp. 1397–1409, 2011.

[3] N. G. M. Gomes, M. G. Campos, J. M. C. Órfão, and C. A. F. Ribeiro, "Plants with neurobiological activity as potential targets for drug discovery," *Progress in Neuro-Psychopharmacology & Biological Psychiatry*, vol. 33, no. 8, pp. 1372–1389, 2009.

[4] WHO, *WHO Monographs on Selected Medicinal Plants—Volume 2*, WHO, Geneva, Switzerland, 2004, http://apps.who.int/medicinedocs/en/d/Js4927e/18.html#Js4927e.18.

[5] M. Bayat, A. A. Tameh, M. H. Ghahremani et al., "Neuroprotective properties of *Melissa officinalis* after hypoxic-ischemic injury both *in vitro* and *in vivo*," *DARU Journal of Pharmaceutical Sciences*, vol. 20, article 42, 2012.

[6] J. P. Kamdem, A. Adeniran, A. A. Boligon et al., "Antioxidant activity, genotoxicity and cytotoxicity evaluation of lemon balm (*Melissa officinalis* L.) ethanolic extract: Its potential role in neuroprotection," *Industrial Crops and Products*, vol. 51, pp. 26–34, 2013.

[7] J.-T. Lin, Y.-C. Chen, Y.-C. Lee, C.-W. R. Hou, F.-L. Chen, and D.-J. Yang, "Antioxidant, anti-proliferative and cyclooxygenase-2 inhibitory activities of ethanolic extracts from lemon balm (*Melissa officinalis* L.) leaves," *LWT—Food Science and Technology*, vol. 49, no. 1, pp. 1–7, 2012.

[8] G. Guginski, A. P. Luiz, M. D. Silva et al., "Mechanisms involved in the antinociception caused by ethanolic extract obtained from the leaves of *Melissa officinalis* (lemon balm) in mice," *Pharmacology Biochemistry & Behavior*, vol. 93, no. 1, pp. 10–16, 2009.

[9] N. Perry, G. Court, N. Bidet, J. Court, and E. Perry, "European herbs with cholinergic activities: potential in dementia therapy," *International Journal of Geriatric Psychiatry*, vol. 11, no. 12, pp. 1063–1069, 1996.

[10] E. K. Perry, A. T. Pickering, W. W. Wang, P. J. Houghton, and N. S. L. Perry, "Medicinal plants and Alzheimer's disease: from ethnobotany to phytotherapy," *Journal of Pharmacy and Pharmacology*, vol. 51, no. 5, pp. 527–534, 1999.

[11] M.-J. R. Howes, N. S. L. Perry, and P. J. Houghton, "Plants with traditional uses and activities, relevant to the management of Alzheimer's disease and other cognitive disorders," *Phytotherapy Research*, vol. 17, no. 1, pp. 1–18, 2003.

[12] I. Orhan and M. Aslan, "Appraisal of scopolamine-induced antiamnesic effect in mice and *in vitro* antiacetylcholinesterase and antioxidant activities of some traditionally used Lamiaceae plants," *Journal of Ethnopharmacology*, vol. 122, no. 2, pp. 327–332, 2009.

[13] S. Akhondzadeh, M. Noroozian, M. Mohammadi, S. Ohadinia, A. H. Jamshidi, and M. Khani, "*Melissa officinalis* extract in the treatment of patients with mild to moderate Alzheimer's disease: a double blind, randomised, placebo controlled trial," *Journal of Neurology Neurosurgery and Psychiatry*, vol. 74, no. 7, pp. 863–866, 2003.

[14] D. O. Kennedy, A. B. Scholey, N. T. J. Tildesley, E. K. Perry, and K. A. Wesnes, "Modulation of mood and cognitive performance following acute administration of *Melissa officinalis* (lemon balm)," *Pharmacology Biochemistry & Behavior*, vol. 72, no. 4, pp. 953–964, 2002.

[15] D. O. Kennedy, G. Wake, S. Savelev et al., "Modulation of mood and cognitive performance following acute administration of single doses of *Melissa officinalis* (Lemon balm) with human CNS nicotinic and muscarinic receptor-binding properties," *Neuropsychopharmacology*, vol. 28, no. 10, pp. 1871–1881, 2003.

[16] D. O. Kennedy and E. L. Wightman, "Herbal extracts and phytochemicals: plant secondary metabolites and the enhancement of human brain function," *Advances in Nutrition*, vol. 2, no. 1, pp. 32–50, 2011.

[17] R. P. Pereira, A. A. Boligon, A. S. Appel et al., "Chemical composition, antioxidant and anticholinesterase activity of *Melissa officinalis*," *Industrial Crops and Products*, vol. 53, pp. 34–45, 2014.

[18] M. Soodi, N. Naghdi, H. Hajimehdipoor, S. Choopani, and E. Sahraei, "Memory-improving activity of *Melissa officinalis* extract in naïve and scopolamine-treated rats," *Research in Pharmaceutical Sciences*, vol. 9, no. 2, pp. 107–114, 2014.

[19] K. Dastmalchi, V. Ollilainen, P. Lackman et al., "Acetylcholinesterase inhibitory guided fractionation of *Melissa officinalis* L.," *Bioorganic & Medicinal Chemistry*, vol. 17, no. 2, pp. 867–871, 2009.

[20] W. Chaiyana and S. Okonogi, "Inhibition of cholinesterase by essential oil from food plant," *Phytomedicine*, vol. 19, no. 8-9, pp. 836–839, 2012.

[21] K. Dastmalchi, H. J. D. Dorman, P. P. Oinonen, Y. Darwis, I. Laakso, and R. Hiltunen, "Chemical composition and in vitro antioxidative activity of a lemon balm (*Melissa officinalis* L.) extract," *LWT—Food Science and Technology*, vol. 41, no. 3, pp. 391–400, 2008.

[22] P. Pereira, D. Tysca, P. Oliveira, L. F. D. S. Brum, J. N. Picada, and P. Ardenghi, "Neurobehavioral and genotoxic aspects of rosmarinic acid," *Pharmacological Research*, vol. 52, no. 3, pp. 199–203, 2005.

[23] M. Ozarowski, P. L. Mikolajczak, A. Bogacz et al., "*Rosmarinus officinalis* L. leaf extract improves memory impairment and affects acetylcholinesterase and butyrylcholinesterase activities in rat brain," *Fitoterapia*, vol. 91, pp. 261–271, 2013.

[24] G. P. Kumar and F. Khanum, "Neuroprotective potential of phytochemicals," *Pharmacognosy Reviews*, vol. 6, no. 12, pp. 81–90, 2012.

[25] M. Stobiecki, A. Staszków, A. Piasecka, P. M. Garcia-Lopez, F. Zamora-Natera, and P. Kachlicki, "LC-MSMS profiling of flavonoid conjugates in wild mexican lupine, *Lupinus reflexus*," *Journal of Natural Products*, vol. 73, no. 7, pp. 1254–1260, 2010.

[26] A. Wojakowska, A. Piasecka, P. M. García-López et al., "Structural analysis and profiling of phenolic secondary metabolites of

Mexican lupine species using LC-MS techniques," *Phytochemistry*, vol. 92, pp. 71–86, 2013.

[27] A. Gryszczynska, B. Opala, Z. Lowicki et al., "Bioactive compounds determination in the callus and hydroalcoholic extracts from *Salvia miltiorrhiza* and *Salvia przewalskii*—preliminary study on their anti-alcoholic activity effects," *Phytochemistry Letters*, vol. 11, pp. 399–403, 2015.

[28] K. Slinkart and V. L. Singleton, "Total phenol analysis: automation and comparison with manual method," *American Journal of Enology and Viticulture*, vol. 28, no. 1, pp. 49–55, 1977.

[29] P. J. R. Boissier, J. Tardy, and J. C. Diverres, "Une nouvelle méthode simple pour explorer l'action 'tranquillisante': le test de la cheminée," *Medicina Experimentalis*, vol. 3, no. 1, pp. 81–84, 1960.

[30] R. Ader, J. A. Weijnen, and P. Moleman, "Retention of a passive avoidance response as a function of the intensity and duration of electric shock," *Psychonomic Science*, vol. 26, no. 3, pp. 125–128, 1972.

[31] E. M. Blalock, K.-C. Chen, K. Sharrow et al., "Gene microarrays in hippocampal aging: statistical profiling identifies novel processes correlated with cognitive impairment," *Journal of Neuroscience*, vol. 23, no. 9, pp. 3807–3819, 2003.

[32] K. Isomae, S. Morimoto, H. Hasegawa, K. Morita, and J. Kamei, "Effects of T-82, a novel acetylcholinesterase inhibitor, on impaired learning and memory in passive avoidance task in rats," *European Journal of Pharmacology*, vol. 465, no. 1-2, pp. 97–103, 2003.

[33] J. Patora and B. Klimek, "Flavonoids from lemon balm (*Melissa officinalis* L., Lamiaceae)," *Acta Poloniae Pharmaceutica-Drug Research*, vol. 59, no. 2, pp. 139–143, 2002.

[34] L. Barros, M. Dueñas, M. I. Dias, M. J. Sousa, C. Santos-Buelga, and I. C. F. R. Ferreira, "Phenolic profiles of cultivated, in vitro cultured and commercial samples of *Melissa officinalis* L. infusions," *Food Chemistry*, vol. 136, no. 1, pp. 1–8, 2013.

[35] T. L. Miron, M. Herrero, and E. Ibáñez, "Enrichment of antioxidant compounds from lemon balm (*Melissa officinalis*) by pressurized liquid extraction and enzyme-assisted extraction," *Journal of Chromatography A*, vol. 1288, pp. 1–9, 2013.

[36] Y. Lu, L. Y. Foo, and H. Wong, "Sagecoumarin, a novel caffeic acid trimer from *Salvia officinalis*," *Phytochemistry*, vol. 52, no. 6, pp. 1149–1152, 1999.

[37] S. Abuhamdah, L. Huang, M. S. J. Elliott et al., "Pharmacological profile of an essential oil derived from *Melissa officinalis* with anti-agitation properties: focus on ligand-gated channels," *Journal of Pharmacy and Pharmacology*, vol. 60, no. 3, pp. 377–384, 2008.

[38] G. Wake, J. Court, A. Pickering, R. Lewis, R. Wilkins, and E. Perry, "CNS acetylcholine receptor activity in European medicinal plants traditionally used to improve failing memory," *Journal of Ethnopharmacology*, vol. 69, no. 2, pp. 105–114, 2000.

[39] S.-H. Ryu, C. Katona, B. Rive, and G. Livingston, "Persistence of and changes in neuropsychiatric symptoms in Alzheimer disease over 6 months: the LASER-AD study," *American Journal of Geriatric Psychiatry*, vol. 13, no. 11, pp. 976–983, 2005.

[40] L. N. Gitlin, H. C. Kales, and C. G. Lyketsos, "Nonpharmacologic management of behavioral symptoms in dementia," *Journal of the American Medical Association*, vol. 308, no. 19, pp. 2020–2029, 2012.

[41] Á. Könczöl, J. Müller, E. Földes et al., "Applicability of a blood-brain barrier specific artificial membrane permeability assay at the early stage of natural product-based CNS drug discovery," *Journal of Natural Products*, vol. 76, no. 4, pp. 655–663, 2013.

[42] Y.-J. Zhang, L. Wu, Q.-L. Zhang, J. Li, F.-X. Yin, and Y. Yuan, "Pharmacokinetics of phenolic compounds of Danshen extract in rat blood and brain by microdialysis sampling," *Journal of Ethnopharmacology*, vol. 136, no. 1, pp. 129–136, 2011.

[43] X. Li, C. Yu, Y. Lu et al., "Pharmacokinetics, tissue distribution, metabolism, and excretion of depside salts from *Salvia miltiorrhiza* in rats," *Drug Metabolism and Disposition*, vol. 35, no. 2, pp. 234–239, 2007.

[44] H. Xu, Y. Li, X. Che, H. Tian, H. Fan, and K. Liu, "Metabolism of *salvianolic acid* a and antioxidant activities of its methylated metabolites," *Drug Metabolism and Disposition*, vol. 42, no. 2, pp. 274–281, 2014.

[45] D. H. Kim, S. J. Park, J. M. Kim et al., "Cognitive dysfunctions induced by a cholinergic blockade and Aβ 25-35 peptide are attenuated by salvianolic acid B," *Neuropharmacology*, vol. 61, no. 8, pp. 1432–1440, 2011.

[46] G.-H. Du, Y. Qiu, and J.-T. Zhang, "Salvianolic acid B protects the memory functions against transient cerebral ischemia in mice," *Journal of Asian Natural Products Research*, vol. 2, no. 2, pp. 145–152, 2000.

[47] G. Du and J. Zhang, "Protective effects of salvianolic acid A against impairment of memory induced by cerebral ischemia-reperfusion in mice," *Chinese Medical Journal*, vol. 110, no. 1, pp. 65–68, 1997.

[48] J. Anwar, R. M. Spanevello, G. Thomé et al., "Effects of caffeic acid on behavioral parameters and on the activity of acetylcholinesterase in different tissues from adult rats," *Pharmacology Biochemistry and Behavior*, vol. 103, no. 2, pp. 386–394, 2012.

[49] Y. W. Lee, D. H. Kim, S. J. Jeon et al., "Neuroprotective effects of salvianolic acid B on an Aβ25-35 peptide-induced mouse model of Alzheimer's disease," *European Journal of Pharmacology*, vol. 704, no. 1-3, pp. 70–77, 2013.

[50] J. Zhong, M.-K. Tang, Y. Zhang, Q.-P. Xu, and J.-T. Zhang, "Effect of salvianolic acid B on neural cells damage and neurogenesis after brain ischemia-reperfusion in rats," *Yao Xue Xue Bao*, vol. 42, no. 7, pp. 716–721, 2007.

[51] P. Zhuang, Y. Zhang, G. Cui et al., "Direct stimulation of adult neural stem/progenitor cells in vitro and neurogenesis *in vivo* by salvianolic acid B," *PLoS ONE*, vol. 7, no. 4, Article ID e35636, 2012.

[52] M. Tang, W. Feng, Y. Zhang, J. Zhong, and J. Zhang, "Salvianolic acid B improves motor function after cerebral ischemia in rats," *Behavioural Pharmacology*, vol. 17, no. 5-6, pp. 493–498, 2006.

[53] Q. Li, L.-P. Han, Z.-H. Li, J.-T. Zhang, and M.-K. Tang, "Salvianolic acid B alleviate the disruption of blood-brain barrier in rats after cerebral ischemia-reperfusion by inhibiting MAPK pathway," *Yao Xue Xue Bao*, vol. 45, no. 12, pp. 1485–1490, 2010.

[54] Y.-L. Lin, H.-J. Tsay, T.-H. Lai, T.-T. Tzeng, and Y.-J. Shiao, "Lithospermic acid attenuates 1-methyl-4-phenylpyridine-induced neurotoxicity by blocking neuronal apoptotic and neuroinflammatory pathways," *Journal of Biomedical Science*, vol. 22, article 37, 2015.

[55] M.-K. Tang and J.-T. Zhang, "Salvianolic acid B inhibits fibril formation and neurotoxicity of amyloid beta-protein *in vitro*," *Acta Pharmacologica Sinica*, vol. 22, no. 4, pp. 380–384, 2001.

[56] S. S. K. Durairajan, Q. Yuan, L. Xie et al., "Salvianolic acid B inhibits Aβ fibril formation and disaggregates preformed fibrils and protects against Aβ-induced cytotoxicty," *Neurochemistry International*, vol. 52, no. 4-5, pp. 741–750, 2008.

[57] F. D. Pinheiro Fernandes, A. P. Fontenele Menezes, J. C. de Sousa Neves et al., "Caffeic acid protects mice from memory deficits

induced by focal cerebral ischemia," *Behavioural Pharmacology*, vol. 25, no. 7, pp. 637–647, 2014.

[58] S.-J. Tsai, C.-Y. Chao, and M.-C. Yin, "Preventive and therapeutic effects of caffeic acid against inflammatory injury in striatum of MPTP-treated mice," *European Journal of Pharmacology*, vol. 670, no. 2-3, pp. 441–447, 2011.

[59] J. H. Kim, Q. Wang, J. M. Choi, S. Lee, and E. J. Cho, "Protective role of caffeic acid in an $A\beta_{25-35}$-induced Alzheimer's disease model," *Nutrition Research and Practice*, vol. 9, no. 5, pp. 480–488, 2015.

[60] G. Liang, B. Shi, W. Luo, and J. Yang, "The protective effect of caffeic acid on global cerebral ischemia-reperfusion injury in rats," *Behavioral and Brain Functions*, vol. 11, no. 1, article 18, 2015.

[61] D. Y. Yoo, J. H. Choi, W. Kim et al., "Effects of luteolin on spatial memory, cell proliferation, and neuroblast differentiation in the hippocampal dentate gyrus in a scopolamine-induced amnesia model," *Neurological Research*, vol. 35, no. 8, pp. 813–820, 2013.

[62] Y. Liu, X. Tian, L. Gou, L. Sun, X. Ling, and X. Yin, "Luteolin attenuates diabetes-associated cognitive decline in rats," *Brain Research Bulletin*, vol. 94, pp. 23–29, 2013.

[63] S.-M. Liu, Z.-H. Yang, and X.-B. Sun, "Simultaneous determination of six *Salvia miltiorrhiza* gradients in rat plasma and brain by LC-MS/MS," *Zhongguo Zhongyao Zazhi*, vol. 39, no. 9, pp. 1704–1708, 2014.

[64] M. A. Papandreou, A. Dimakopoulou, Z. I. Linardaki et al., "Effect of a polyphenol-rich wild blueberry extract on cognitive performance of mice, brain antioxidant markers and acetylcholinesterase activity," *Behavioural Brain Research*, vol. 198, no. 2, pp. 352–358, 2009.

[65] M.-S. García-Ayllón, O. Cauli, M.-X. Silveyra et al., "Brain cholinergic impairment in liver failure," *Brain*, vol. 131, no. 11, pp. 2946–2956, 2008.

[66] G. K. Ferreira, M. Carvalho-Silva, C. L. Gonçalves et al., "L-Tyrosine administration increases acetylcholinesterase activity in rats," *Neurochemistry International*, vol. 61, no. 8, pp. 1370–1374, 2012.

[67] R. Vassar, P.-H. Kuhn, C. Haass et al., "Function, therapeutic potential and cell biology of BACE proteases: current status and future prospects," *Journal of Neurochemistry*, vol. 130, no. 1, pp. 4–28, 2014.

[68] R. Vassar, "The β-secretase, BACE: a prime drug target for Alzheimer's disease," *Journal of Molecular Neuroscience*, vol. 17, no. 2, pp. 157–170, 2001.

[69] D. T. R. Coulson, N. Beyer, J. G. Quinn et al., "BACE1 mRNA expression in Alzheimer's disease postmortem brain tissue," *Journal of Alzheimer's Disease*, vol. 22, no. 4, pp. 1111–1122, 2010.

[70] S. Vladimir-Knežević, B. Blažeković, M. Kindl, J. Vladić, A. D. Lower-Nedza, and A. H. Brantner, "Acetylcholinesterase inhibitory, antioxidant and phytochemical properties of selected medicinal plants of the lamiaceae family," *Molecules*, vol. 19, no. 1, pp. 767–782, 2014.

[71] F. Marcelo, C. Dias, A. Martins et al., "Molecular recognition of rosmarinic acid from *Salvia sclareoides* extracts by acetylcholinesterase: a new binding site detected by NMR spectroscopy," *Chemistry—A European Journal*, vol. 19, no. 21, pp. 6641–6649, 2013.

[72] G. Johnson and S. W. Moore, "Why has butyrylcholinesterase been retained? Structural and functional diversification in a duplicated gene," *Neurochemistry International*, vol. 61, no. 5, pp. 783–797, 2012.

[73] R. J. Grayer, M. R. Eckert, N. C. Veitch et al., "The chemotaxonomic significance of two bioactive caffeic acid esters, nepetoidins A and B, in the Lamiaceae," *Phytochemistry*, vol. 64, no. 2, pp. 519–528, 2003.

[74] A. M. D. El-Mousallamy, U. W. Hawas, and S. A. M. Hussein, "Teucrol, a decarboxyrosmarinic acid and its $4'$-O-triglycoside, teucroside from *Teucrium pilosum*," *Phytochemistry*, vol. 55, no. 8, pp. 927–931, 2000.

[75] I. Fecka and S. Turek, "Determination of water-soluble polyphenolic compounds in commercial herbal teas from Lamiaceae: peppermint, melissa, and sage," *Journal of Agricultural and Food Chemistry*, vol. 55, no. 26, pp. 10908–10917, 2007.

[76] L. W. Sumner, A. Amberg, D. Barrett et al., "Proposed minimum reporting standards for chemical analysis Working Group (CAWG) Metabolomics Standards Initiative (MSI)," *Metabolomics*, vol. 3, pp. 211–221, 2007.

Berberine Inhibition of Fibrogenesis in a Rat Model of Liver Fibrosis and in Hepatic Stellate Cells

Ning Wang,[1] Qihe Xu,[2] Hor Yue Tan,[1] Ming Hong,[1] Sha Li,[1] Man-Fung Yuen,[3] and Yibin Feng[1]

[1]School of Chinese Medicine, Li Ka Shing Faculty of Medicine, The University of Hong Kong, Pokfulam, Hong Kong
[2]Centre for Integrative Chinese Medicine and Department of Renal Medicine, Faculty of Life Sciences and Medicine, King's College London, London SE5 9NU, UK
[3]Division of Gastroenterology and Hepatology, Queen Mary Hospital and Department of Medicine, Li Ka Shing Faculty of Medicine, The University of Hong Kong, Pokfulam, Hong Kong

Correspondence should be addressed to Yibin Feng; yfeng@hku.hk

Academic Editor: Victor Kuete

Aim. To examine the effect of berberine (BBR) on liver fibrosis and its possible mechanisms through direct effects on hepatic stellate cells (HSC). *Methods.* The antifibrotic effect of BBR was determined in a rat model of bile duct ligation- (BDL-) induced liver fibrosis. Multiple cellular and molecular approaches were introduced to examine the effects of BBR on HSC. *Results.* BBR potently inhibited hepatic fibrosis induced by BDL in rats. It exhibited cytotoxicity to activated HSC at doses nontoxic to hepatocytes. High doses of BBR induced apoptosis of activated HSC, which was mediated by loss of mitochondrial membrane potential and Bcl-2/Bax imbalance. Low doses of BBR suppressed activation of HSC as evidenced by the inhibition of α-smooth muscle actin (α-SMA) expression and cell motility. BBR did not affect Smad2/3 phosphorylation but significantly activated $5'$ AMP-activated protein kinase (AMPK) signalling, which was responsible for the transcriptional inhibition by BBR of profibrogenic factors α-SMA and collagen in HSC. *Conclusion.* BBR is a promising agent for treating liver fibrosis through multiple mechanisms, at least partially by directly targeting HSC and by inhibiting the AMPK pathway. Its value as an antifibrotic drug in patients with liver disease deserves further investigation.

1. Introduction

Hepatic fibrosis is a common pathology in various progressive chronic liver diseases [1]. Fibrogenesis in liver, which often accompanies disease progression from hepatitis to cancerous transformation [2], is an abnormal process in which the organ develops excessive accumulation of extracellular matrix proteins in response to chronic injury [3]. Activation of hepatic stellate cells (HSC) is critical in the fibrogenic process of the liver and activated HSC are known as the main sources of a pathogenic extracellular matrix proteins in liver fibrosis [4, 5]. It is believed that effective treatment of hepatic fibrosis will be both crucial for the prevention of chronic liver failure and beneficial for the prevention of liver cancerous diseases [6]; however, there is still no standard treatment for liver fibrosis [7].

Berberine (BBR) is a natural alkaloid extracted from Coptidis Rhizoma (Huang Lian in Chinese), an herbal drug commonly used in traditional Chinese medicine for treating patients with inflammatory diseases. The major pharmacological actions of BBR may include antimicrobial [8], anti-inflammatory [9], antioxidative [10], and antitumoral activities [11]. Our previous studies have revealed the therapeutic effects of Coptidis Rhizoma and BBR on hepatocellular carcinoma, by inducing apoptotic and autophagic cell death at high doses [12] and by repressing tumor cell motility at lower doses [13]. These observations suggested that BBR be of potential value for treating liver malignancies [14]. Furthermore, it was also found by our group that extract of Coptidis Rhizoma exerted potent protective effect on acute and chronic liver damage in an experimental animal model of liver injury, significantly improving liver function and tissue structure [15, 16]. We further reported that, BBR, a major active compound extracted from Coptidis Rhizoma also protected animal from acute hepatic damage [17, 18]. BBR is able to reduce sustained and chronic liver injury in various animal models of hepatic damage [19]. We have proposed that BBR as an antifibrotic drug and its mechanisms of action are worth further investigation [20].

In this study, we aimed to investigate the in vitro and in vivo antifibrotic effect of BBR and its potential mechanisms with focus on HSC. The antifibrotic activity of BBR was evaluated in bile duct ligation-induced hepatic fibrosis model in rats. The action of BBR on activated HSC was investigated at both nontoxic and toxic levels. Understanding the action and mechanism of BBR in inhibiting hepatic fibrosis may shed light on the further development of antifibrotic treatment.

2. Materials and Methods

2.1. Chemicals and Reagents. BBR hydrochloride and Compound C, an AMPK inhibitor, were purchased from Sigma-Aldrich (USA).

2.2. Animals. Male SD rats of 220~250 g body weight were purchased from Guangdong Medical Laboratory Animal Centre, Guangzhou, Guangdong Province, China. Animals were housed at $25 \pm 2°C$, with a 12 h light cycle, starting at 06:00, and were provided free access to standard laboratory chow and water. All experiments were approved by the ethics committee of the University of Hong Kong and complied with international guidelines.

2.3. Animal Model. Bile duct ligation (BDL) was applied to rats to induce extrahepatic cholestasis-related liver fibrosis. Briefly, under anaesthesia with ether, rats were subjected to ligation of the common bile duct with 3-0 silk and sectioned between the ligatures. The abdominal midline was then closed with catgut. Rats in a sham control group had their bile duct exposed with neither ligation nor sectioning. All rats were caged at 24°C with 12 h : 12 h light-dark cycle and were provided free access to food and water for 7 days before the study. All operated rats except sham controls were randomised into different groups.

2.4. Animal Treatment. Rats in sham and model groups received 10 mL/kg of distilled water per day by oral administration. Rats in BBR treatment group received 120 mg/kg/day BBR dissolved in distilled water orally. All treatment lasted for seven weeks.

2.5. Biochemical Analysis. At the end of the experiment, animals were sacrificed by i.p. injection of 200 mg/kg pentobarbitone. Blood was collected and serum was separated by centrifugation at 3000 g for 5 min. Serum AST, ALT, and TBil were quantified by a biochemical autoanalyzer. The tissue hydroxyproline (HyP) level was examined with a HyP detection kit (Jiancheng Bioengineering Institute, Nanjing, China) following the manufacturer's instructions.

2.6. Histological Analysis. Livers collected from different groups of rats were rinsed with PBS and fixed in 4% buffered formaldehyde for 24 h. Paraffin-embedded tissues were cut into 5 μm sections and stained with hematoxylin and eosin (H&E). To evaluate chronic liver injury by a semiquantitative scoring, five phases of liver injury were defined as follows: S0: no observable scaring; S1: no extended portal area scaring; S2: fibrotic portal area with intact lobule structure; S3: fibrosis with broken lobule structure and no cirrhosis; and S4: cirrhosis. Fibrotic area within 1.5 mm^2 of each section was measured. Images were captured under light microscope (Leica Microsystems Digital Imaging, Germany) with CCD camera at the magnification of 10×10 (Leica DFC 280, Germany).

2.7. Cells and Cell Culture. The human hepatocyte cell line L-02 and human HSC line hHS were obtained from Sun Yat-Sen University (Guangdong, China). The cells were cultured in Dulbecco's Modified Eagle medium with high glucose (4.5 g/L) with supplements of 10% Foetal Bovine Serum (FBS) and 1% penicillin/streptomycin and incubated in a humidified atmosphere containing 5% CO_2 at 37°C.

2.8. Cell Viability Assay. Cell viability assay was performed to examine the cytotoxicity of BBR to HSC cells. Briefly, cells were cultured in 96-well cell culture plate in DMEM supplemented with 10% FBS. Each well contained 10,000 cells for attachment overnight. A series of concentrations of BBR were added to the cells to incubate. Then, 10 μL of 3-(4,5-dimethylthiazol-2-yl)-2,5-diphenyltetrazolium bromide (MTT, 5 mg/mL, Sigma, USA) was added to each well 4 h before the end of treatment and the incubation was continued at 37°C. The medium was then discarded and 100 μL DMSO was added to dissolve the crystals with gentle pipetting. The absorbance was read at 575 nm on a Multiskan MS Microplate Reader (Labsystems, Finland).

2.9. Annexin V and Propidium Iodide (PI) Staining. Annexin V and PI double staining was introduced to analyze cell apoptosis and necrosis. In brief, cells were trypsinized, collected, and centrifuged. Cells were stained using the Annexin V and PI double staining kit (Sigma-Aldrich, USA) in binding buffer containing 100 mM HEPES/NaOH, 1.4 mM NaCl, and 25 mM $CaCl_2$, pH 7.5. Five μL 50 μg/mL FITC-conjugated Annexin V and 10 μL 100 μg/mL PI were added and samples were incubated in dark at room temperature for 15 min. The cell suspension was then detected by flow cytometer (Epics XL, Beckman Coulter, USA). Results were analyzed with the FlowJo software (USA).

2.10. Transwell Migration Assay. hHSC motility upon BBR treatment was examined in Millicell-PCF Cell Culture Insert (24-well, 8.0 μm, Millipore). Briefly, the inserts were standing in 24-well cell culture plate. 5×10^4 cells in 100 μL serum-free medium were added to the insert, while 0.5 mL 10% FBS DMEM containing indicated concentrations of BBR was added to each well of the 24-well plate. This was followed by incubation in 5% CO_2 at 37°C for 24 hr. The noninvading cells on the upper surface were removed by cotton swabs.

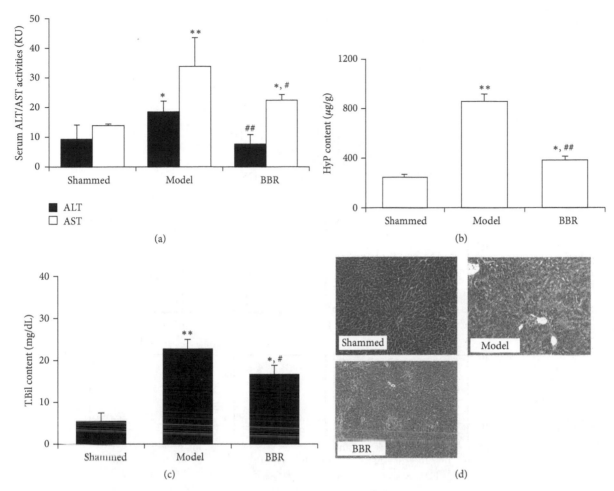

FIGURE 1: BBR attenuated hepatic fibrosis induced by BDL in rats. The common bile duct of rat was ligated with 3-0 silk and sectioned between the ligatures. Rats in sham-operated control group had their bile duct exposed without ligation or section. Rats were randomised and received either PBS or BBR (120 mg/kg/day orally) for seven weeks. At the end of the study, rats were sacrificed and the serum and liver were collected. (a) BBR reduced serum ALT and AST in BDL rats. (b) BBR reduced the HyP content in the liver. (c) BBR reduced serum total bile acid (T.Bil) in rats with BDL. (d) Histological analysis revealed that the fibrosis was inhibited by BBR treatment. $^{*}p < 0.05$ and $^{**}p < 0.01$ versus normal group; $^{\#}p < 0.05$ and $^{\#\#}p < 0.01$ versus the model group.

The cells that invaded across the transmembrane to the lower surface of the membrane were fixed by ice cool 100% ethanol and stained by 2% crystal violet (Sigma-Aldrich, USA). Photographs of the stained migrated cells (3 random fields per culture) were taken under an inverted microscope at 400× and the mean number of cells of the 3 fields was recorded.

2.11. JC-1 Staining. The measurement of mitochondrial membrane potential was conducted with JC-1 staining. Cells were seeded in 35 mm glass-bottom dishes and treated with BBR. Cells were then stained with $10\,\mu g/mL$ JC-1 (Invitrogen, USA) in dark for 30 min and visualized under a fluorescence microscope. Intense red fluorescence indicates the integrity of mitochondrial membrane, while increased green fluorescence represents loss of mitochondrial membrane potential.

2.12. Immunofluorescence. Cells were seeded in 35 mm glass-bottom dishes and treated with BBR. The cells were then fixed with 4% paraformaldehyde in PBS followed by incubation with blocking buffer (5% normal goat serum and 0.03% Triton X-100 in PBS). Then, cells were incubated with antibody against α-SMA at 4°C overnight followed by wash. Alexa Fluor-conjugated secondary antibody (Invitrogen, USA) was added and cells were incubated in dark for 60 min. Cell nuclei were stained with 4′,6-diamidino-2-phenylindole (DAPI). The cells were observed under fluorescence microscope (Carl Zeiss, USA) and images were captured with a CCD camera (400× magnification).

2.13. Reverse-Transcription Quantitative Polymerase Chain Reaction (RT-qPCR). Total RNA was extracted with total RNA purification kit (Norgen, Canada). cDNA was generated with first-strand cDNA synthesis kit (Roche, USA) using the collected RNA as template. The quantitative PCR was conducted with SYBR Green I master mix (Roche, USA) on LightCycler 480 (Roche, USA). The primer sequences of target genes were listed in Table 1.

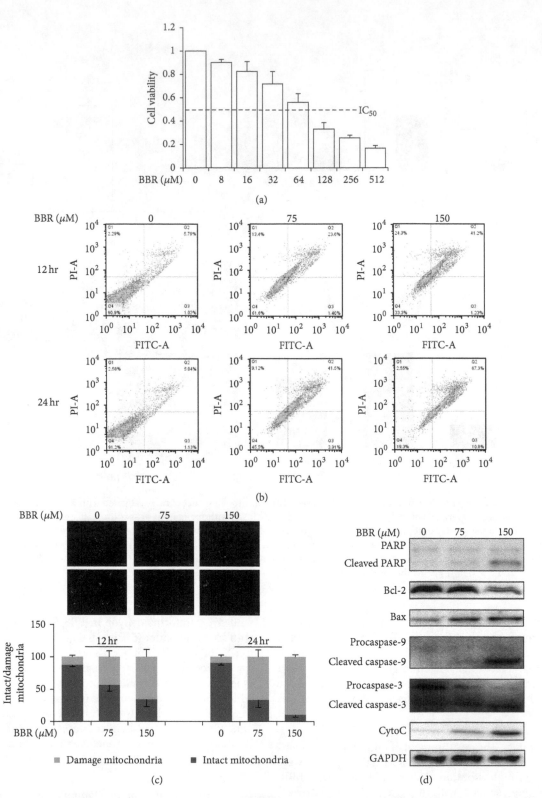

FIGURE 2: BBR induced apoptosis in constitutively activated hHSC. (a) Constitutively activated hHSC in 96-well plate were treated with BBR for 24 hr and cytotoxicity of BBR was determined by MTT assay. The IC$_{50}$ of BBR on hHSC was roughly 75 μM. (b) hHSC were treated with BBR for 12 hr or 24 hr. Apoptosis and necrosis were analyzed by Annexin V/PI dual staining and flow cytometry. (c) BBR-treated hHSC were stained with JC-1 (10 μg/mL). Significant increase of green fluorescence with loss of red fluorescence indicated the relapse of mitochondrial membrane integrity. (d) BBR regulated Bcl-2/Bax ratio in hHSC. The cells were treated with BBR for 24 hr and cell lysates were subjected to Western blot hybridization. Increase of cleaved caspase-3 and caspase-9 and PARP indicated BBR induced apoptosis, while cyto C released from mitochondria exhibited loss of membrane integrity. Upregulation of Bax with Bcl-2 inhibition was observed in BBR-treated cells.

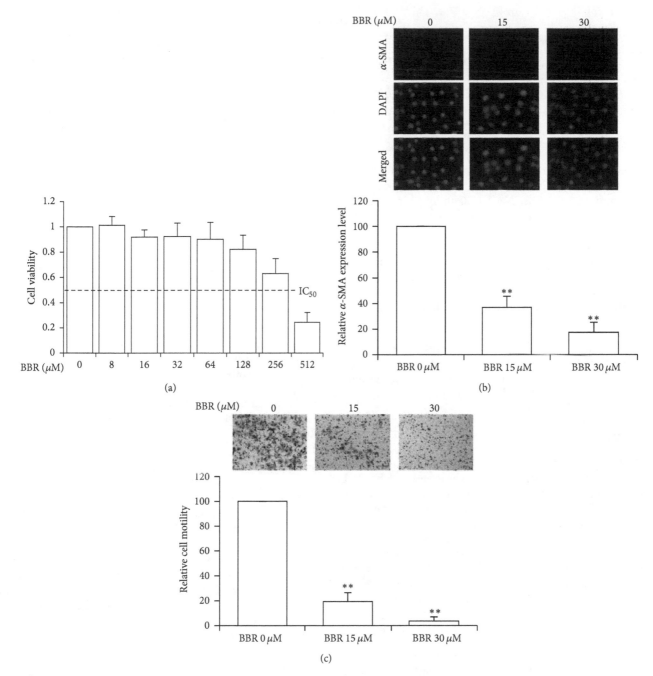

FIGURE 3: Nontoxic BBR suppressed the activity of hHSC. (a) The normal hepatocyte cell line L-02 in 96-well plates was treated with BBR for 24 hr and cell viability was determined by MTT assay. The IC_{50} of BBR on L-02 cells was around 250 μM. (b) BBR suppressed hHSC migration. Cells in serum-free medium were seeded onto the Transwell and medium containing 10% FBS was used as attractant to initiate cell migration. After different doses of BBR were added, the cells were cultured for 24 hr, fixed with 4% paraformaldehyde, and then stained with 2% crystal violet. Three images were captured for each well and the representative images are shown. BBR treatment significantly reduced cell motility. (c) BBR downregulated α-SMA expression in constitutively activated hHSC. Cells were treated with BBR for 24 hr and then fixed with 4% paraformaldehyde. The expression of α-SMA was stained (red) and nuclei were stained with Hoechst 33342 (blue). Three images were captured per treatment group and the representative image of each group is shown. BBR treatment significantly reduced α-SMA expression in constitutively activated hHSC. $^{**}p < 0.01$ versus control.

2.14. *Immunoblotting.* Cells were lysed with the Radioimmunoprecipitation Assay (RIPA) Buffer with the cOmplete Cocktail Proteinase Inhibitor (Roche, USA) and phosphatase inhibitor (1 mM Na_3VO_4 and 1 mM NaF) on ice for 30 min followed by centrifugation at 14,000 rpm at 4°C for 15 min. Supernatants were transferred and protein concentrations were determined by BSA assay (Bio-Rad, USA). Equal yield of protein was separated on SDS-PAGE and transferred onto

TABLE 1: Primer sequence.

	Forward	Reverse
TGFB1	TGAACCGGCCTTTCCTGCTTCTCATG	GCGGAAGTCAATGTACAGCTGCCGC
ACTA2	CCGACCGAATGCAGAAGGA	ACAGAGTATTTGCGCTCCGAA
COL1A1	CAGCCGCTTCACCTACAGC	TTTTGTATTCAATCACTGTCTTGCC
COL4A3	GCTGTCAACACCAGCTCTGA	CGGTGCACCTGCTAATGTAA
ACTB	CCAACCGCCAGAAGATGA	CCAGAGGCGTACAGGGATAG

a polyvinylidene fluoride membrane (PVDF, Bio-Rad). The membrane was then blocked in buffer containing 5% BSA, Tris (10 mmol/L, pH 7.4), NaCl (150 mmol/L, and Tween 20 (1%) at room temperature for 1 hr with gentle shaking. The membrane was then incubated with primary antibodies at 4°C overnight followed by incubation with appropriate secondary antibody (Abcam, UK) at room temperature for 1 hr. The immunoreactivities were detected using ECL advanced kit (GE Healthcare, UK) and visualized using a chemiluminescence imaging system (Bio-Rad, USA).

2.15. Statistical Analysis. Data were expressed as mean ± standard deviation of means (SD) and statistical comparisons were conducted using one-way ANOVA. p value lower than 0.05 was considered statistically significant.

3. Results

3.1. BBR Suppressed BDL-Induced Hepatic Fibrosis in Rats. In the present study, hepatic fibrosis was induced by BDL in rats to induce extrahepatic cholestasis. Significant serum ALT and AST elevation was observed in BDL rats and BBR treatment remarkably reduced serum ALT and AST (Figure 1(a)). Content of HyP in the liver, as a biomarker of hepatic fibrosis, was measured, and BBR potently reduced the liver content of HyP consistently (Figure 1(b)) and reduced serum total bile acid level (Figure 1(c)). Histological analysis revealed that administration of BBR attenuated the hepatic fibrosis induced by BDL in rats (Figure 1(d)). Overall scores of liver fibrosis in different groups are shown in Table 2.

3.2. Toxic Doses of BBR Induced Mitochondrial Apoptosis of HSC through Altering Bcl-2/Bax Ratio and Subsequent Caspase Activation. To explore possible mechanisms of the antifibrotic effect of BBR, we focused on the HSC, which are activated during fibrogenic process. hHSC, a constitutively activated human HSC line, was used to evaluate the cytotoxicity of BBR. High dose of BBR exhibited toxic effects to hHSC (IC$_{50}$ 75 μM, Figure 2(a)). Toxic dose of BBR could initiate apoptosis of hHSC (Figure 2(b)). This effect may be due to the increased permeability of mitochondrial membrane in hHSC with exposure of toxic dose of BBR (Figure 2(c)), which was indicated by the loss of mitochondrial membrane integrity. Expression of Bcl-2 was significantly downregulated upon BBR treatment, leading to Bcl-2/Bax imbalance and mitochondrial membrane polarization (Figure 2(d)). This observation was further confirmed by the release of

cytochrome C into cytoplasm, which initiated caspase activation subsequently (Figure 2(d)). These results suggest that toxic dose of BBR may induce mitochondrial apoptosis in hHSC.

3.3. Nontoxic Doses of BBR Suppress HSC Activation by Inhibiting α-SMA Expression and Cell Migration. The toxic dose of BBR on normal hepatic cell line L-02 was examined to evaluate its possible adverse effect. It was shown that the IC$_{50}$ value of BBR on L-02 cells was about 250 μM, indicating that high doses of BBR may exhibit some toxic action to normal hepatocytes (Figure 3(a)). Further examining the effect of BBR on HSC at nontoxic doses, we found that BBR significantly downregulated the expression of α-SMA, the biomarker of HSC activation, indicating that BBR might inactivate the activated hHSC at nontoxic doses (Figure 3(b)). Furthermore, BBR significantly downregulated hHSC motility (Figure 3(c)).

3.4. BBR Repressed α-SMA and Collagen mRNA Expression without Altering Smad2/3 Phosphorylation. The TGF-β/Smad signalling plays an important role in HSC activation in liver fibrosis [21]. As BBR was reported to suppress TGF-β expression in the plasma of patients with lung cancer who were undergoing radiotherapy [22], the expression of TGF-β was analyzed in our study to prove if similar action of BBR could be found. However, in our study, we observed no significant reduction of TGF-β expression in BBR-treated hHSC (Figure 4(a)). Neither did BBR suppress Smad2/3 phosphorylation (Figure 4(b)). However, BBR dose-dependently inhibited the mRNA expression of α-SMA (ACTA2), collagen 1A (COL1A1), and collagen IV (COL4A3) (Figure 4(c)).

3.5. AMPK Activation Is Responsible for the Smad2/3 Inhibition by BBR in HSC. Activation of AMPK signalling by BBR was observed in hHSC (Figure 5(a)). Previous studies have exhibited the role of AMPK activation in the treatment against oxidative stress-induced liver injury [23] and it was shown that AMPK activity is critical for the experimental therapy of hepatic fibrosis as well [24]. In our study, further examination was made to explore the role of AMPK activation in BBR's inhibitory effect of experimental hepatic fibrosis. BBR suppression of α-SMA, COL1A1, and COL4A3 mRNA in hHSC was potently attenuated by the presence of Compound C, an AMPK inhibitor (Figure 5(b)), suggesting that BBR suppression of these mRNAs might be attributed to AMPK activation in hHSC. A critical role for AMPK in

TABLE 2: Histological analysis of the effect of BBR on BDL-induced liver fibrosis in rats.

Group	Sample (n)	Fibrosis stage					Fibrotic area within 1.5 mm^2
		S0	S1	S2	S3	S4	
Shammed	6	6	0	0	0	0	0.007 ± 0.005
Model	6	0	1	1	3	1	$0.079 \pm 0.025^{**}$
BBR (120 mg/kg)	6	0	3	2	1	0	$0.032 \pm 0.024^{*,\#}$

*: $p < 0.05$, **: $p < 0.01$ versus shammed group; #: $p < 0.05$ versus model group.

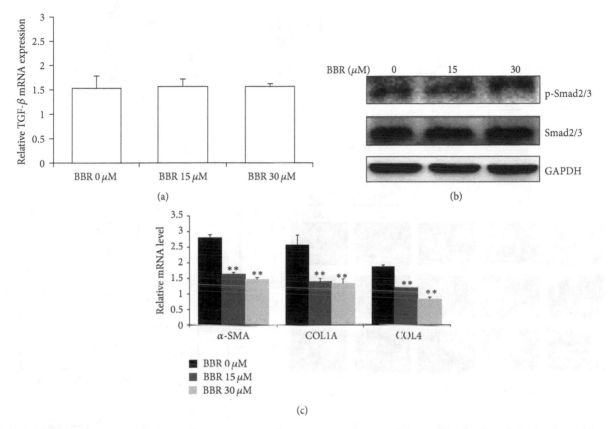

FIGURE 4: BBR suppressed α-SMA, without affecting Smad2/3 phosphorylation. (a) BBR did not affect the TGF-β production in hHSC. The expression of TGF-β mRNA transcript was analyzed with RT-qPCR. No significant difference between treatment and nontreatment group was observed. (b) BBR did not inhibit Smad2/3 phosphorylation in hHSC. Immunoblotting analysis using specific antibodies revealed no significant difference between treatment and nontreatment group in the phosphorylation of Smad2/3. (c) BBR suppressed the expression of profibrogenic factors. The downstream targets of Smad2/3, fibrogenic α-Sma, Col1a1, and Col4a3 were analyzed by RT-qPCR. Significant reduction of α-SMA, Col1A1, and Col4a3 mRNAs was observed in BBR-treated cells in a dose-dependent manner. $^{**}p < 0.01$ versus control.

BBR repression of hHSC activation was further confirmed by the fact that BBR repression of α-SMA expression and hHSC motility were both prevented by Compound C (Figures 5(c) and 5(d)).

4. Discussion

Critical role of HSC activation in the early development of liver fibrosis has been revealed by previous studies [25]. The activation of HSC initiates its proliferation as well as the production of extracellular matrix (ECM) proteins such as α-SMA and collagens [6]. Attempts have been made to explore the use of BBR in the therapy for fibrosis-related hepatic diseases. Previous studies have shown that BBR could be used for the treatment against hypertyraminemia in patients with liver cirrhosis [26], which was correlated with BBR's capacity of reducing blood lipid in hyperlipidemic patients [27]. Experimental studies have been also conducted, the results of which exhibit the potential of BBR in ameliorating hepatic fibrosis with various mechanisms [28, 29]. In particular, it was shown that the antioxidative activity of BBR contributes to improvement of experimental hepatic fibrosis via stimulating matrix metalloproteinase-2 (MMP-2) [30]. Our findings further showed that apoptosis of HSC could be initiated by toxic doses of BBR, and Bcl-2/Bax-mediated mitochondrial membrane potential loss may be involved in induction of HSC apoptosis by BBR. Interestingly, we found that nontoxic doses of BBR downregulated the activation of

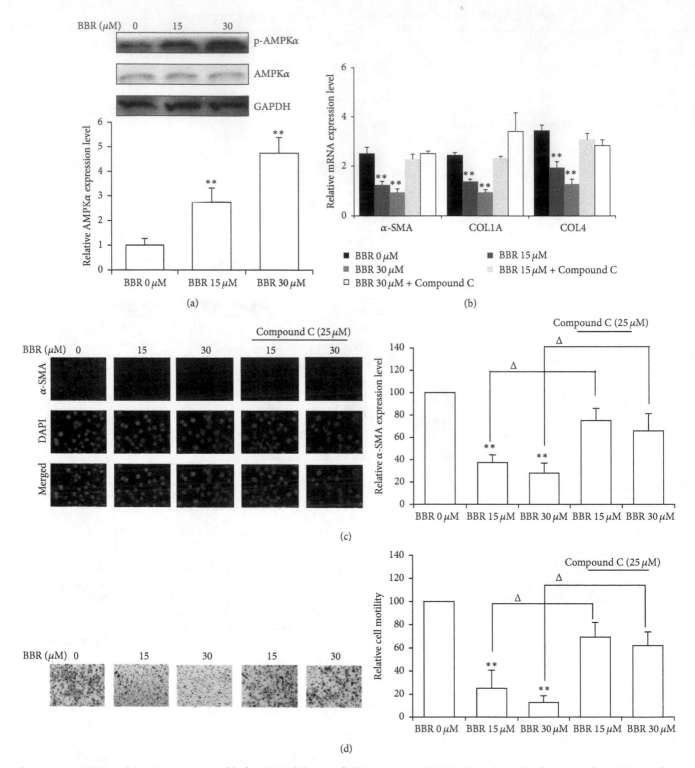

FIGURE 5: Activation of AMPK was responsible for BBR inhibition of HSC activation. (a) BBR dose-dependently activated AMPK signalling in HSC. (b) Suppression of AMPK with Compound C attenuated inhibition of α-SMA, Col1A1, and Col4a3 transcripts by BBR. Cells were treated with BBR alone or in combination with AMPK inhibitor Compound C (25 μM) for 24 hr and then RNA was collected. Expression of α-SMA, Col1A1, and Col4a3 mRNA transcripts was analyzed with RT-qPCR. Significant restoration of α-SMA, Col1A1, and Col4a3 mRNA expression was found when BBR was given in combination with Compound C. (c) Inhibition of AMPK reactivated BBR-treated hHSC. Significant reduction of α-SMA distribution was observed in BBR-treated cells, while recovery of α-SMA was found when BBR was given in combination with AMPK inhibitor Compound C (25 μM). (d) hHSC motility was recovered, when cells were treated with BBR in the presence of Compound C (25 μM). $^{**}p < 0.01$ versus control. $^{\Delta}p < 0.05$ versus the same treatment in the absence of Compound C.

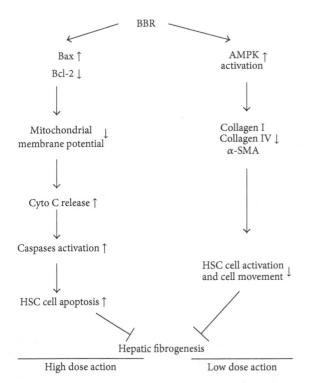

FIGURE 6: Proposed mechanisms of BBR regulation of HSC.

HSC, suppressing production of ECM proteins, preventing deregulation of hepatic architecture and protecting hepatocytes from hepatocellular dysfunction (Figure 6) [31].

It has been previously shown that the activity of AMPK signalling is a critical factor in the prevention of hepatic fibrogenesis. In AMPK-deficient mice, the fibrogenesis and liver fibrosis could be enhanced dramatically, and initiation of AMPK could suppress HSC proliferation and collagen expression [31]. The preventive effect of AMPK on hepatic fibrosis was further evidenced by the fact that an adipocytokine adiponectin could disrupt leptin-mediated hepatic fibrosis through the activation of AMPK in HSC [24]. A recent study showed that berberine can replenish the activity of AMPK in the liver of carbon tetrachloride- (CCl_4) treated mice [32]; however, whether activation of AMPK by berberine is responsible for the improvement of experimental fibrosis remains not clear. Furthermore, whether activation of AMPK by berberine can suppress activated hepatic stellate cells, which majorly mediates fibrogenesis in the liver, was not studied. In our study, we observed that hepatic fibrosis induced by BDL could be attenuated by BBR, which in hHSC activates AMPK signalling and inhibits hHSC migration and α-SMA production. Inhibition of AMPK by Compound C potently reduced the inhibitory effect on hHSC activation, which was evidenced by the fact that cell motility and α-SMA expression were restored in BBR-treated cells in the presence of Compound C. These findings support a central role of AMPK activation in BBR's effect on HSC activation and subsequent fibrogenesis.

We noticed that BBR has no effect on the signal transduction of TGF-β/Smad. BBR neither suppresses the TGF-β expression in HSC nor inhibits Smad2/3 phosphorylation. However, the expression of profibrogenic factors α-SMA, COL1A1, and COL4A3 was inhibited by BBR and this effect could be attenuated by inhibition of AMPK by Compound C. These observations indicate that activation of AMPK could repress fibrogenesis without affecting Smad2/3 phosphorylation. A previous study showed that transcription activity mediated by Smad2/3 requires cooperation of transcription coactivators CBP and p300, which initiate the N-terminal acetylation of Smad2/3 [33, 34]. Phosphorylated AMPK was reported to bind with p300, initiate its proteasomal degradation, and consequently inhibit Smad2/3 transcription activity without affecting their phosphorylation [35]. Deletion of p300 has been found to suppress fibrogenic collagen type I and α-SMA expression and lead to fibrogenesis inhibition [35, 36]. Our findings on the critical role for BBR activation of AMPK in HSC shed light on the antifibrotic action of BBR and support its potential value for the treatment of fibrosis in liver disease.

5. Conclusion

BBR is a promising agent for treating liver fibrosis through multiple mechanisms, at least partially by directly targeting HSC and by inhibiting the AMPK pathway. Its value as an antifibrotic drug in patients with liver disease deserves further investigation.

Competing Interests

The authors declare that they have no competing interests.

Authors' Contributions

Ning Wang did the experiments and drafted the paper. Qihe Xu provided guidance on fibrosis models and antifibrotic assays. All authors revised and commented on the paper and discussed the paper. Yibin Feng conceived and designed the project and finalized the paper.

Acknowledgments

This research was partially supported by the research council of the University of Hong Kong (Project Codes: 104002889 and 104003422), Wong's donation (Project Code: 200006276), the donation of Gaia Family Trust, New Zealand (Project Code: 200007008), National Natural Science Foundation of China (Project Code: 81302808), and the Research Grant Committee (RGC) of Hong Kong (RGC General Research Fund, Project Code: 10500362).

References

[1] G. Shiha, S. K. Sarin, A. E. Ibrahim et al., "Liver fibrosis: consensus recommendations of the Asian Pacific association for the study of the liver (APASL)," *Hepatology International*, vol. 3, no. 2, pp. 323–333, 2009.

[2] M. Kukla, "Angiogenesis: a phenomenon which aggravates chronic liver disease progression," *Hepatology International*, vol. 7, no. 1, pp. 4–12, 2013.

[3] H. Hayashi and T. Sakai, "Animal models for the study of liver fibrosis: new insights from knockout mouse models," *American Journal of Physiology—Gastrointestinal and Liver Physiology*, vol. 300, no. 5, pp. G729–G738, 2011.

[4] S. L. Friedman, "Mechanisms of hepatic fibrogenesis," *Gastroenterology*, vol. 134, no. 6, pp. 1655–1669, 2008.

[5] V. Hernandez-Gea and S. L. Friedman, "Pathogenesis of liver fibrosis," *Annual Review of Pathology: Mechanisms of Disease*, vol. 6, pp. 425–456, 2011.

[6] S. L. Friedman, "Hepatic stellate cells: protean, multifunctional, and enigmatic cells of the liver," *Physiological Reviews*, vol. 88, no. 1, pp. 125–172, 2008.

[7] K. Cheng and R. I. Mahato, "Gene modulation for treating liver fibrosis," *Critical Reviews in Therapeutic Drug Carrier Systems*, vol. 24, no. 2, pp. 93–146, 2007.

[8] G. Lei, H. Dan, L. Jinhua, Y. Wei, G. Song, and W. Li, "Berberine and itraconazole are not synergistic in vitro against aspergillus fumigatus isolated from clinical patients," *Molecules*, vol. 16, no. 11, pp. 9218–9233, 2011.

[9] X.-H. Wang, S.-M. Jiang, and Q.-W. Sun, "Effects of berberine on human rheumatoid arthritis fibroblast-like synoviocytes," *Experimental Biology and Medicine*, vol. 236, no. 7, pp. 859–866, 2011.

[10] S. Kim, Y. Kim, J. E. Kim, K. H. Cho, and J. H. Chung, "Berberine inhibits TPA-induced MMP-9 and IL-6 expression in normal human keratinocytes," *Phytomedicine*, vol. 15, no. 5, pp. 340–347, 2008.

[11] J. Tang, Y. Feng, S. Tsao, N. Wang, R. Curtain, and Y. Wang, "Berberine and Coptidis rhizoma as novel antineoplastic agents: a review of traditional use and biomedical investigations," *Journal of Ethnopharmacology*, vol. 126, no. 1, pp. 5–17, 2009.

[12] N. Wang, Y. Feng, M. Zhu et al., "Berberine induces autophagic cell death and mitochondrial apoptosis in liver cancer cells: the cellular mechanism," *Journal of Cellular Biochemistry*, vol. 111, no. 6, pp. 1426–1436, 2010.

[13] N. Wang, Y. Feng, E. P. W. Lau et al., "F-actin reorganization and inactivation of Rho signaling pathway involved in the inhibitory effect of Coptidis Rhizoma on hepatoma cell migration," *Integrative Cancer Therapies*, vol. 9, no. 4, pp. 354–364, 2010.

[14] Y. Feng, N. Wang, M. Zhu, Y. Feng, H. Li, and S. Tsao, "Recent progress on anticancer candidates in patents of herbal medicinal products," *Recent Patents on Food, Nutrition and Agriculture*, vol. 3, no. 1, pp. 30–48, 2011.

[15] X. Ye, Y. Feng, Y. Tong et al., "Hepatoprotective effects of Coptidis rhizoma aqueous extract on carbon tetrachloride-induced acute liver hepatotoxicity in rats," *Journal of Ethnopharmacology*, vol. 124, no. 1, pp. 130–136, 2009.

[16] Y. Feng, N. Wang, X. Ye et al., "Hepatoprotective effect and its possible mechanism of Coptidis rhizoma aqueous extract on carbon tetrachloride-induced chronic liver hepatotoxicity in rats," *Journal of Ethnopharmacology*, vol. 138, no. 3, pp. 683–690, 2011.

[17] Y. Feng, K.-Y. Siu, X. Ye et al., "Hepatoprotective effects of berberine on carbon tetrachloride-induced acute hepatotoxicity in rats," *Chinese Medicine*, vol. 5, article 33, 2010.

[18] X. Zhao, J. Zhang, N. Tong, Y. Chen, and Y. Luo, "Protective effects of berberine on doxorubicin-induced hepatotoxicity in mice," *Biological and Pharmaceutical Bulletin*, vol. 35, no. 5, pp. 796–800, 2012.

[19] N. Wang, Y. Feng, F. Cheung et al., "A comparative study on the hepatoprotective action of bear bile and coptidis rhizoma aqueous extract on experimental liver fibrosis in rats," *BMC Complementary and Alternative Medicine*, vol. 12, article 239, 2012.

[20] Y. Feng, K.-F. Cheung, N. Wang, P. Liu, T. Nagamatsu, and Y. Tong, "Chinese medicines as a resource for liver fibrosis treatment," *Chinese Medicine*, vol. 4, article 16, 2009.

[21] E. Piek, C.-H. Heldin, and P. T. Dijke, "Specificity, diversity, and regulation in TGF-β superfamily signaling," *The FASEB Journal*, vol. 13, no. 15, pp. 2105–2124, 1999.

[22] Y. Liu, H. Yu, C. Zhang et al., "Protective effects of berberine on radiation-induced lung injury via intercellular adhesion molecular-1 and transforming growth factor-beta-1 in patients with lung cancer," *European Journal of Cancer*, vol. 44, no. 16, pp. 2425–2432, 2008.

[23] Y. W. Kim, S. M. Lee, S. M. Shin et al., "Efficacy of sauchinone as a novel AMPK-activating lignan for preventing iron-induced oxidative stress and liver injury," *Free Radical Biology and Medicine*, vol. 47, no. 7, pp. 1082–1092, 2009.

[24] J. A. Handy, N. K. Saxena, P. Fu et al., "Adiponectin activation of AMPK disrupts leptin-mediated hepatic fibrosis via suppressors of cytokine signaling (SOCS-3)," *Journal of Cellular Biochemistry*, vol. 110, no. 5, pp. 1195–1207, 2010.

[25] R. Bataller and D. A. Brenner, "Liver fibrosis," *The Journal of Clinical Investigation*, vol. 115, no. 2, pp. 209–218, 2005.

[26] A. Watanabe, T. Obata, and H. Nagashima, "Berberine therapy of hypertyraminemia in patients with liver cirrhosis," *Acta Medica Okayama*, vol. 36, no. 4, pp. 277–281, 1982.

[27] W. Zhao, R. Xue, Z.-X. Zhou, W.-J. Kong, and J.-D. Jiang, "Reduction of blood lipid by berberine in hyperlipidemic patients with chronic hepatitis or liver cirrhosis," *Biomedicine and Pharmacotherapy*, vol. 62, no. 10, pp. 730–731, 2008.

[28] B.-J. Zhang, D. Xu, Y. Guo, J. Ping, L.-B. Chen, and H. Wang, "Protection by and anti-oxidant mechanism of berberine against rat liver fibrosis induced by multiple hepatotoxic factors," *Clinical and Experimental Pharmacology and Physiology*, vol. 35, no. 3, pp. 303–309, 2008.

[29] X. Sun, X. Zhang, H. Hu et al., "Berberine inhibits hepatic stellate cell proliferation and prevents experimental liver fibrosis," *Biological and Pharmaceutical Bulletin*, vol. 32, no. 9, pp. 1533–1537, 2009.

[30] R. Domitrović, H. Jakovac, V. V. Marchesi, and B. Blažeković, "Resolution of liver fibrosis by isoquinoline alkaloid berberine in CCl_4-intoxicated mice is mediated by suppression of oxidative stress and upregulation of MMP-2 expression," *Journal of Medicinal Food*, vol. 16, no. 6, pp. 518–528, 2013.

[31] A. M. Gressner and R. Weiskirchen, "Modern pathogenetic concepts of liver fibrosis suggest stellate cells and TGF-β as major players and therapeutic targets," *Journal of Cellular and Molecular Medicine*, vol. 10, no. 1, pp. 76–99, 2006.

[32] J. Li, Y. Pan, M. Kan et al., "Hepatoprotective effects of berberine on liver fibrosis via activation of AMP-activated protein kinase," *Life Sciences*, vol. 98, no. 1, pp. 24–30, 2014.

[33] Y. Inoue, Y. Itoh, K. Abe et al., "Smad3 is acetylated by p300/CBP to regulate its transactivation activity," *Oncogene*, vol. 26, no. 4, pp. 500–508, 2007.

[34] A. W. Tu and K. Luo, "Acetylation of Smad2 by the co-activator p300 regulates activin and transforming growth factor β response," *The Journal of Biological Chemistry*, vol. 282, no. 29, pp. 21187–21196, 2007.

[35] J.-Y. Lim, M.-A. Oh, W. H. Kim, H.-Y. Sohn, and S. I. Park, "AMP-activated protein kinase inhibits TGF-β-induced fibrogenic responses of hepatic stellate cells by targeting transcriptional coactivator p300," *Journal of Cellular Physiology*, vol. 227, no. 3, pp. 1081–1089, 2012.

[36] S. Yavrom, L. Chen, S. Xiong, J. Wang, R. A. Rippe, and H. Tsukamoto, "Peroxisome proliferator-activated receptor γ suppresses proximal α1(I) collagen promoter via inhibition of p300-facilitated NF-I binding to DNA in hepatic stellate cells," *The Journal of Biological Chemistry*, vol. 280, no. 49, pp. 40650–40659, 2005.

The Relieving Effects of BrainPower Advanced, a Dietary Supplement, in Older Adults with Subjective Memory Complaints: A Randomized, Double-Blind, Placebo-Controlled Trial

Jingfen Zhu,[1] Rong Shi,[2] Su Chen,[3] Lihua Dai,[4] Tian Shen,[1] Yi Feng,[1] Pingping Gu,[5] Mina Shariff,[6] Tuong Nguyen,[6] Yeats Ye,[7] Jianyu Rao,[8] and Guoqiang Xing[9,10]

[1] Department of Community Health and Family Medicine, School of Public Health, Shanghai Jiao Tong University, Shanghai 200025, China
[2] School of Public Health, Shanghai University of TCM, Shanghai 201203, China
[3] Si-Tang Community Health Service Center of Shanghai, Shanghai 200431, China
[4] Department of Emergency Medicine, Xin Hua Hospital Affiliated to Shanghai Jiao Tong University School of Medicine, Shanghai 200092, China
[5] Southern California Kaiser Sunset, 4867 Sunset Boulevard, Los Angeles, CA 90027, USA
[6] Department of Research, DRM Resources, 1683 Sunflower Avenue, Costa Mesa, CA 92626, USA
[7] Maryland Population Research Center, University of Maryland, College Park, MD 20742, USA
[8] Department of Pathology and Laboratory Medicine, David Geffen School of Medicine, University of California at Los Angeles, Los Angeles, CA 90095, USA
[9] Imaging Institute of Rehabilitation and Development of Brain Function, North Sichuan Medical University, Nanchong Central Hospital, Nanchong 637000, China
[10] Lotus Biotech.com LLC, John Hopkins University-MCC, 9601 Medical Center Drive, Rockville, MD 20850, USA

Correspondence should be addressed to Rong Shi; shirong61@163.com and Guoqiang Xing; gxing99@yahoo.com

Academic Editor: Jairo Kennup Bastos

Subjective memory complaints (SMCs) are common in older adults that can often predict further cognitive impairment. No proven effective agents are available for SMCs. The effect of BrainPower Advanced, a dietary supplement consisting of herbal extracts, nutrients, and vitamins, was evaluated in 98 volunteers with SMCs, averaging 67 years of age (47–88), in a randomized, double-blind, placebo-controlled trial. Subjective hypomnesis/memory loss (SML) and attention/concentration deficits (SAD) were evaluated before and after 12-week supplementation of BrainPower Advanced capsules ($n = 47$) or placebo ($n = 51$), using a 5-point memory questionnaire (1 = no/slight, 5 = severe). Objective memory function was evaluated using 3 subtests of visual/audio memory, abstraction, and memory recall that gave a combined total score. The BrainPower Advanced group had more cases of severe SML (severity ≥ 3) (44/47) and severe SAD (43/47) than the placebo group (39/51 and 37/51, < 0.05, < 0.05, resp.) before the treatment. BrainPower Advanced intervention, however, improved a greater proportion of the severe SML (29.5%)(13/44) ($P < 0.01$) and SAD (34.9%)(15/43)($P < 0.01$) than placebo (5.1% (2/39) and 13.5% (5/37), resp.). Thus, 3-month BrainPower Advanced supplementation appears to be beneficial to older adults with SMCs.

1. Introduction

Memory is the ability of an individual to record, retain, and recall sensory stimuli, events, and information over short and long periods of time. Deficits in memory function can compromise one's quality of life and ability to work.

Hypomnesis/forgetfulness/memory decline can occur with aging or as results of subhealth conditions [1]. Complaints about memory impairment, or subjective memory complaints (SMCs), are common in elderly people but are rarely detected by clinicians using objective memory function tests due to the subtle and heterogeneous nature of SMC [2–5]. SMCs are a criterion of mild cognitive impairment (MCI), which is common in older adults and in people who have experienced subhealth conditions [6–12].

MCI is an intermediary status between normal aging and prodromal memory decline [6, 13]. Individuals with MCI appear to have intact general cognitive function and activities of daily living, but their memory is impaired for normal age. The prevalence of MCI is estimated at 3%–19% in adults older than 65 years and 15% in adults older than 75 years [14–18]. Less than half of people with MCI are stable or able to reverse back to normal memory function again within 5 years [19–21].

SMC and MCI are often associated with a decline in episodic memory (a recollection of specific past events) [22–24], which is most frequently found in those with the amnesic subtype MCI [22–28]. Positron emission tomography (PET) brain image studies show that people with SMC are characterized with elevated brain beta-amyloid [25–27]. Increased amyloid deposition has an early and subclinical impact on cognition that precedes hypometabolism [28] and impairs blood vessel functions [29] that could contribute to increased inflammation in amnestic mild cognitive impairment [30].

Latent insufficiency of cerebrovascular circulation and loss of phospholipid asymmetry may underlie early manifestation of SMC and MCI [31] and could be a risk factor for episodic nonspecific complaints of mild cognitive deficit, regional hypoperfusion, and hypometabolism [32–38].

Episodic memory processes depend on the integrity of the medial temporal lobe, hippocampus, the posterior parietal cortex, and lateral prefrontal cortex (PFC) [33–35]. Imaging studies have shown an asymmetric hemispheric encoding/retrieval (HERA) pattern in young adults where the left PFC and temporo-occipital cortex are involved in encoding and the right PFC is involved in retrieval of the stored information [36–39]. During normal aging, PFC activation becomes less asymmetric during memory tasks. Normal or high-performing older adults balance age-related neural decline through neuroplasticity, which reorganizes neurocognitive networks. The subnormal or low-performing older adults use a network similar to young adults, but inefficiently [36, 40].

Abnormal cholinergic and glutamatergic neurotransmissions are thought to be involved in SMC and MCI [41–43]. Cognitive decline in older adults is associated with a loss of cholinergic function (cholinergic hypofunction) including a reduction in choline acetyltransferase (ChAT), muscarinic and nicotinic acetylcholine receptor binding sites, and concentrations of acetylcholine in the synaptic clefts [43, 44]. Glutamatergic overstimulation (excitotoxicity) of the postsynaptic NMDA receptors could also lead to memory impairment [45].

Currently, there are no effective and safe pharmaceutical drugs for SMC and MCI. Prevention of the progression of the symptomatic development could be the best strategy [46]. Although acetylcholinesterase inhibitors (AChEIs) and N-methyl D-aspartate (NMDA) receptor antagonists have been used for treatment of people with varying degree of memory deficits, their effects on cognition and memory improvement are often negative [47–54]. A portion of people with MCI, however, may respond favorably to AChEIs (15%–35%) and NMDA receptor antagonists (30%) [55–57], but usually after high doses or long treatment, and with potential adverse effects, such as nausea, vomiting, diarrhea, headache, hypertension, and hepatotoxicity [58–64].

A variety of plant-derived compounds have been studied as potential enhancers of memory and cognitive function [65] with potential mechanisms on (1) modulation of neuronal membrane integrity; (2) modulation of the cholinergic system through inhibition of acetylcholinesterase (AChE) or stimulation of muscarinic and nicotinic receptors; (3) neuroprotection against NMDA receptor excitotoxicity; (4) anti-inflammatory and antioxidant activities; (5) improved cerebral blood flow and microperfusion.

Table 1 lists some herbal extracts and compounds that are active ingredients of BrainPower Advanced, the formulation used in this pilot study. BrainPower Advanced is a dietary supplement formulated to support healthy memory and cognitive function in adults. Its key ingredients include extracts of *Ginkgo biloba* (flavonoids, terpenoids, and terpene lactones), *Camellia sinensis* leaf (tea polyphenols), *Catharanthus roseus* (vinpocetine), kola nut (*Cola nitida*, caffeine), *Huperzia serrata* (hup A and hup B), phosphatidylserine (PS), L-tyrosine, L-pyroglutamic acid, acetyl-L-carnitine, choline bitartrate, L-glutamine, L-phenylalanine, L-cysteine, vitamin B6, and vitamin B12 (Table 1).

PS is a key integrative phospholipid component of neuronal cell membranes and represents 15% of the total phospholipid pool. PS acts to maintain membrane integrity and neuroplasticity, buffer oxidative stress, facilitate neurotransmitter release, and increase brain glucose metabolism [66–69]. Phospholipid deficits in neuronal membranes are involved in age-related brain-structural and cognitive decline. A decline of PS and other phospholipids in neuronal membranes has been associated with memory impairment and cognitive deficits whereas dietary PS and phospholipid supplements have prevented or reversed such deficits [70–75]. PS supplementation improved learning capacity and memory in rodents [76, 77] and improved physical and mental performance such as long-term memory and recognition in elderly people with cognitive decline [73, 78–80], in stressed young adults [81], and in children with attention deficit hyperactivity disorder [82].

Vinpocetine (ethyl apovincaminate) is synthesized from the alkaloid vincamine, an extract from the leaf of the lesser periwinkle plant (*Catharanthus roseus*). Vinpocetine has been used widely in Japan and Europe for the treatment of cognitive decline since the late 1970s. Vinpocetine can improve cerebral blood flow and glucose metabolism in the thalamus and basal ganglia and the occipital, parietal, and temporal cortex [83–86]. Previous studies have confirmed that vinpocetine can inhibit beta-amyloid-induced activation of NF-κB, inflammation, and cytokine production and interferes with many stages of the ischemic cascade: ATP depletion, activation of voltage-sensitive Na(+) and Ca(++)

TABLE 1: Information of the key ingredients of BrainPower Advanced.

Ingredients	Main active compounds	Effects and possible mechanisms of actions
Phosphatidylserine	Phosphatidylserine	Improves cognitive performance in elderly adults with memory deficits
		Enhances cognitive performance in school children and adults
		Restores impaired neuronal calcium and glucose uptake and metabolism in aged brain
		Precursor of neuronal membrane phospholipid that is responsible for neuroplasticity, learning, and memory
		Neuroprotection
Catharanthus roseus	Vinpocetine	Enhance memory function in young healthy volunteers and in animals
		Protect against ischemia by improving blood perfusion and cerebral blood flow
		Increase glucose and oxygen consumption, cerebral ATP, and cAMP levels
		Improve cerebral microcirculation by inhibiting platelet aggregation
		Reduce red blood cell deformability and cerebral vascular resistance
		Enhance neurotransmitter production, release, and concentration in the brain
		Block voltage-gated sodium channels and potentiate the neuroprotective effect of adenosine in hypoxia
Huperzia serrata (whole plant)	Huperzine A, Huperzine B	Inhibitor of AChE and NMDAR
		Inhibitor of b-amyloid neurotoxicity
		Strong antioxidative, antiapoptotic, and neuroprotective activities
		Improve cognition in healthy people
		Reverse or attenuate cognitive deficits in older adults
Ginkgo biloba	Flavonoids, Terpenoids, Terpene lactones (ginkgolides and bilobalide)	Large dose may improve cognition, daily living activities, and mood
		Dose-dependent and specific enhancing effects on memory, cognitive performance, and alertness in healthy adults
		Delay cognitive decline in elderly population
		Potentiate the cognitive-enhancing effects of phosphatidylserine
		Memory improving effect in older people with memory deficits
		Increase blood supply, vasodilation, reduce blood viscosity, balance neurotransmitter systems, and reduce free radicals
		Inhibitor of platelet activating factor
Vitamin B6	Pyridoxal, pyridoxamine, and pyridoxine	Homocysteine remethylation cofactor
		Reduce blood homocysteine level which is a risk factor for cerebrovascular disease and neuron toxicity
Vitamin B12		Required for the methylation of homocysteine to methionine and needed for myelin, neurotransmitters, and membrane phospholipids for maintaining the integrity of the central nervous system
		Protects against brain atrophy
		Protects mood and memory function
L-Tyrosine	L-Tyrosine	Promotes protein utilization and enhances IgG antibody induction
L-Pyroglutamic acid	L-Pyroglutamic acid	Makes N-terminal modification in neuronal peptides, hormones and peptides, and analogue/reservoir of glutamate
Green tea extract (Camellia sinensis, leaf)	Tea polyphenols (epigallocatechin gallate)	Free-radical scavengers, strong antioxidants, and neuroprotection
		Anti-inflammatory; improve vasodilation and normal blood pressure, normal glucose, and lipid metabolism
Acetyl-L-carnitine	Acetyl-L-carnitine	Regulates neuroplasticity, membrane function, and neurotransmitter release; reduces pain and depression activity at cholinergic neurons; membrane stabilization; and enhancing mitochondrial function
Cola nut extract (kola nitida)	Caffeine, Theobromine, Theophylline	Decrease brain beta-amyloid
Choline bitartrate		A precursor of acetylcholine, a cholinergic neurotransmitter that declines with advancing age
		Improves auditory and visual word recognition at a dose of 12 g per day for 2 weeks
L-Glutamine		Reduces beta-amyloid and H_2O_2-induced stress and DNA damage
L-Phenylalanine		An essential amino acid that can be converted to tyrosine and other excitatory neurotransmitters (dopamine, norepinephrine, and epinephrine)
L-Cysteine		A precursor of the antioxidant glutathione and a flavor

channels, and glutamate and free-radical release (antioxidant activity) [87–91]. Vinpocetine treatment for 18 months significantly improved cognitive functions, overall health status, and quality of life in people with chronic cerebral hypoperfusion [92]. Vinpocetine is considered prophylactic for MCI [92–94].

Huperzine A (hup A), is a quinolizidine-related alkaloid isolated from *Huperzia serrata* (Thunb.) Trevis. Hup A is a competitive, reversible, and well-tolerated inhibitor of AChE that is more potent than current memory-promoting agents (donepezil, rivastigmine, and galantamine) [95–98]. Hup A is also a competitive NMDA receptor inhibitor and an antagonist of Aβ-induced neurotoxicity [99–108]. It has significant antioxidative, antiapoptotic, and neuroprotective effects [100]. Hup A has been used for enhancing memory and mental function in healthy people [101] and in animal models of cognitive deficits [97] without showing any obvious serious adverse effects [102]. Other studies suggest, however, that hup A has limited effects on cognition. One recent multicenter, randomized, placebo-controlled trial showed that a dose of 0.4 mg daily, but not 0.2 mg daily, of hup A was effective in improving cognition in people with moderate cognition decline [103].

The active components of the leaf extract of *Ginkgo biloba* (EGb) consist of flavonoids, terpenoids, and terpene lactones (ginkgolides and bilobalide). EGb has long been used in traditional Chinese medicine [104, 105]. EGb has also been prescribed for memory and concentration complaints in Germany and France since the 1960s [106, 107]. EGb protects neuronal cell membranes and mitochondria from free-radical damage [108]; reduces the aggregation and toxicity of beta-amyloid [109, 110]; promotes hippocampal neurogenesis [111–116]; decreases blood viscosity [117, 118]; enhances microperfusion [119]; improves neurotransmission of glutamatergic [120–122], dopaminergic, and cholinergic systems [123, 124]; and improves learning and memory in animal models [125–129].

Recent meta-analyses of multiple randomized, controlled trials suggest that EGb may be effective for reversing or delaying age-related memory deficits [130–135]. However, two recent large-scale studies, conducted in more than 6000 participants aged 70 years and over [136, 137], failed to confirm such effects. One explanation is that, due to the particularly long incubation phase of severe memory decline (20–30 years), a quick reduction in the incidence of severe memory deficits by EGb is unrealistic, or EGb is only effective in subjects at early stages of memory decline such as SMC and/or MCI, but not in advanced stage of memory deficits. To support this, short-term and acute EGb administration could be used to enhance specific memory and cognitive functions in cognitively intact older, middle-aged, and younger healthy volunteers [138]. In addition, coadministration of EGb and PS improved secondary memory and the speed of memory task performance [125, 126].

Other studies show that deficits or dysregulation in brain metabolism is linked with aging-related cognition decline and that decline could be reversed through nutrients and vitamin supplements such as acetyl-L-carnitine, vitamin B6, and vitamin B12 [139–151]. L-Tyrosine is a precursor to L-dopa and catecholamines, an imbalance of which may be involved in cognitive dysfunction [127, 128].

The preventive effects of coffee, tea, and caffeine consumption on late-life cognitive decline and dementia have been extensively reviewed recently [129]. Besides the well-known short-term enhancing effects, some studies examined the long-term effects and showed that coffee, tea, and caffeine consumption could protect against late-life cognitive impairment/decline and dementia. These findings, however, are still considered preliminary [129].

Green tea (*Camellia sinensis*) extract enhances parietofrontal connectivity during working memory processing [152] and protects against okadaic acid-induced acute learning and memory impairments in rats [153]. A recent review suggests that the green tea constituent theanine could have therapeutic effects against psychiatric and neurodegenerative disorders including mild cognitive impairment and dementia through multiple mechanisms such as inhibition of NMDA-induced neurotoxicity, enhanced brain GABA and glycine content, and enhanced BDNF-related neuroprotection [154]. Most of these mechanistic studies, however, were done on animals.

Coadministration of multiple medicinal herbal ingredients is a common practice in traditional Chinese medicine. The main goal of such practices is to potentiate the bioavailability, activity, and efficacy of the key therapeutic ingredients and to minimize or antagonize potential toxicities associated with the ingredients.

The objective of this exploratory, randomized, placebo-controlled trial was to evaluate the safety and effectiveness of short-term administration of BrainPower Advanced, a multi-ingredient dietary supplement, on SMCs in older adults.

2. Methods

2.1. Samples and Participants Recruitment. This study was conducted between December 15, 2011, and April 10, 2012, at the Si Tang Community Health Service Center in Baoshan district in Shanghai, China. Community volunteers of older adults were recruited by self-referral in response to media coverage and word of mouth. All study procedures were conducted in accordance with the Helsinki Declaration of 1975 and were approved by the Shanghai Jiao Tong University Medical Center Institutional Review Board. Informed consent was obtained from all participants prior to enrollment into the study.

Subjects who met the following criteria were eligible for the study: *inclusion criteria*: (1) healthy males or females at least 50 years of age; (2) having self-reported hypomnesis, forgetfulness, memory loss, or impaired attention/concentration as determined by a standard medical examination questionnaire; *exclusion criteria*: (1) having been diagnosed with neurological diseases such as Alzheimer's Disease, Parkinson's Disease, migraine, and epilepsy; (2) having taken any medication likely to affect brain and nervous system function such as L-dopa, MAO inhibitors, modafinil, and amphetamine, within 30 days before the start of the trial; (3) having a history of severe cerebral-cardiovascular events (myocardial infarction, cerebrovascular disorder, acute coronary syndrome, or other cerebrovascular diseases); (4) other severe medical conditions (severe diseases of the liver, kidneys, or lungs; malignant tumors; motor impairment; dysphonia; visual impairment; etc.).

2.2. Randomization and Blindness. Participants were randomly assigned to the BrainPower Advanced treatment group or placebo treatment group. The randomization was performed using a predetermined randomization code which was generated by a random number generator. The numbers generated were placed in sealed envelopes and a serial number was assigned to each envelope according to the sequence of allocation of the randomized number. Each envelope was then opened sequentially according to the admission sequence of subjects.

Trial participants and community doctors were both blinded from the treatment (double-blind trial). Of the 101 enrolled participants, 98 participants completed the 12-week follow-up, including 47 subjects in the BrainPower Advanced group and 51 subjects in the placebo group. Three subjects withdrew from the study (2 due to symptoms of diarrhea and 1 due to family objection).

The participants received similar-looking capsules in color-coded bottles (white bottles for BrainPower Advanced and yellow bottles for placebo). Neither the subjects nor the medical doctors, including the study principal investigator (Rong Shi), knew the specific color code until the end of the study. Both the BrainPower Advanced capsules and the placebo (which was mainly composed of flour) were manufactured and supplied by Robinson Pharma, Inc. (Costa Mesa, California, USA).

Each participant was instructed to take 2 capsules with meals daily for 12 weeks and a new batch of supplements was dispensed every 4 weeks during follow-up sessions. Changes in subjective hypomnesis/memory loss and attention/concentration deficits were recorded using a self-administrated medical questionnaire. Memory function capacity was evaluated using a subset of tester-administered memory tests before and after the 12-week intervention. All participants were followed up each month in order to check compliance and adverse effects.

2.3. Evaluation of Subjective Memory Complaints. Two aspects of subjective memory complaints, that is, subjective hypomnesis/forgetfulness/memory loss (SML) and subjective attention/concentration deficits (SAD), were screened using a self-administered 5-point scale (1 = no symptoms or occasional slight symptoms complaints; 2 = slight/mild symptom complaints; 3 = moderate severe symptom complaints; 4 = severe symptom complaints; 5 = very severe symptom complaints) included in a medical questionnaire that included the demographics and medication history of the participants. Because relatively few participants scored 1 and 2 points in the memory questionnaire, participants who scored 1 and 2 points were combined as the "slight symptom" group, and participants who scored 3, 4, and 5 points were combined as the "severe symptom" group for further statistical analysis.

2.4. Evaluation of Objective Memory Function. The short-term working memory of the participants was evaluated using three simple tester-administered subtests constructed and validated for the Chinese population [155].

(1) Visual/Auditory Memory (1 Point for Each Correct Answer, a Maximal Total of 5 Points). Subjects were allowed to watch 5 film clips in 5 minutes (1 minute per film clip). The films were selected from a pool of popular old Chinese films that all participants should have been familiar with. The subjects were then asked to recall the correct order and content of the films based on the movie listings provided by the tester.

(2) Abstracting (1 Point for Each Correct Answer, a Maximal Total of 5 Points). Subjects were shown 5 different pictures/images of cartoon characters (such as a policeman, soldier, medical doctor, nurse, taxi driver, bus driver, school teacher, university professor, cook, waitress, and tour guide) on a computer screen and were asked to recall them immediately.

(3) Memory Recall (1 Point for Each Correct Answer, a Maximal Total of 5 Points). Subjects were shown 5 consecutive pictures of famous historical landscapes located in different Chinese cities and were asked to recall the pictures' contents and their locations.

2.5. Statistics Analysis. EpiData 3.02 software was used for the establishment of the database. SPSS 20.0 software was used for statistical analysis. Group data were presented as the mean ± s.d. Mean differences of the variables between the BrainPower Advanced and placebo groups were compared using Student's t-test for variables with normal distribution or using nonparametric tests for variables with nonnormal distributions. Ridit scoring test, which is a nonparameter test for comparing two or more sets of ordered qualitative data, was used for evaluating the changes in the symptom severity score of SML and SAD in response to the intervention. The alpha level of $P > 0.05$ was chosen as being statistically significant. All P values reported were 2-sided.

3. Results

3.1. Participants' Characteristics. The baseline characteristics of age and gender and histories of alcohol intake, disease, and medication of the participants are shown in Table 2. There were 14 males (29.8%) and 33 females (70.2%) in the BrainPower Advanced group and 17 males (33.3%) and 34 females (66.7%) in the placebo group. The gender distribution between the two groups was not significantly different ($\chi^2 = 0.142$, $P > 0.05$), with females accounting for more than two-thirds of the total participants. The overall average age of all participants was 67.1 ± 10.5, with no significant difference found between the BrainPower Advanced group (69.1 ± 9.5 years) and the placebo group (65.2 ± 11.1 years) ($t = 1.839$, $P > 0.05$). The BrainPower Advanced and placebo groups also showed similar patterns of alcohol intake history ($\chi^2 = 0.542$, $P > 0.05$). However, a greater proportion of the participants in the BrainPower Advanced group had disease

TABLE 2: Demographics and medical history of the participants (N = 98).

	Treatment	Male	Female	Subtotal
Gender, N (% of subtotal)	BrainPower	14 (29.8%)	33 (70.2%)	47 (100%)
	Placebo	17 (33.3%)	34 (66.7%)	51 (100%)
	Combined	31 (31.6%)	69 (68.4)	98 (100%)
Age, year (mean ± s.d.)	BrainPower	69.68 ± 9.52	68.80 ± 9.60	
	Placebo	64.03 ±10.73	65.81 ± 11.41	
	Combined	69.07 ± 9.48	65.22 ± 11.1	67.07 ± 10.49
Age, year (range)	BrainPower	52.87–82.80	53.18–84.86	
	Placebo	47.28–83.47	49.03–88.43	
	Combined	52.87–84.46	47.28–88.43	47.28–88.43
History of chronic disease, yes/total (%)	BrainPower	39/47 (83.0%)		
	Placebo	31/51 (60.8%)		
	Combined	70/98 (71.4%)		
History of alcohol use, yes/total (%)	BrainPower	5/47 (10.6%)		
	Placebo	8/51 (15.7%)		
	Combined	13/98 (13.3%)		
History of medication, yes/total (%)	BrainPower	35/47 (74.5%)		
	Placebo	23/51 (45.1%)		
	Combined	58/98 (59.2%)		

TABLE 3: Mean values of symptom severity of subjective hypomnesis/memory loss (SML) and subjective attention deficit (SAD) (mean ± s.d.) before and after 12 weeks of BrainPower Advanced and placebo intervention.

Self-reported deficits	Intervention	Before intervention	After intervention	Relative to baseline (= 1)
Subjective hypomnesis/memory loss (SML)	BrainPower	3.77 + 0.89	2.94 + 0.94	0.779840849
	Placebo	3.43 + 1.19	2.88 + 0.77	0.839650146
Subjective concentration/attention deficit (SAD)	BrainPower	3.62 + 0.99	2.68 + 0.89	0.740331492
	Placebo	3.25 + 1.35	2.92 + 0.94	0.898461538

history (39/47, 83%) and medication history (35/47, 74.5%) compared to the placebo group (31/51, 60.8%, χ^2 = 5.904, $P < 0.05$ and 23/51, 45.1%, χ^2 = 8.734, $P < 0.01$, resp.).

3.2. Subjective Memory Complaints (SMC). The mean value, distribution pattern, and the differences between the Brain-Power Advanced group and placebo group in the severity level of subjective hypomnesis/forgetfulness/memory loss (SML) and subjective attention/concentration deficit (SAD) before and after the 12-week intervention are shown in Tables 3, 4(a), and 5(a).

The baseline symptom severities of SML and SAD in the BrainPower Advanced group (3.77 ± 0.89; 3.62 ± 0.99, resp.) were about 10% greater than those of the placebo group (3.43 ± 1.19; 3.25 ± 1.35, resp.) (Table 3). These differences in SML and SAD between the two groups disappeared after the 12-week intervention, primarily due to a greater proportion of the BrainPower Advanced group showing greater reduction of symptom severity than the placebo group (Tables 4(b) and 5(b)). The placebo group had more participants that showed worsened symptom severity than the BrainPower Advanced group.

Ridit scoring test shows a significant and differential reduction in the SML (mean ± s.d. = 0.418 ± 0.236 versus 0.575 ± 0.299, $P < 0.01$) and SAD symptom severity (means = 0.424 ± 0.229 versus 0.612 ± 0.283, $P < 0.01$) after BrainPower Advanced and placebo treatment. Table 4(b) shows that a total of 34 people reported reduced SML symptom severity after BrainPower Advanced intervention (2 people by 3 points, 12 people by 2 points, and 20 people by 1 point), 12 people reported no change, and 1 person reported worsened symptom severity (by 1 point). In comparison, only 23 people reported reduced SML severity after placebo intervention (1 person by 3 points, 10 people by 2 points, and 12 people by 1 point), 15 people reported no change in symptom severity, and 13 people reported worsened symptom severity (10 people by 1 point, 2 people by 2 points, and 1 person by 3 points).

Similarly, Table 5(b) shows that a total of 36 people reported different reductions in SAD symptom severity after BrainPower Advanced intervention (2 people by 3 points, 14 people by 2 points, and 20 people by 1 point), 9 people reported no change, and 2 people reported worsened symptom severity (by 1 point) (Table 5(b)). After placebo intervention, 20 people reported different reductions in SAD symptom severity (2 people by 3 points, 8 people by 2 points, and 10 people by 1 point), 15 people reported no change, and 16 people reported worsened symptoms (11 people by 1 point, 3 people by 2 points, and 2 people by 3 points).

TABLE 4: (a) Distribution of symptom severity levels (5-point scale) of subjective hypomnesis/memory loss (SML) in older adults before and after BrainPower Advanced or placebo interventions. (b) Ridit scoring test of the ranked data showed that more subjects showed reduced (−) SML symptoms and far fewer subjects showed worsened SML symptoms (+) after BrainPower Advanced intervention than after placebo intervention, $P < 0.01$. (c) McNemar's test of the combined data (2 scales: 1-2 and 3–5) of subjective memory loss (SML) shows that BrainPower Advanced intervention, but not placebo intervention, significantly reversed the proportion of severe SML in the older adults. It was noted, however, that BrainPower Advanced group had more severe cases and fewer mild cases of SML than the placebo group before the intervention.

(a)

	Group	Distribution of SML symptom severity				
		1, none or slight	2, mild	3, moderate	4, severe	5, very severe
Before intervention	BrainPower group	0 (0%)	3 (6.4%)	16 (34.0%)	17 (36.2%)	11 (23.4%)
	Placebo group	5 (9.8%)	7 (13.7%)	7 (13.7%)	25 (49.0%)	7 (13.7%)
	Total	5 (5.1%)	10 (10.2%)	23 (23.5%)	42 (42.9%)	18 (18.4%)
After intervention	BrainPower group	2 (4.3%)	14 (29.8%)	18 (38.3%)	11 (23.4%)	2 (4.3%)
	Placebo group	2 (3.9%)	12 (23.5%)	27 (52.9%)	10 (19.6%)	0 (0%)
	Total	4 (4.1%)	26 (26.5%)	45 (45.9%)	21 (21.4%)	2 (2.0%)

(b)

Symptom score change	BrainPower group		Placebo group		Total	
	N	%	N	%	N	%
−3	2	4.3	1	2.0	3	3.1
−2	12	25.5	10	19.6	22	22.4
−1	20	42.6	12	23.5	32	32.7
0	12	25.5	15	29.4	27	27.6
+1	1	2.1	10	19.6	11	11.2
+2	0	0.0	2	3.9	2	2.0
+3	0	0.0	1	2.0	1	1.0
Total	47	100.0	51.0	100.0	98	100.0

(c)

Treatment group	Before intervention		After intervention		P value of McNemar's test
	No or slight	Severe	No or slight	Severe	
BrainPower group	3 (6.4%)	44 (93.6%)	16 (34.0%)	31 (66.0%)	0.001
Placebo group	12 (23.5%)	39 (76.5%)	14 (27.5%)	37 (72.5%)	0.791
Pearson χ^2	5.547		0.5		
P	0.019		0.479		

Because the symptom severity scores are nominal variables and because only few participants of the BrainPower Advanced group scored 1 and 2 points (Tables 4(a) and 5(a)) of SML and SAD, participants with the severity scores of 1 and 2 were combined as the "slight symptom" group and participants with the severity scores of 3, 4, and 5 were combined as the "severe symptom" group for further chi-square test (Tables 4(c) and 5(c)).

It was noted that a greater proportion of the BrainPower Advanced group (44/47, 93.6%) than the placebo group (39/51, 76.5%) had severe SML symptoms (severity scores $\geqslant$ 3), or a smaller proportion of the BrainPower Advanced group had slight SML symptoms (severity scores $\leqslant$ 2) (3/47, 6.4%) than the placebo group (12/51, 23.5%) (Pearson χ^2 = 5.547, $P = 0.019$) before the start of the intervention (Tables 4(a) and 4(c)). Similar pretreatment differences in severe SAD distribution existed between the BrainPower Advanced (43/47, 91.5%) and placebo groups (37/51, 72.5%) (severity

scores $\geqslant$ 3) (Pearson χ^2 = 5.852, $P = 0.016$) (Tables 5(a) and 5(c)).

After the intervention, however, the BrainPower Advanced group had fewer cases of severe SML (31) and SAD (28) than the placebo group (37 for SML and 32 for SAD, resp.) and the difference in SML and SAD between the BrainPower Advanced and placebo groups was no longer significant (Pearson χ^2 = 0.5, $P = 0.479$; χ^2 = 0.104, $P = 0.748$, resp.) (Tables 4(c) and 5(c)).

Placebo group analysis of the combined data showed that the proportion of people with severe SML showed little change after placebo intervention (reduced by 2 people, from 39 to 37, $P > 0.05$) whereas the proportion of people with severe SML dropped significantly after BrainPower Advanced intervention (reduced by 13 people, from 44 to 31, $P < 0.001$) (Table 4(c)). Similarly, the proportion of severe SAD did not change significantly after placebo intervention (reduced by 5 people, from 37 to 32, $P > 0.05$) whereas

TABLE 5: (a) Distribution of subjective attention deficit (SAD) symptom severity (using a 5-point questionnaire) in older adults before and after BrainPower Advanced or placebo intervention. (b) Ridit scoring test of the ranked data showed that more people in the BrainPower Advanced group showed reduced SAD (−) and fewer people in the BrainPower Advanced group showed no change or worsened SAD than people in the placebo group after the interventions ($P < 0.01$). (c) McNemar's test of the combined data (2 scales) of subjective attention deficit (SAD) shows that BrainPower Advanced intervention, but not placebo intervention, reversed a significantly greater proportion of severe SAD in the older adults. It was noted, however, that BrainPower Advanced group had more severe cases and fewer mild cases of SAD than the placebo group before the intervention.

(a)

| | Group | \multicolumn{5}{c}{Distribution of SAD symptom severity} |
		1, none or slight	2, mild	3, moderate	4, severe	5, very severe
Before intervention	BrainPower group	1 (2.1%)	3 (6.4%)	16 (34.0%)	19 (40.4%)	8 (17.0%)
	Placebo group	7 (13.7%)	7 (13.7%)	8 (15.7%)	22 (43.1%)	7 (13.7%)
	Total	8 (8.2%)	10 (10.2%)	24 (24.5%)	41 (41.8%)	15 (15.3%)
After intervention	BrainPower group	4 (8.5%)	15 (31.9%)	21 (44.7%)	6 (12.8%)	1 (2.1%)
	Placebo group	2 (3.9%)	17 (33.3%)	16 (31.4%)	15 (29.4%)	1 (2.0%)
	Total	6 (6.1%)	32 (32.7%)	37 (37.8%)	21 (21.4%)	2 (2.0%)

(b)

| Symptom score change | BrainPower group | | Placebo group | | Total | |
	N	%	N	%	N	%
−3	2	4.3	2	3.9	4	4.1
−2	14	29.8	8	15.7	22	22.4
−1	20	42.6	10	19.6	30	30.6
0	9	19.1	15	29.4	14	14.3
+1	2	4.3	11	21.6	13	13.3
+2	0	0.0	3	5.9	3	3.1
+3	0	0.0	2	3.9	2	2.0
Total	47	100.0	51	100.0	98	100.0

(c)

| Treatment group | Before intervention | | After intervention | | P value of McNemar's test |
	No or slight	Severe	No or slight	Severe	
BrainPower group	4 (8.5%)	43 (91.5%)	19 (40.4%)	28 (59.6%)	0.001
Placebo group	14 (27.5%)	37 (72.5%)	19 (37.3%)	32 (62.7%)	0.302
Pearson χ^2	5.852		0.104		
P	0.016		0.748		

the proportion of severe SAD decreased significantly after BrainPower Advanced intervention (reduced by 15 people, from 43 to 28, $P < 0.001$) (Table 5(c)).

3.3. Memory Function Test Scores. The memory function test focused on 3 subareas: visual/auditory impression memory, abstract thinking, and immediate memory recall. The subtest scores and the combined total test scores are shown in Tables 6(a) and 6(b), respectively. The BrainPower Advanced group had about 10% lower baseline scores than placebo group in audio/visual memory (2.28 ± 1.06 versus 2.51 ± 0.81), abstract thinking (2.40 ± 1.08 versus 2.73 ± 1.08), and combined total memory function scores (6.85 ± 2.46 versus 7.37 ± 2.32), but similar scores in memory retrieval (2.17 ± 1.15 versus 2.18 ± 1.14). These baseline differences disappeared after the 12-week intervention (3.43 ± 0.83 versus $3.41 \pm$ 1.00, 3.45 ± 0.75 versus 3.47 ± 0.92, 9.66 ± 1.85 versus 9.39 ± 1.98, and 2.81 ± 0.92 versus 2.47 ± 0.83, resp.). Both the BrainPower Advanced and the placebo groups produced significant improvements (129%–150%) ($P < 0.01$, each) of the subtests and combined total scores in the older adults, with the BrainPower Advanced group producing better improvements (1.50-, 1.35-, 1.43-, and 1.29-fold relative to the baseline values of audio/visual memory, abstract thinking, memory retrieval, and combined total function test scores) than the placebo group (1.35-, 1.27-, 1.13-, and 1.27-fold, resp.) (Tables 6(a) and 6(b)).

Ridit scoring test showed that the improvement in the combined total scores of the memory function subtests was significantly better after the BrainPower Advanced intervention (mean = 0.56 ± 0.287) than after the placebo intervention (0.445 ± 0.276) ($P < 0.05$) (Table 6(c)).

TABLE 6: (a) Subtest scores (mean ± s.d.) of memory function test before and after the interventions between BrainPower Advanced and placebo groups. (b) Comparison of the combined total memory function test scores between BrainPower Advanced and placebo groups shows no differences between the two groups before or after the interventions. However, BrainPower Advanced and placebo interventions both improved the combined total scores significantly ($P < 0.01$ each). (c) Different impacts of BrainPower Advanced and placebo interventions on the improvement of memory function tests. Ridit scoring test of the ranked data showed a better improvement after BrainPower Advanced intervention than after placebo interventions ($P < 0.05$).

(a)

Memory function subtest scores		Before intervention	After intervention	Improvement relative to baseline (= 1)	t	P
Audio/visual memory	BrainPower	2.28 ± 1.06	3.43 ± 0.83	1.50	−8.247	<0.001
	Placebo	2.51 ± 0.81	3.41 ± 1.00	1.36	−5.014	<0.001
	t	−1.232	0.074			
	P	0.221	0.941			
Abstracting ability	BrainPower	2.40 ± 1.08	3.45 ± 0.75	1.44	−6.602	<0.001
	Placebo	2.73 ± 1.08	3.47 ± 0.92	1.27	−4.791	<0.001
	t	−1.474	0.081			
	P	0.144	0.889			
Memory retrieval	BrainPower	2.17 ± 1.15	2.81 ± 0.92	1.29	−3.526	0.001
	Placebo	2.18 ± 1.14	2.47 ± 0.83	1.13	−1.820	0.075
	t	−.027	0.410			
	P	0.979	0.060			

(b)

	Before intervention	After intervention	t	P
BrainPower	6.85 ± 2.46	9.66 ± 1.85	8.478	<0.001
Placebo	7.37 ± 2.32	9.39 ± 1.98	6.988	<0.001
t	−1.08	0.692		
P	0.283	0.491		

(c)

Score change	BrainPower intervention		Placebo control		Total	
	N	%	N	%	N	%
−5	1	2.1	0	0	1	1
−3	0	0	1	2	1	1
−2	1	2.1	2	3.9	3	3.1
−1	1	2.1	5	9.8	6	6.1
0	2	4.3	2	3.9	4	4.1
+1	6	12.8	5	9.8	11	11.2
+2	7	14.9	17	33.3	24	24.5
+3	12	25.5	8	15.7	20	20.4
+4	9	19.1	5	9.8	14	14.3
+5	2	4.3	5	9.8	7	7.1
+6	4	8.5	0	0	4	4.1
+7	2	4.3	1	2	3	3.1
Total	47	100.0	51	100.0	98	100.0

4. Discussion

In this exploratory randomized, double-blind, placebo-controlled study, we evaluated the effectiveness of a proprietary dietary supplement, BrainPower Advanced, in older adults with SMCs. The results show that BrainPower Advanced intervention for 12 weeks was safe and effective in improving the symptoms of SMC in older adults.

SMCs are defined as self-awareness of memory loss that can be assessed by a simple "yes" or "no" questionnaire but are often not detected by clinicians using objective memory scales [2]. SMC is also a predictor of mild cognitive impairment (MCI) and of future cognitive decline [156, 157]. There are studies showing that people with SMC are 3–6 times more likely to develop MCI than people without SMC [158–162].

Because SMCs are often reversible, improvement of SMC would represent a good opportunity to intervene prodromal MCI and cognitive decline. So far, no proven agents are available for SMC. BrainPower Advanced is a dietary supplement based on polyherbal extracts, nutrients, and vitamins. Previous studies have shown that the active ingredients of BrainPower Advanced could potentially improve cognitive function in different age groups of healthy people in the presence or absence of SMCs through various mechanisms including anti-inflammation, improved cerebral blood flow and perfusion, and improved glucose/energy metabolism (Table 1).

In the present study, BrainPower Advanced treatment reversed 13 of the 44 (29.5%) cases of severe SML and 15 of the 43 (34.9%) cases of severe SAD. In contrast, placebo treatment reversed only 2 of the 39 (5.1%) cases of severe SML ($P > 0.05$) and 5 of the 37 (13.5%) cases of severe SAD ($P > 0.05$). Furthermore, a greater proportion of the participants showed various degrees of symptom improvement after BrainPower Advanced intervention (72.3%, 34/47 for SML and 76.6%, 36/47 for SAD) than after placebo treatment (49%, 25/51 for SML and 39.2%, 20/51 for SAD).

In contrast, a greater proportion of participants in the placebo group reported worsened symptoms of SML (25.5%, 13/51) and SAD (31.4%, 16/51) or no change in SML (29.4%, 15/51) and SAD (29.4%, 15/51) compared to the BrainPower Advanced group that reported worsened SML (2.1%, 1/47) and SAD (2%, 2/47) or no change in SML (25.5%, 12/47) and SAD (19.1%, 9/47) after the intervention.

The 29.5% reversion rate (13/44) of severe SML and 34.9% reversion rate (15/43) of severe SAD by BrainPower Advanced are comparable to the reported 15%–35% response rate of MCI to AChEIs treatment and the 30% response rate of MCI to NMDA receptor antagonist treatment [139]. Given that there is no standard anti-SMC treatment yet, the current results are very promising [140–142].

These results suggest that BrainPower Advanced is not only effective in reducing a significant portion (about 30%) of severe SMC and in reducing symptom severity in about 70% of the subjects with SMCs, but also effective in reducing the progression or worsening of SMCs. It is noted, however, that 25.5% of the people with severe SML showed no response to BrainPower Advanced intervention.

In this study, no significant differences were found in visual/auditory memory, abstract thinking, and memory retrieval and in the combined total memory function testing scores between the BrainPower Advanced and placebo groups before or after the intervention. Both BrainPower Advanced and placebo interventions resulted in significantly improved memory function performance, albeit with the BrainPower Advanced group showing better improvement than the placebo group at a nonsignificant level.

Because both placebo and BrainPower Advanced intervention enhanced the performance scores of the memory function tests, this raised the possibility that factors other than the intervention per se may be responsible for the improvement. One such possibility is that the postintervention memory test score was unintendedly "enhanced" by the preintervention test. Like any learning activity, practice or repetition of the same learning task would improve performance and produce better scores. This may not mean that the memory was "getting better" but simply reflecting the remembered answers from the last test. There are suggestions that the same memory tests should not be given within a short period of time (3–6 months) or that only the tests taken the first time should be taken seriously as a true measure of memory abilities.

It is the current view that SMC is a subjective experience that cannot be reliably measured by objective memory scales due to the subtle and heterogeneous nature of SMC [2–5]. Nevertheless, more accurate diagnosis of SMC and/or MCI could be corroborated by informants and by using different questionnaires and memory scales before and after an intervention such as the use of Mini-Mental State Examination (MMSE), Six-Item Screener, Subjective Memory Rating Scale (SMRS) and Deterioration Cognitive Observee (DECO) [143], Memory Complaint Questionnaire (MAC-Q), and Subjective Cognitive Decline Questionnaire (SCD-Q) [144]. The updated Wechsler Memory Scale (WMS) also has a battery of subtests for evaluating multiple aspects of learning and memory including immediate and delayed memory for visual working memory and auditory memory [145–148].

There are other limitations of this study. The sample size is too small to detect potential performance differences in the memory function tests. Despite the randomization process, more participants in the BrainPower Advanced group had a history of disease and medication use than the placebo group. Due to the multi-ingredient nature of BrainPower Advanced, it was difficult to determine whether any single ingredient (*Ginkgo biloba*, *Camellia sinensis*, vinpocetine, kola nut, hup A, PS, L-tyrosine, L-pyroglutamic acid, acetyl-L-carnitine, choline bitartrate, L-glutamine, L-phenylalanine, L-cysteine, vitamin B6, or vitamin B12) was primarily responsible for BrainPower Advanced overall effects or, more likely, whether it was a synergistic combination of the ingredients working together that produced the observed results. Because SMCs are heterogeneous and potentially affected by a range of genetic and epigenetic factors including lifestyle [149], daily activity/exercise [150, 151], APOE genotype [163], affective status [164–166], education achievements [11, 167], inflammation, and alcohol use, controlling these factors would allow better understanding of BrainPower Advanced intervention in further studies [168].

5. Conclusion

Twelve-week BrainPower Advanced intervention was effective and safe in reducing the progression of symptom severity in older adults with severe SML and SAD. As no proven agents are currently available in reversing or delaying the progression of SMC in the increasing aging population, further well-controlled, large-scale studies could validate if long-term dietary supplementation of combined polyherbal ingredients, nutrients, and vitamins could be an alternative prophylactic strategy for older adults with SMCs.

Disclosure

The sponsor had no role in the design or analysis of this study or the interpretation of the findings. Mina Shariff and Tuong Nguyen are employees of DRM Resources.

Competing Interests

Jingfen Zhu, Guoqiang Xing, Su Chen, Lihua Dai, Tian Shen, Yi Feng, Yeats Ye, Jianyu Rao, and Rong Shi have declared that they have no competing or potential conflict of interests in the study.

Authors' Contributions

Jingfen Zhu, Guoqiang Xing, and Su Chen have contributed equally to this work. All authors have read the paper and had full access to the study data.

Acknowledgments

The authors thank Reza Emaddudin for proofreading the paper. This study was sponsored by DRM Resources (Costa Mesa, California, USA).

References

[1] T. Hänninen, K. Koivisto, K. J. Reinikainen et al., "Prevalence of ageing-associated cognitive decline in an elderly population," *Age and Ageing*, vol. 25, no. 3, pp. 201–205, 1996.

[2] K. Abdulrab and R. Heun, "Subjective memory impairment. A review of its definitions indicates the need for a comprehensive set of standardised and validated criteria," *European Psychiatry*, vol. 23, no. 5, pp. 321–330, 2008.

[3] A. Pearman and M. Storandt, "Self-discipline and self-consciousness predict subjective memory in older adults," *Journals of Gerontology B Psychological Sciences and Social Sciences*, vol. 60, no. 3, pp. P153–P157, 2005.

[4] B. E. Snitz, L. A. Morrow, E. G. Rodriguez, K. A. Huber, and J. A. Saxton, "Subjective memory complaints and concurrent memory performance in older patients of primary care providers," *Journal of the International Neuropsychological Society*, vol. 14, no. 6, pp. 1004–1013, 2008.

[5] B. E. Snitz, L. Yu, P. K. Crane, C.-C. H. Chang, T. F. Hughes, and M. Ganguli, "Subjective cognitive complaints of older adults at the population level: an item response theory analysis," *Alzheimer Disease and Associated Disorders*, vol. 26, no. 4, pp. 344–351, 2012.

[6] A. Burns and M. Zaudig, "Mild cognitive impairment in older people," *The Lancet*, vol. 360, no. 9349, pp. 1963–1965, 2002.

[7] R. O. Roberts, D. S. Knopman, Y. E. Geda, R. H. Cha, V. L. Roger, and R. C. Petersen, "Coronary heart disease is associated with non-amnestic mild cognitive impairment," *Neurobiology of Aging*, vol. 31, no. 11, pp. 1894–1902, 2010.

[8] R. Grambaite, E. Hessen, E. Auning, D. Aarsland, P. Selnes, and T. Fladby, "Correlates of subjective and mild cognitive impairment: depressive symptoms and CSF biomarkers," *Dementia and Geriatric Cognitive Disorders Extra*, vol. 3, pp. 291–300, 2013.

[9] M. M. Mielke, R. Savica, H. J. Wiste et al., "Head trauma and in vivo measures of amyloid and neurodegeneration in a population-based study," *Neurology*, vol. 82, no. 1, pp. 70–76, 2014.

[10] A. Sajjad, S. S. Mirza, M. L. P. Portegies et al., "Subjective memory complaints and the risk of stroke," *Stroke*, vol. 46, no. 1, pp. 170–175, 2015.

[11] A. Alagoa João, J. Maroco, S. Ginó, T. Mendes, A. de Mendonça, and I. P. Martins, "Education modifies the type of subjective memory complaints in older people," *International Journal of Geriatric Psychiatry*, vol. 31, no. 2, pp. 153–160, 2016.

[12] S. F. Rowell, J. S. Green, B. A. Teachman, and T. A. Salthouse, "Age does not matter: memory complaints are related to negative affect throughout adulthood," *Aging & Mental Health*, 2015.

[13] R. C. Petersen, "Early diagnosis of Alzheimer's disease: is MCI too late?" *Current Alzheimer Research*, vol. 6, no. 4, pp. 324–330, 2009.

[14] J. Bischkopf, A. Busse, and M. C. Angermeyer, "Mild cognitive impairment—a review of prevalence, incidence and outcome according to current approaches," *Acta Psychiatrica Scandinavica*, vol. 106, no. 6, pp. 403–414, 2002.

[15] A. Busse, J. Bischkopf, S. G. Riedel-Heller, and M. C. Angermeyer, "Subclassifications for mild cognitive impairment: prevalence and predictive validity," *Psychological Medicine*, vol. 33, no. 6, pp. 1029–1038, 2003.

[16] F. Panza, C. Capurso, A. D'Introno, A. M. Colacicco, A. Capurso, and V. Solfrizzi, "Prevalence rates of mild cognitive impairment subtypes and progression to dementia," *Journal of the American Geriatrics Society*, vol. 54, no. 9, pp. 1474–1475, 2006.

[17] F. Panza, C. Capurso, A. D'Introno, A. M. Colacicco, A. Capurso, and V. Solfrizzi, "Mild cognitive impairment: risk of Alzheimer disease and rate of cognitive decline," *Neurology*, vol. 68, no. 12, pp. 964–965, 2007.

[18] S. Gauthier, B. Reisberg, M. Zaudig et al., "Mild cognitive impairment," *The Lancet*, vol. 367, no. 9518, pp. 1262–1270, 2006.

[19] K. Meguro, K. Akanuma, M. Meguro, S. Yamaguchi, H. Ishii, and M. Tashiro, "Prevalence and prognosis of prodromal Alzheimer's disease as assessed by magnetic resonance imaging and f-fluorodeoxyglucose-positron emission tomography in a community: reanalysis from the Osaki-Tajiri project," *Psychogeriatrics*, 2015.

[20] S. J. B. Vos, F. Verhey, L. Frölich et al., "Prevalence and prognosis of alzheimer's disease at the mild cognitive impairment stage," *Brain*, vol. 138, no. 5, pp. 1327–1338, 2015.

[21] A. Ward, S. Tardiff, C. Dye, and H. M. Arrighi, "Rate of conversion from prodromal Alzheimer's disease to Alzheimer's dementia: a systematic review of the literature," *Dementia and Geriatric Cognitive Disorders Extra*, vol. 3, no. 1, pp. 320–332, 2013.

[22] D. G. Darby, A. Brodtmann, R. H. Pietrzak et al., "Episodic memory decline predicts cortical amyloid status in community-dwelling older adults," *Journal of Alzheimer's Disease*, vol. 27, no. 3, pp. 627–637, 2011.

[23] S. Erk, A. Spottke, A. Meisen, M. Wagner, H. Walter, and F. Jessen, "Evidence of neuronal compensation during episodic memory in subjective memory impairment," *Archives of General Psychiatry*, vol. 68, no. 8, pp. 845–852, 2011.

[24] K. A. Gifford, D. Liu, S. M. Damon et al., "Subjective memory complaint only relates to verbal episodic memory performance in mild cognitive impairment," *Journal of Alzheimer's Disease*, vol. 44, no. 1, pp. 309–318, 2015.

[25] A. Forsberg, H. Engler, O. Almkvist et al., "PET imaging of amyloid deposition in patients with mild cognitive impairment," *Neurobiology of Aging*, vol. 29, no. 10, pp. 1456–1465, 2008.

[26] B. E. Snitz, L. A. Weissfeld, A. D. Cohen et al., "Subjective cognitive complaints, personality and brain amyloid-beta in cognitively normal older adults," *The American Journal of Geriatric Psychiatry*, vol. 23, no. 9, pp. 985–993, 2015.

[27] Y. Y. Lim, K. A. Ellis, K. Harrington et al., "Cognitive decline in adults with amnestic mild cognitive impairment and high amyloid-β: prodromal Alzheimer's disease?" *Journal of Alzheimer's Disease*, vol. 33, no. 4, pp. 1167–1176, 2013.

[28] S. M. Landau, M. A. Mintun, A. D. Joshi et al., "Amyloid deposition, hypometabolism, and longitudinal cognitive decline," *Annals of Neurology*, vol. 72, no. 4, pp. 578–586, 2012.

[29] E. E. Smith and S. M. Greenberg, "β-Amyloid, blood vessels, and brain function," *Stroke*, vol. 40, no. 7, pp. 2601–2606, 2009.

[30] S. Karim, S. Hopkins, N. Purandare et al., "Peripheral inflammatory markers in amnestic mild cognitive impairment," *International Journal of Geriatric Psychiatry*, vol. 29, no. 3, pp. 221–226, 2014.

[31] M. L. Bader Lange, G. Cenini, M. Piroddi et al., "Loss of phospholipid asymmetry and elevated brain apoptotic protein levels in subjects with amnestic mild cognitive impairment and Alzheimer disease," *Neurobiology of Disease*, vol. 29, no. 3, pp. 456–464, 2008.

[32] D. Hadjiev, "Asymptomatic ischemic cerebrovascular disorders and neuroprotection with vinpocetine," *Ideggyogyaszati Szemle*, vol. 56, no. 5-6, pp. 166–172, 2003.

[33] G. Douaud, R. A. L. Menke, A. Gass et al., "Brain microstructure reveals early abnormalities more than two years prior to clinical progression from mild cognitive impairment to Alzheimer's disease," *Journal of Neuroscience*, vol. 33, no. 5, pp. 2147–2155, 2013.

[34] S. L. Leal and M. A. Yassa, "Perturbations of neural circuitry in aging, mild cognitive impairment, and Alzheimer's disease," *Ageing Research Reviews*, vol. 12, no. 3, pp. 823–831, 2013.

[35] L. Zhuang, P. S. Sachdev, J. N. Trollor et al., "Microstructural white matter changes, not hippocampal atrophy, detect early amnestic mild cognitive impairment," *PLoS ONE*, vol. 8, no. 3, Article ID e58887, 2013.

[36] R. Cabeza, C. L. Grady, L. Nyberg et al., "Age-related differences in neural activity during memory encoding and retrieval: a positron emission tomography study," *The Journal of Neuroscience*, vol. 17, no. 1, pp. 391–400, 1997.

[37] D. A. Loewenstein, A. Acevedo, E. Potter et al., "Severity of medial temporal atrophy and amnestic mild cognitive impairment: selecting type and number of memory tests," *The American Journal of Geriatric Psychiatry*, vol. 17, no. 12, pp. 1050–1058, 2009.

[38] M. Okamoto, Y. Wada, Y. Yamaguchi et al., "Process-specific prefrontal contributions to episodic encoding and retrieval of tastes: a functional NIRS study," *NeuroImage*, vol. 54, no. 2, pp. 1578–1588, 2011.

[39] G. Prendergast, E. Limbrick-Oldfield, E. Ingamells, S. Gathercole, A. Baddeley, and G. G. R. Green, "Differential patterns of prefrontal MEG activation during verbal & visual encoding and retrieval," *PLoS ONE*, vol. 8, no. 12, Article ID e82936, 2013.

[40] R. Manenti, M. Cotelli, and C. Miniussi, "Successful physiological aging and episodic memory: a brain stimulation study," *Behavioural Brain Research*, vol. 216, no. 1, pp. 153–158, 2011.

[41] B. P. Lockhart and P. J. Lestage, "Cognition enhancing or neuroprotective compounds for the treatment of cognitive disorders: why? when? which?" *Experimental Gerontology*, vol. 38, no. 1-2, pp. 119–128, 2003.

[42] M. A. Taffe, M. R. Weed, T. Gutierrez, S. A. Davis, and L. H. Gold, "Differential muscarinic and NMDA contributions to visuo-spatial paired-associate learning in rhesus monkeys," *Psychopharmacology*, vol. 160, no. 3, pp. 253–262, 2002.

[43] E. L. Schaeffer and W. F. Gattaz, "Cholinergic and glutamatergic alterations beginning at the early stages of Alzheimer disease: participation of the phospholipase A_2 enzyme," *Psychopharmacology*, vol. 198, no. 1, pp. 1–27, 2008.

[44] G. L. Wenk, "Neuropathologic changes in Alzheimer's disease: potential targets for treatment," *Journal of Clinical Psychiatry*, vol. 67, supplement 3, pp. 3–7, 2006.

[45] P. T. Francis, "Glutamatergic systems in Alzheimer's disease," *International Journal of Geriatric Psychiatry*, vol. 18, no. 1, pp. S15–S21, 2003.

[46] C. McVeigh and P. Passmore, "Vascular dementia: prevention and treatment," *Clinical Interventions in Aging*, vol. 1, no. 3, pp. 229–235, 2006.

[47] K. M. Cosman, L. L. Boyle, and A. P. Porsteinsson, "Memantine in the treatment of mild-to-moderate Alzheimer's disease," *Expert Opinion on Pharmacotherapy*, vol. 8, no. 2, pp. 203–214, 2007.

[48] O. Peters, D. Lorenz, A. Fesche et al., "A combination of galantamine and memantine modifies cognitive function in subjects with amnestic MCI," *Journal of Nutrition, Health and Aging*, vol. 16, no. 6, pp. 544–548, 2012.

[49] S. Salloway, S. Correia, and S. Richardson, "Key lessons learned from short-term treatment trials of cholinesterase inhibitors for amnestic MCI," *International Psychogeriatrics*, vol. 20, no. 1, pp. 40–46, 2008.

[50] R. C. Petersen, R. G. Thomas, M. Grundman et al., "Vitamin E and donepezil for the treatment of mild cognitive impairment," *The New England Journal of Medicine*, vol. 352, no. 23, pp. 2379–2388, 2005.

[51] H. H. Feldman, S. Ferris, B. Winblad et al., "Effect of rivastigmine on delay to diagnosis of Alzheimer's disease from mild cognitive impairment: the InDDEx study," *The Lancet Neurology*, vol. 6, no. 6, pp. 501–512, 2007.

[52] J. T. O'Brien, A. Burns, and Group BAPDC, "Clinical practice with anti-dementia drugs: a revised (second) consensus statement from the British Association for Psychopharmacology," *Journal of Psychopharmacology*, vol. 25, no. 8, pp. 997–1019, 2011.

[53] T. C. Russ, "Cholinesterase inhibitors should not be prescribed for mild cognitive impairment," *Evidence-Based Medicine*, vol. 19, no. 3, article 101, 2014.

[54] T. C. Russ and J. R. Morling, "Cholinesterase inhibitors for mild cognitive impairment," *Cochrane Database of Systematic Reviews*, vol. 9, Article ID CD009132, 2012.

[55] A. Servello, P. Andreozzi, F. Bechini et al., "Effect of ache and BuChE inhibition by rivastigmin in a group of old-old elderly patients with cerebrovascular impairment (SIVD type)," *Minerva Medica*, vol. 105, no. 2, pp. 167–174, 2014.

[56] R. M. Lane and T. Darreh-Shori, "Understanding the beneficial and detrimental effects of donepezil and rivastigmine to improve their therapeutic value," *Journal of Alzheimer's Disease*, vol. 44, no. 4, pp. 1039–1039, 2015.

[57] P. R. Heckman, C. Wouters, and J. Prickaerts, "Phospho-diesterase inhibitors as a target for cognition enhancement in aging and Alzheimer's disease: a translational overview," *Current Pharmaceutical Design*, vol. 21, no. 3, pp. 317–331, 2014.

[58] M. Singer, B. Romero, E. Koenig, H. Förstl, and H. Brunner, "Nightmares in patients with Alzheimer's disease caused by donepezil. Therapeutic effect depends on the time of intake," *Nervenarzt*, vol. 76, no. 9, pp. 1128–1129, 2005.

[59] N. Mimica and P. Presečki, "Side effects of approved antidementives," *Psychiatria Danubina*, vol. 21, no. 1, pp. 108–113, 2009.

[60] P. Gareri, D. Putignano, A. Castagna et al., "Retrospective study on the benefits of combined memantine and cholinesterase inhibitor treatment in aged patients affected with Alzheimer's disease: the memage study," *Journal of Alzheimer's Disease*, vol. 41, no. 2, pp. 633–640, 2014.

[61] M. D. Nguyen and R. L. Salbu, "Donepezil 23 mg: a brief insight on efficacy and safety concerns," *Consultant Pharmacist*, vol. 28, no. 12, pp. 800–803, 2013.

[62] P. Anand and B. Singh, "A review on cholinesterase inhibitors for Alzheimer's disease," *Archives of Pharmacal Research*, vol. 36, no. 4, pp. 375–399, 2013.

[63] S. G. Di Santo, F. Prinelli, F. Adorni, C. Caltagirone, and M. Musicco, "A meta-analysis of the efficacy of donepezil, rivastigmine, galantamine, and memantine in relation to severity of Alzheimer's disease," *Journal of Alzheimer's Disease*, vol. 35, no. 2, pp. 349–361, 2013.

[64] S. Mehta, K. Chandersekhar, G. Prasadrao et al., "Safety and efficacy of donepezil hydrochloride in patients with mild to moderate Alzheimer's disease: findings of an observational study," *Indian Journal of Psychiatry*, vol. 54, no. 4, pp. 337–343, 2012.

[65] P. Russo, A. Frustaci, A. Del Bufalo, M. Fini, and A. Cesario, "Multitarget drugs of plants origin acting on Alzheimer's disease," *Current Medicinal Chemistry*, vol. 20, no. 13, pp. 1686–1693, 2013.

[66] G. Pepeu, I. M. Pepeu, and L. Amaducci, "A review of phosphatidylserine pharmacological and clinical effects. Is phosphatidylserine a drug for the ageing brain?" *Pharmacological Research*, vol. 33, no. 2, pp. 73–80, 1996.

[67] H.-Y. Kim, B. X. Huang, and A. A. Spector, "Phosphatidylserine in the brain: metabolism and function," *Progress in Lipid Research*, vol. 56, no. 1, pp. 1–18, 2014.

[68] M. A. Starks, S. L. Starks, M. Kingsley, M. Purpura, and R. Jäger, "The effects of phosphatidylserine on endocrine response to moderate intensity exercise," *Journal of the International Society of Sports Nutrition*, vol. 5, article 11, 2008.

[69] P. V. Escribá, X. Busquets, J. Inokuchi et al., "Membrane lipid therapy: modulation of the cell membrane composition and structure as a molecular base for drug discovery and new disease treatment," *Progress in Lipid Research*, vol. 59, pp. 38–53, 2015.

[70] T. Crook, W. Petrie, C. Wells, and D. C. Massari, "Effects of phosphatidylserine in Alzheimer's disease," *Psychopharmacology Bulletin*, vol. 28, no. 1, pp. 61–66, 1992.

[71] T. H. Crook, J. Tinklenberg, J. Yesavage et al., "Effects of phosphatidylserine in age-associated memory impairment," *Neurology*, vol. 41, no. 5, pp. 644–649, 1991.

[72] S. Schreiber, "An open trial of plant-source derived phosphatydilserine for treatment of age-related cognitive decline," *Israel Journal of Psychiatry and Related Sciences*, vol. 37, no. 4, pp. 302–307, 2000.

[73] A. Kato-Kataoka, M. Sakai, R. Ebina, C. Nonaka, T. Asano, and T. Miyamori, "Soybean-derived phosphatidylserine improves memory function of the elderly Japanese subjects with memory complaints," *Journal of Clinical Biochemistry and Nutrition*, vol. 47, no. 3, pp. 246–255, 2010.

[74] K. Yurko-Mauro, "Cognitive and cardiovascular benefits of docosahexaenoic acid in aging and cognitive decline," *Current Alzheimer Research*, vol. 7, no. 3, pp. 190–196, 2010.

[75] Y. Richter, Y. Herzog, Y. Lifshitz, R. Hayun, and S. Zchut, "The effect of soybean-derived phosphatidylserine on cognitive performance in elderly with subjective memory complaints: a pilot study," *Clinical Interventions in Aging*, vol. 8, pp. 557–563, 2013.

[76] H.-J. Park, S. Y. Lee, H. S. Shim, J. S. Kim, K. S. Kim, and I. Shim, "Chronic treatment with squid phosphatidylserine activates glucose uptake and ameliorates TMT-induced cognitive deficit in rats via activation of cholinergic systems," *Evidence-Based Complementary and Alternative Medicine*, vol. 2012, Article ID 601018, 8 pages, 2012.

[77] B. Lee, B.-J. Sur, J.-J. Han et al., "Oral administration of squid lecithin-transphosphatidylated phosphatidylserine improves memory impairment in aged rats," *Progress in Neuro-Psychopharmacology and Biological Psychiatry*, vol. 56, pp. 1–10, 2015.

[78] L. Amaducci, "Phosphatidylserine in the treatment of Alzheimer's disease: results of a multicenter study," *Psychopharmacology Bulletin*, vol. 24, no. 1, pp. 130–134, 1988.

[79] L. Amaducci, T. H. Crook, A. Lippi et al., "Use of phosphatidylserine in Alzheimer's disease," *Annals of the New York Academy of Sciences*, vol. 640, pp. 245–249, 1991.

[80] T. Cenacchi, T. Bertoldin, C. Farina et al., "Cognitive decline in the elderly: a double-blind, placebo-controlled multicenter study on efficacy of phosphatidylserine administration," *Aging Clinical and Experimental Research*, vol. 5, no. 2, pp. 123–133, 1993.

[81] M. I. Kingsley, M. Miller, L. P. Kilduff, J. McEneny, and D. Benton, "Effects of phosphatidylserine on exercise capacity during cycling in active males," *Medicine and Science in Sports and Exercise*, vol. 38, no. 1, pp. 64–71, 2006.

[82] S. Hirayama, K. Terasawa, R. Rabeler et al., "The effect of phosphatidylserine administration on memory and symptoms of attention-deficit hyperactivity disorder: a randomised, double-blind, placebo-controlled clinical trial," *Journal of Human Nutrition and Dietetics*, vol. 27, supplement 2, pp. 284–291, 2014.

[83] N. Tamaki, T. Kusunoki, and S. Matsumoto, "The effect of vinpocetine on cerebral blood flow in patients with cerebrovascular disorders," *Therapia Hungarica*, vol. 33, no. 1, pp. 13–21, 1985.

[84] N. Tamaki and S. Matsumoto, "Agents to improve cerebrovascular circulation and cerebral metabolism—vinpocetine," *Nippon Rinsho*, vol. 43, no. 2, pp. 376–378, 1985.

[85] P. Bönöczk, G. Panczel, and Z. Nagy, "Vinpocetine increases cerebral blood flow and oxygenation in stroke patients: a near infrared spectroscopy and transcranial Doppler study," *European Journal of Ultrasound*, vol. 15, no. 1-2, pp. 85–91, 2002.

[86] G. Szilágyi, Z. Nagy, L. Balkay et al., "Effects of vinpocetine on the redistribution of cerebral blood flow and glucose metabolism in chronic ischemic stroke patients: a PET study," *Journal of the Neurological Sciences*, vol. 229-230, pp. 275–284, 2005.

[87] C. Pereira, P. Agostinho, P. I. Moreira, A. I. Duarte, M. S. Santos, and C. R. Oliveira, "Neuroprotection strategies: effect

of vinpocetinein in vitro oxidative stress models," *Acta Medica Portuguesa*, vol. 16, no. 6, pp. 401–406, 2003.

[88] C. Pereira, P. Agostinho, and C. R. Oliveira, "Vinpocetine attenuates the metabolic dysfunction induced by amyloid β-peptides in PC12 cells," *Free Radical Research*, vol. 33, no. 5, pp. 497–506, 2000.

[89] E. I. Solntseva, I. V. Bukanova, and V. G. Skrebitskiĭ, "Memory and potassium channels," *Uspekhi Fiziologicheskikh Nauk*, vol. 34, no. 4, pp. 16–25, 2003.

[90] R. T. Liu, A. Wang, E. To et al., "Vinpocetine inhibits amyloid-beta induced activation of NF-κB, NLRP3 inflammasome and cytokine production in retinal pigment epithelial cells," *Experimental Eye Research*, vol. 127, pp. 49–58, 2014.

[91] L. Zhang and L. Yang, "Anti-inflammatory effects of vinpocetine in atherosclerosis and ischemic stroke: a review of the literature," *Molecules*, vol. 20, no. 1, pp. 335–347, 2015.

[92] A. Valikovics, A. Csányi, and L. Németh, "Study of the effects of vinpocetin on cognitive functions," *Ideggyogyaszati Szemle*, vol. 65, no. 3-4, pp. 115–120, 2012.

[93] S. Z. Szatmari and P. J. Whitehouse, "Vinpocetine for cognitive impairment and dementia," *Cochrane Database of Systematic Reviews*, no. 1, Article ID CD003119, 2003.

[94] A. Valikovics, "Investigation of the effect of vinpocetine on cerebral blood flow and cognitive functions," *Ideggyógyászati Szemle*, vol. 60, no. 7-8, pp. 301–310, 2007.

[95] Y. Q. Liang and X. C. Tang, "Comparative effects of huperzine A, donepezil and rivastigmine on cortical acetylcholine level and acetylcholinesterase activity in rats," *Neuroscience Letters*, vol. 361, no. 1-3, pp. 56–59, 2004.

[96] Y.-Q. Liang and X.-C. Tang, "Comparative studies of huperzine A, donepezil, and rivastigmine on brain acetylcholine, dopamine, norepinephrine, and 5-hydroxytryptamine levels in freely-moving rats," *Acta Pharmacologica Sinica*, vol. 27, no. 9, pp. 1127–1136, 2006.

[97] R. Wang, H. Yan, and X.-C. Tang, "Progress in studies of huperzine A, a natural cholinesterase inhibitor from Chinese herbal medicine," *Acta Pharmacologica Sinica*, vol. 27, no. 1, pp. 1–26, 2006.

[98] S.-H. Xing, C.-X. Zhu, R. Zhang, and L. An, "Huperzine A in the treatment of Alzheimer's disease and vascular dementia: a meta-analysis," *Evidence-Based Complementary and Alternative Medicine*, vol. 2014, Article ID 363985, 10 pages, 2014.

[99] G. T. Ha, R. K. Wong, and Y. Zhang, "Huperzine a as potential treatment of Alzheimer's disease: an assessment on chemistry, pharmacology, and clinical studies," *Chemistry and Biodiversity*, vol. 8, no. 7, pp. 1189–1204, 2011.

[100] N. Zhu, J. Lin, K. Wang, M. Wei, Q. Chen, and Y. Wang, "Huperzine a protects neural stem cells against Aβ-induced apoptosis in a neural stem cells and microglia co-culture system," *International Journal of Clinical and Experimental Pathology*, vol. 8, no. 6, pp. 6425–6433, 2015.

[101] Z.-Q. Xu, X.-M. Liang, Juan-Wu, Y.-F. Zhang, C.-X. Zhu, and X.-J. Jiang, "Treatment with huperzine a improves cognition in vascular dementia patients," *Cell Biochemistry and Biophysics*, vol. 62, no. 1, pp. 55–58, 2012.

[102] J. Li, H. M. Wu, R. L. Zhou, G. J. Liu, and B. R. Dong, "Huperzine a for Alzheimer's disease," *Cochrane database of Systematic Reviews*, no. 2, Article ID CD005592, 2008.

[103] M. S. Rafii, S. Walsh, J. T. Little et al., "A phase II trial of huperzine A in mild to moderate Alzheimer disease," *Neurology*, vol. 76, no. 16, pp. 1389–1394, 2011.

[104] R. Ihl, "Gingko biloba extract EGb 761®: clinical data in dementia," *International Psychogeriatrics*, vol. 24, supplement 1, pp. S35–S40, 2012.

[105] S. Kasper, "Clinical data in early intervention," *International Psychogeriatrics*, vol. 24, supplement 1, pp. S41–S45, 2012.

[106] M. J. Serby, C. Yhap, and E. Y. Landron, "A study of herbal remedies for memory complaints," *Journal of Neuropsychiatry and Clinical Neurosciences*, vol. 22, no. 3, pp. 345–347, 2010.

[107] H.-J. Gertz and M. Kiefer, "Review about Ginkgo biloba special extract EGb 761 (Ginkgo)," *Current Pharmaceutical Design*, vol. 10, no. 3, pp. 261–264, 2004.

[108] S. Stoll, K. Scheuer, O. Pohl, and W. E. Müller, "Ginkgo biloba extract (EGb 761) independently improves changes in passive avoidance learning and brain membrane fluidity in the aging mouse," *Pharmacopsychiatry*, vol. 29, no. 4, pp. 144–149, 1996.

[109] C.-S. Liu, J.-F. Hu, N.-H. Chen, and J.-T. Zhang, "Comparison of the inhibitory activities of salvianolic acid B and *Ginkgo biloba* extract EGb 761 on neurotoxicity of beta-amyloid peptide," *Yao Xue Xue Bao*, vol. 41, no. 8, pp. 706–711, 2006.

[110] F. Longpré, P. Garneau, Y. christen, and C. Ramassamy, "Protection by EGb 761 against β-amyloid-induced neurotoxicity: Involvement of NF-κB, SIRT1, and MAPKs pathways and inhibition of amyloid fibril formation," *Free Radical Biology and Medicine*, vol. 41, no. 12, pp. 1781–1794, 2006.

[111] O. M. E. Abdel-Salam, "Stem cell therapy for Alzheimer's disease," *CNS and Neurological Disorders-Drug Targets*, vol. 10, no. 4, pp. 459–485, 2011.

[112] N. M. Osman, A. S. Amer, and S. Abdelwahab, "Effects of Ginko biloba leaf extract on the neurogenesis of the hippocampal dentate gyrus in the elderly mice," *Anatomical Science International*, 2015.

[113] L. Sun, W. Zhuang, X. Xu, J. Yang, J. Teng, and F. Zhang, "The effect of injection of EGb 761 into the lateral ventricle on hippocampal cell apoptosis and stem cell stimulation in situ of the ischemic/reperfusion rat model," *Neuroscience Letters*, vol. 555, pp. 123–128, 2013.

[114] F. Tchantchou, P. N. Lacor, Z. Cao et al., "Stimulation of neurogenesis and synaptogenesis by bilobalide and quercetin via common final pathway in hippocampal neurons," *Journal of Alzheimer's Disease*, vol. 18, no. 4, pp. 787–798, 2009.

[115] F. Tchantchou, Y. Xu, Y. Wu, Y. Christen, and Y. Luo, "EGb 761 enhances adult hippocampal neurogenesis and phosphorylation of CREB in transgenic mouse model of Alzheimer's disease," *The FASEB Journal*, vol. 21, no. 10, pp. 2400–2408, 2007.

[116] D. Y. Yoo, Y. Y. Nam, W. Kim et al., "Effects of ginkgo biloba extract on promotion of neurogenesis in the hippocampal dentate gyrus in C57BL/6 mice," *Journal of Veterinary Medical Science*, vol. 73, no. 1, pp. 71–76, 2011.

[117] R. F. Santos, J. C. F. Galduróz, A. Barbieri, M. L. V. Castiglioni, L. Y. Ytaya, and O. F. A. Bueno, "Cognitive performance, SPECT, and blood viscosity in elderly non-demented people using Ginkgo biloba," *Pharmacopsychiatry*, vol. 36, no. 4, pp. 127–133, 2003.

[118] S.-Y. Huang, C. Jeng, S.-C. Kao, J. J.-H. Yu, and D.-Z. Liu, "Improved haemorrheological properties by *Ginkgo biloba* extract (Egb 761) in type 2 diabetes mellitus complicated with retinopathy," *Clinical Nutrition*, vol. 23, no. 4, pp. 615–621, 2004.

[119] P. Koltringer, O. Eber, G. Klima et al., "Microcirculation under therapy of parenteral Ginkgo biloba extract," *Wiener Klinische Wochenschrift*, vol. 101, no. 6, pp. 198–200, 1989.

[120] M. Esposito and M. Carotenuto, "Ginkgolide B complex efficacy for brief prophylaxis of migraine in school-aged children: an open-label study," *Neurological Sciences*, vol. 32, no. 1, pp. 79–81, 2011.

[121] E. Nooshinfar, R. Lashgari, A. Haghparast, and S. Sajjadi, "NMDA receptors are involved in Ginkgo extract-induced facilitation on memory retention of passive avoidance learning in rats," *Neuroscience Letters*, vol. 432, no. 3, pp. 206–211, 2008.

[122] S. R. Veerman, P. Schulte, M. Begemann, and L. de Haan, "Non-glutamatergic clozapine augmentation strategies: a review and meta-analysis," *Pharmacopsychiatry*, vol. 47, no. 7, pp. 231–238, 2014.

[123] W. H. Cong, J. X. Liu, and L. Xu, "Effects of extracts of ginseng and ginkgo biloba on hippocampal acetylcholine and monoamines in pdap-pv717i transgenic mice," *Zhongguo Zhong Xi Yi Jie He Za Zhi*, vol. 27, no. 9, pp. 810–813, 2007.

[124] J. Kehr, S. Yoshitake, S. Ijiri, E. Koch, M. Nöldner, and T. Yoshitake, "Ginkgo biloba leaf extract (EGb 761®) and its specific acylated flavonol constituents increase dopamine and acetylcholine levels in the rat medial prefrontal cortex: possible implications for the cognitive enhancing properties of EGb 761®," *International Psychogeriatrics*, vol. 24, supplement 1, pp. S25–S34, 2012.

[125] R. Kaschel, "Specific memory effects of Ginkgo biloba extract EGb 761 in middle-aged healthy volunteers," *Phytomedicine*, vol. 18, no. 14, pp. 1202–1207, 2011.

[126] D. O. Kennedy, P. A. Jackson, C. F. Haskell, and A. B. Scholey, "Modulation of cognitive performance following single doses of 120 mg Ginkgo biloba extract administered to healthy young volunteers," *Human Psychopharmacology*, vol. 22, no. 8, pp. 559–566, 2007.

[127] J. Kulisevsky, "Role of dopamine in learning and memory: implications for the treatment of cognitive dysfunction in patients with Parkinson's disease," *Drugs and Aging*, vol. 16, no. 5, pp. 365–379, 2000.

[128] C. Chen, Y.-F. Zhu, and K. Wilcoxen, "An improved synthesis of selectively protected L-dopa derivatives from L-tyrosine," *Journal of Organic Chemistry*, vol. 65, no. 8, pp. 2574–2576, 2000.

[129] F. Panza, V. Solfrizzi, M. R. Barulli et al., "Coffee, tea, and caffeine consumption and prevention of late-life cognitive decline and dementia: a systematic review," *Journal of Nutrition, Health and Aging*, vol. 19, no. 3, pp. 313–328, 2015.

[130] J. Birks and J. Grimley Evans, "*Ginkgo biloba* for cognitive impairment and dementia," *Cochrane Database of Systematic Reviews*, no. 1, Article ID CD003120, 2009.

[131] S. Gauthier and S. Schlaefke, "Efficacy and tolerability of Ginkgo biloba extract EGb 761® in dementia: a systematic review and meta-analysis of randomized placebo-controlled trials," *Journal of Clinical Interventions in Aging*, vol. 9, pp. 2065–2077, 2014.

[132] S. Kasper and H. Schubert, "Ginkgo biloba extract EGb 761 in the treatment of dementia: evidence of efficacy and tolerability," *Fortschritte der Neurologie-Psychiatrie*, vol. 77, no. 9, pp. 494–506, 2009.

[133] S. Weinmann, S. Roll, C. Schwarzbach, C. Vauth, and S. N. Willich, "Effects of *Ginkgo biloba* in dementia: systematic review and meta-analysis," *BMC Geriatrics*, vol. 10, article 14, 2010.

[134] T. Charemboon and K. Jaisin, "Ginkgo biloba for prevention of dementia: a systematic review and meta-analysis," *Journal of the Medical Association of Thailand*, vol. 98, no. 5, pp. 508–513, 2015.

[135] G. Yang, Y. Wang, J. Sun, K. Zhang, and J. Liu, "Ginkgo biloba for mild cognitive impairment and alzheimer's disease: a systematic review and meta-analysis of randomized controlled trials," *Current Topics in Medicinal Chemistry*, vol. 16, no. 5, pp. 520–528, 2015.

[136] B. E. Snitz, E. S. O'Meara, M. C. Carlson et al., "*Ginkgo biloba* for preventing cognitive decline in older adults: a randomized trial," *The Journal of the American Medical Association*, vol. 302, no. 24, pp. 2663–2670, 2009.

[137] H. Amieva, C. Meillon, C. Helmer, P. Barberger-Gateau, and J. F. Dartigues, "*Ginkgo biloba* extract and long-term cognitive decline: a 20-year follow-up population-based study," *PLoS ONE*, vol. 8, no. 1, Article ID e52755, 2013.

[138] J. A. Mix and W. D. Crews Jr., "An examination of the efficacy of *Ginkgo biloba* extract EGb 761 on the neuropsychologic functioning of cognitively intact older adults," *The Journal of Alternative and Complementary Medicine*, vol. 6, no. 3, pp. 219–229, 2000.

[139] R. S. Doody, J. L. Cummings, and M. R. Farlow, "Reviewing the role of donepezil in the treatment of Alzheimer's disease," *Current Alzheimer Research*, vol. 9, no. 7, pp. 773–781, 2012.

[140] H. MacPherson, K. A. Ellis, A. Sali, and A. Pipingas, "Memory improvements in elderly women following 16 weeks treatment with a combined multivitamin, mineral and herbal supplement: a randomized controlled trial," *Psychopharmacology*, vol. 220, no. 2, pp. 351–365, 2012.

[141] H. Macpherson, R. Silberstein, and A. Pipingas, "Neurocognitive effects of multivitamin supplementation on the steady state visually evoked potential (SSVEP) measure of brain activity in elderly women," *Physiology and Behavior*, vol. 107, no. 3, pp. 346–354, 2012.

[142] V. Solfrizzi and F. Panza, "Plant-based nutraceutical interventions against cognitive impairment and dementia: meta-analytic evidence of efficacy of a standardized *Gingko biloba* extract," *Journal of Alzheimer's Disease*, vol. 43, no. 2, pp. 605–611, 2015.

[143] S. Ramlall, J. Chipps, A. I. Bhigjee, and B. J. Pillay, "Screening a heterogeneous elderly South African population for cognitive impairment: the utility and performance of the mini-mental state examination, six item screener, subjective memory rating scale and deterioration cognitive observee," *African Journal of Psychiatry*, vol. 16, no. 6, pp. 445–455, 2013.

[144] L. Rami, M. A. Mollica, C. Garcfa-Sanchez et al., "The subjective cognitive decline questionnaire (SCD-Q): a validation study," *Journal of Alzheimer's Disease*, vol. 41, no. 2, pp. 453–466, 2014.

[145] L. A. Rabin, W. B. Barr, and L. A. Burton, "Assessment practices of clinical neuropsychologists in the United States and Canada: a survey of INS, NAN, and APA division 40 members," *Archives of Clinical Neuropsychology*, vol. 20, no. 1, pp. 33–65, 2005.

[146] B. L. Brooks, G. L. Iverson, J. A. Holdnack, and H. H. Feldman, "Potential for misclassification of mild cognitive impairment: a study of memory scores on the Wechsler Memory Scale-III in healthy older adults," *Journal of the International Neuropsychological Society*, vol. 14, no. 3, pp. 463–478, 2008.

[147] C. P. D'Amato and R. L. Denney, "The diagnostic utility of the rarely missed index of the wechsler memory scale-third edition in detecting response bias in an adult male incarcerated setting," *Archives of Clinical Neuropsychology*, vol. 23, no. 5, pp. 553–561, 2008.

[148] A. M. Seelye, D. B. Howieson, K. V. Wild, M. M. Moore, and J. A. Kaye, "Wechsler memory scale-III faces test performance in patients with mild cognitive impairment and mild Alzheimer's disease," *Journal of Clinical and Experimental Neuropsychology*, vol. 31, no. 6, pp. 682–688, 2009.

[149] H. R. Sohrabi, K. A. Bates, M. Rodrigues et al., "The relationship between memory complaints, perceived quality of life and mental health in apolipoprotein eε4 carriers and non-carriers," *Journal of Alzheimer's Disease*, vol. 17, no. 1, pp. 69–79, 2009.

[150] P.-L. Lee, "The relationship between memory complaints, activity and perceived health status," *Scandinavian Journal of Psychology*, vol. 55, no. 2, pp. 136–141, 2014.

[151] K. E. Zuniga, M. J. Mackenzie, A. Kramer, and E. McAuley, "Subjective memory impairment and well-being in community-dwelling older adults," *Psychogeriatrics*, vol. 16, no. 1, pp. 20–26, 2016.

[152] A. Schmidt, F. Hammann, B. Wölnerhanssen et al., "Green tea extract enhances parieto-frontal connectivity during working memory processing," *Psychopharmacology*, vol. 231, pp. 3879–3888, 2014.

[153] H. Li, X. Wu, Q. Wu et al., "Green tea polyphenols protect against okadaic acid-induced acute learning and memory impairments in rats," *Nutrition*, vol. 30, no. 3, pp. 337–342, 2014.

[154] A. L. Lardner, "Neurobiological effects of the green tea constituent theanine and its potential role in the treatment of psychiatric and neurodegenerative disorders," *Nutritional Neuroscience*, vol. 17, no. 4, pp. 145–155, 2014.

[155] S. Xu and Z. Wu, "The construction of the 'clinical memory teste'," *Acta Psychologica Sinica*, vol. 8, pp. 100–108, 1986.

[156] A. F. Jacinto, S. M. D. Brucki, C. S. Porto, M. D. A. Martins, and R. Nitrini, "Subjective memory complaints in the elderly: a sign of cognitive impairment?" *Clinics*, vol. 69, no. 3, pp. 194–197, 2014.

[157] C. Jonker, L. J. Launer, C. Hooijer, and J. Lindeboom, "Memory complaints and memory impairment in older individuals," *Journal of the American Geriatrics Society*, vol. 44, no. 1, pp. 44–49, 1996.

[158] E. L. Abner, R. J. Kryscio, A. M. Caban-Holt, and F. A. Schmitt, "Baseline subjective memory complaints associate with increased risk of incident dementia: the preadvise trial," *The Journal of Prevention of Alzheimer's Disease*, vol. 2, pp. 11–16, 2015.

[159] J.-M. Kim, R. Stewart, S.-W. Kim, S.-J. Yang, I.-S. Shin, and J.-S. Yoon, "A prospective study of changes in subjective memory complaints and onset of dementia in South Korea," *American Journal of Geriatric Psychiatry*, vol. 14, no. 11, pp. 949–956, 2006.

[160] T. Luck, S. G. Riedel-Heller, M. Luppa et al., "Risk factors for incident mild cognitive impairment—results from the german study on ageing, cognition and dementia in primary care patients (AgeCoDe)," *Acta Psychiatrica Scandinavica*, vol. 121, no. 4, pp. 260–272, 2010.

[161] M. Rönnlund, A. Sundström, R. Adolfsson, and L.-G. Nilsson, "Subjective memory impairment in older adults predicts future dementia independent of baseline memory performance: evidence from the Betula prospective cohort study," *Alzheimer's & Dementia*, vol. 11, no. 11, pp. 1385–1392, 2015.

[162] A. B. Zonderman and T. Grimmer, "Risk of mild cognitive impairment: the olmsted county mci risk score," *Neurology*, vol. 84, no. 14, pp. 1392–1393, 2015.

[163] V. K. Ramanan, S. L. Risacher, K. Nho et al., "APOE and BCHE as modulators of cerebral amyloid deposition: a florbetapir PET genome-wide association study," *Molecular Psychiatry*, vol. 19, no. 3, pp. 351–357, 2014.

[164] M. Arbabi, N. Zhand, S. Eybpoosh, N. Yazdi, S. Ansari, and M. Ramezani, "Correlates of memory complaints and personality, depression, and anxiety in a memory clinic," *Acta Medica Iranica*, vol. 53, no. 5, pp. 270–275, 2015.

[165] T. Zandi, "Relationship between subjective memory complaints, objective memory performance, and depression among older adults," *American Journal of Alzheimer's Disease and other Dementias*, vol. 19, no. 6, pp. 353–360, 2004.

[166] M. Polyakova, N. Sonnabend, C. Sander et al., "Prevalence of minor depression in elderly persons with and without mild cognitive impairment: a systematic review," *Journal of Affective Disorders*, vol. 152–154, no. 1, pp. 28–38, 2014.

[167] M. Montenegro, P. Montejo, M. D. Claver-Martín et al., "Relationship between memory complaints and memory performance, mood and sociodemographic variables in young adults," *Revista de Neurologia*, vol. 57, no. 9, pp. 396–404, 2013.

[168] F. F. Roussotte, B. A. Gutman, S. K. Madsen, J. B. Colby, K. L. Narr, and P. M. Thompson, "The apolipoprotein E epsilon 4 allele is associated with ventricular expansion rate and surface morphology in dementia and normal aging," *Neurobiology of Aging*, vol. 35, no. 6, pp. 1309–1317, 2014.

Antiobesity Effects of the Combined Plant Extracts Varying the Combination Ratio of *Phyllostachys pubescens* Leaf Extract and *Scutellaria baicalensis* Root Extract

Dong-Seon Kim,[1] Seung-Hyung Kim,[2] and Jimin Cha[3]

[1]KM Convergence Research Division, Korea Institute of Oriental Medicine, 1672 Yuseong-daero,
 Yuseong-gu, Daejeon 305-811, Republic of Korea
[2]Institute of Traditional Medicine and Bioscience, Daejeon University, Daejeon 300-716, Republic of Korea
[3]Department of Microbiology, Faculty of Natural Science, Dankook University, Cheonan, Chungnam 330-714, Republic of Korea

Correspondence should be addressed to Jimin Cha; jimincha@dankook.ac.kr

Academic Editor: Evan P. Cherniack

The antiobesity effects of several different combinations of extracts (BS) prepared from two plants, *Phyllostachys pubescens* leaf (bamboo leaf: BL) and *Scutellaria baicalensis* root (SB), were investigated using a high fat diet (HFD) induced obese mouse model. In order to find the most effective mixture among the mixtures of the two plant extracts, experimental preparations were made by combining BL and SB by different proportions of 3 : 1 (BS31), 2 : 1 (BS21), 1 : 1 (BS11), 1 : 2 (BS12), and 1 : 3 (BS13). Body weight, weight of adipose tissues, size of adipocytes, levels of glucose, leptin and adiponectin, and lipid profile in serum, and fat accumulation in liver were investigated. We have found that BS21 is the most effective in antiobesity among the five mixtures investigated, indicated by reduction in body weight gain, total mass of adipose tissue, and the size of adipocyte. In addition, BS21 has shown to be beneficial in serum lipid profile, levels of glucose, leptin, and adiponectin in serum, and fat accumulation in liver. By chromatographic separation of BS21, the two maker compounds, isoorientin and baicalin, were identified and quantified for the standardization of BS21.

1. Introduction

Obesity is a medical condition in which excess body fat has accumulated to the extent that it may cause negative effects on health leading to reduced life expectancy and/or increased serious health problems. It has been increasingly believed that obesity is associated with numerous metabolic disorders, including hyperlipidemia and type 2 diabetes mellitus [1], cardiovascular diseases [2], such as hypertension and atherosclerosis [3], and many other disorders, such as osteoarthritis [4] and certain types of cancer [5]; all of these conditions can seriously increase morbidity and mortality [6]. It has been also recognized that obesity is correlated with psychological functioning [7]. Pharmacological therapies to treat obesity have been reviewed, classified into four categories: fat blockers, antidepressants, stimulants, and diabetes medications [8].

New therapeutic approaches for the treatment of obesity have been proposed, focusing on the control of energy balance [9].

Obesity has a multifactorial nature resulting from genetic, physiological, sociocultural, psychological, and environmental factors that lead to an energy imbalance [10]. It has been recognized that no one medication is effective in every patient with obesity, and the ideal medication has to be accompanied by lifestyle changes, dietary modification, and increased physical activity in order to treat obesity effectively [10].

With an increasing prevalence of being overweight or obesity in all ages, herbal usage to achieve weight loss has become a major focus for improving public health in many countries. Bangpoongtongsungsan (BPT), a traditional herbal medicine composed of 18 crude medicinal herbs, has been used as an antiobesity treatment in overweight patients [11]. In mice fed with a high fat diet (HFD), BPT appeared to decrease the weight of white adipose tissue and the size of adipocytes [12]. It is of note that these medicinal herbs have beneficial effects in obesity without significant side effects, suggesting that these herbs can offer an excellent alternative strategy to develop safe and effective antiobesity drugs [13, 14].

According to the traditional medicine in Korea and China, bamboo leaves have been used to treat palsy and hypertension [15, 16]. Antioxidant and anticoagulant effects of *Phyllostachys pubescens* leaf have been reported [15]. Isoorientin, one of the flavonoids found in *Phyllostachys pubescens* leaf, has been reported to inhibit adipogenesis in 3T3-L1 cells [17]. *Scutellaria baicalensis* root has been traditionally used for diuretic, antidiarrhea, and anti-inflammation effects and recently reported to reduce the food intake, to improve serum lipid profile, and to increase the total antioxidant status in serum [18]. A recent study also suggested that *Scutellaria baicalensis* extract could be used as potent therapeutic agents for the treatment of weight gain and hypertriglyceridemia [19].

In our previous study, we selected several plants to screen for antiobesity effects among the plants known as safe to use for dietary purpose. *Phyllostachys pubescens* leaf (bamboo leaf: BL) and *Scutellaria baicalensis* root (SB) showed the most reliable antiobesity effects among the plants that we investigated. We found that the 1 : 1 (w/w) mixture of the two plants extracts demonstrated synergistic antiobesity effects [20]. In this study, after exploring the antiobesity effects of the two plants, we investigated whether the different combinations of the two plants extracts' mixtures have effects on antiobesity or not. This study was also designed to estimate to what extent the mixtures of different ratios show potency enabling us to develop an antiobesity agent and to find out the most effective mixture and, therefore, to standardize the most effective mixture for commercialization.

2. Materials and Methods

2.1. Preparation of BL Extract and SB Extract and Various Mixtures in Different Ratios of Each Extract. *Phyllostachys pubescens* leaf was collected in Damyang, Korea. *Scutellaria baicalensis* root was purchased as a dried herb from Omniherb Co., Yeoungcheon, Korea, and was authenticated by the Classification and Identification Committee of KIOM (Korea Institute of Oriental Medicine) based upon its microscopic and macroscopic characteristics. The committee was composed of nine experts working in the fields of plant taxonomy, botany, pharmacognosy, or herbology. The voucher specimens (BL-20120727; SB-20120914) were deposited at the herbarium of KIOM.

The same extraction procedure was applied for both plants. 1 kg of the dried plant material was extracted twice with 80% ethanol (v/v) in water at 82°C for 3 hours. The extract was filtered and then evaporated under the reduced pressure in a rotary evaporator. The yields of BL extract and SB extract were 89.1 g and 193 g, respectively. The five BS mixtures were prepared by mixing BL extract and SB extract at the weight ratios of 3 : 1, 2 : 1, 1 : 1, 1 : 2, and 1 : 3 to give BS31, BS21, BS11, BS12, and BS13, respectively.

2.2. Animals and Experimental Diets. Male C57B1/6 mice were purchased from Daehan Biolink Co., Eumsung, Korea, and maintained for 2 weeks with sufficient supply of commercial diet (AIN-76A diet, Ralston Purina, St. Louis, MO, USA) and water prior to the experiments. 10-week-old mice were housed in the air-conditioned SPF animal room having a 12 h light/12 h dark cycle at $25 \pm 2°C$ temperature and $50 \pm 5\%$ humidity. They were allowed to have access to the laboratory diet and water ad libitum. All experimental protocols were conducted according to the guidelines of NIH (National Institutes of Health) and were approved beforehand by the Animal Care Committee of KIOM.

To induce obesity, the mice were fed with the high fat diet (HFD: Rodent Diet D12492, Research Diets, New Brunswick, NJ, USA) consisting of 60% fat, 20% protein, and 20% carbohydrate as was described in the previously published report [21]. The normal diet group was fed with the standard chow diet (Orient Bio Inc., Seongnam, Korea) commercially available. HCA (Garcinia Cambogia) [22] and XNC (Xenical) [23] were used as positive control groups since they were well known and available in public as antiobesity agents. After 2 weeks of adaptation period, the experiments were initiated when the weights of mice reached 28-29 g by feeding with the high fat diet. The mice were then fed for 6 weeks with group specific diets. The mice were randomly divided into nine groups ($n = 7$) and separately fed with the normal diet (ND), the high fat diet (HFD), HFD plus HCA (HCA), HFD plus XNC (XNC), HFD plus BS31 (BS31), HFD plus BS21 (BS21), HFD plus BS11 (BS11), HFD plus BS12 (BS12), and HFD plus BS13 (BS13). 100 mg/kg/day of oral dosage was applied for all the mice in the experimental groups except XNC group, the dosage of which was chosen to be 15.6 mg/kg/day with reference to the dosage range used in the previous report [24]. All the preparations were made by suspending in normal saline and administered orally by using mouse Zonde. ND and HFD control groups were treated with vehicle (normal saline) only.

2.3. Measurement of Body Weight Gain and Food Intake. Body weight gain and the amount of food intake were measured at the same time and the same day of a week during 6 weeks of experimental period. Average body weight gain and average amount of food intake were daily calculated and recorded. FER (food efficiency ratio) was calculated by (total weight gain/total food intake) × 100.

2.4. Serum Assays for Biochemical Parameters. At the end of 6-week experimental period, the mice were fasted for 15 hours prior to sacrifice. Blood samples were centrifuged at 3000 rpm for 15 min at 4°C. The separated serum samples were stored at −70°C. The serum levels of triglyceride, total cholesterol, high density lipoprotein cholesterol (HDL), low density lipoprotein cholesterol (LDL), glucose, alanine aminotransferase (ALT), aspartate aminotransferase (AST), and creatinine were analyzed by automatic biochemical analyzer (Hitachi-720, Hitachi Medical, Japan). The serum concentrations of leptin and adiponectin were assayed with mouse ELISA (enzyme-linked immunosorbent assay) kits (R&D Systems, Minneapolis, MN, USA).

TABLE 1: Effects of BS mixtures on average daily body weight gain in HFD induced obese mice.

	ND	HFD	HCA	XNC	BS31	BS21	BS11	BS12	BS13
Body weight gain (g/day)	0.153 ± 0.008	$0.410 \pm 0.075^{++}$	0.301 ± 0.03	$0.202 \pm 0.03^{**}$	0.280 ± 0.02	$0.200 \pm 0.02^{***}$	0.284 ± 0.02	0.260 ± 0.022	0.270 ± 0.022

ND: normal diet, HFD: high fat diet control, HCA: high fat diet plus 100 mg/kg/day of Garcinia Cambogia, XNC: high fat diet plus 15.6 mg/kg/day of Xenical, BS31: high fat diet plus 100 mg/kg/day of BS31, BS21: high fat diet plus 100 mg/kg/day of BS21, BS11: high fat diet plus 100 mg/kg/day of BS11, BS12: high fat diet plus 100 mg/kg/day of BS12, and BS13: high fat diet plus 100 mg/kg/day of BS13.

Values are expressed as mean ± SEM ($n = 7$). $^{++}p < 0.01$ (compared with ND) and $^{**}p < 0.01$ and $^{***}p < 0.001$ (compared with HFD) express significant differences as determined by Duncan's multiple-range test.

2.5. Measurement of Adipose Tissue Weight and Histological Observation. After the blood collection, liver, kidney, spleen, and inguinal, epididymal, and perirenal adipose tissues were removed from the mice and weighed immediately. For histochemistry, the tissues were fixed in 10% neutral formalin solution for one day and embedded in paraffin. All tissues were sliced to 6 μm in thickness and stained with H&E (hematoxylin and eosin). To measure the size of adipocytes, the area comprising 20 adipocytes in stained sections was measured by light microscope (Olympus BX51, Olympus Optical Co., Japan) with the aid of image analysis program (Image-Pro Plus 5.0, Media Cybernetics, Silver Spring, MD, USA). Histological analysis was performed using the samples of the collected tissues prepared.

2.6. High Performance Liquid Chromatography Analysis for Identifying the Marker Compounds of BS21. HPLC-grade reagents, acetonitrile, and water were obtained from J. T. Baker (Phillipsburg, NJ, USA). All the other chemicals used in this work were of a reagent grade. The samples were analyzed by reverse phase-high performance liquid chromatography of Waters Alliance 2695 system (Waters Co., Milford, MA, USA) coupled with 2996 photodiode array detector. Phenomenex Luna C18 column (250 mm × 4.6 mm × 5 μm, Phenomenex, Torrance, CA, USA) was used for the stationary phase and the mobile phase was composed of 0.1% (v/v) trifluoroacetic aqueous solution (A) and acetonitrile (B). At zero time, the mobile phase consisted of 90% A and 10% B and was held for 10 min. From 10 to 40 min a gradient was applied to 55% A and 35% B, which was followed by a wash with 100% B for 10 min and a 15 min equilibration period at 90% A and 10% B. For the separation, 1.0 mL/min of flow rate and 20 μL of injection volume were kept throughout the analysis that was performed at 40°C.

Identification of the constituents of BS21 was made by comparing retention times and UV spectra for the peaks of HPLC/PDA chromatogram to those of commercially available standards. For each compound, peak area was determined at 350 nm. The calibration curve of the standards ranging from 6.25 to 200 μg/mL (6 levels) for isoorientin and from 12.5 to 400 μg/mL (6 levels) for baicalin revealed a good linearity.

Quantitation of the marker compounds of BS21 was made in comparison to the mixture of external standards of known concentration. Quantitative measurements were made in duplicate before and after the batch samples. The peak areas were used to calculate the contents of the compounds in the samples.

2.7. Statistical Analysis. Differences between groups were assessed by an analysis of variance (ANOVA) followed by Duncan's multiple-range test. All data are presented as mean ± SEM (Standard Error of the Mean). Differences were considered significant when the p values were less than 0.05.

3. Results

3.1. Effects of BS Mixtures on Body Weight, Food Intake, and Food Efficiency Ratio. HFD control group gained significantly more weight compared to ND group, and the positive control groups (HCA and XNC) and BS (mixture of BL extract and SB extract) treated groups gained significantly less weight compared to HFD (Figure 1(a)). Although average daily body weight gain was considerably reduced in all positive control groups and BS treated groups compared to HFD (Table 1), only Xenical (XNC) and BS21 demonstrated statistically significant reduction among them ($p < 0.01$ for XNC and $p < 0.001$ for BS21).

Daily food intake was significantly decreased in HFD control group compared to ND group. However there was only a slight change in daily food intake between HFD control group and the positive control groups or BS treated groups (Figure 1(b)). Food efficiency ratio was significantly increased in HFD control group compared to ND group. BS31 and BS11 groups showed statistically significant reduction in food efficiency ratio compared to HFD control group (Figure 1(c)).

3.2. Effects of BS Mixtures on Serum Lipid Profile. HFD control group showed significant increases in all parameters of the serum lipid profile compared to ND group except HDL-cholesterol (Figure 2). Compared to HFD control group, almost all BS treated groups showed to decrease significantly the levels of triglycerides, total cholesterol, and LDL-cholesterol in serum (Figures 2(a), 2(b), and 2(c)) and to increase significantly HDL-cholesterol level in serum (Figure 2(d)). HCA group showed little effects on the levels of total cholesterol and LDL-cholesterol in serum, while BS groups significantly reduced.

3.3. Effects of BS Mixtures on Energy Balancing Metabolism. Serum glucose level was increased significantly in HFD control group compared to ND group. Only BS21 among BS treated groups showed statistically significant reduction in serum glucose level compared to HFD control group (Figure 3(a)). Serum leptin levels were increased significantly in HFD control group compared to ND group and significantly decreased in BS groups compared to HFD control group

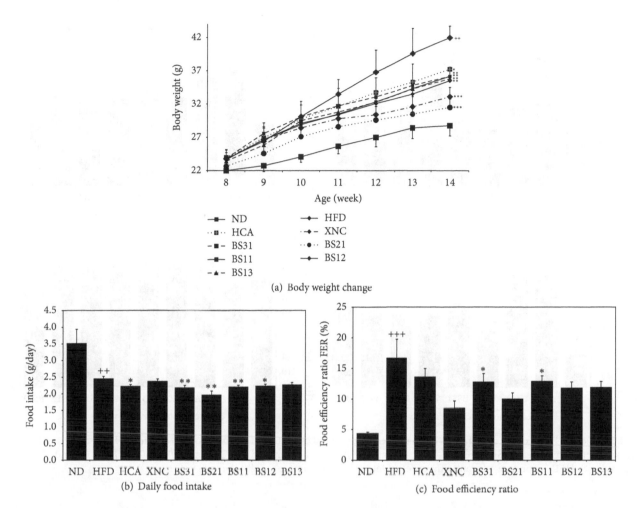

FIGURE 1: Effects of BS mixtures on (a) body weight gain, (b) food intake, and (c) food efficiency ratio in mice consuming high fat diet. The food efficiency ratio is calculated by (daily body weight gain/daily food intake) × 100. ND: normal diet, HFD: high fat diet control, HCA: high fat diet plus 100 mg/kg/day of Garcinia Cambogia, XNC: high fat diet plus 15.6 mg/kg/day of Xenical, BS31: high fat diet plus 100 mg/kg/day of BS31, BS21: high fat diet plus 100 mg/kg/day of BS21, BS11: high fat diet plus 100 mg/kg/day of BS11, BS12: high fat diet plus 100 mg/kg/day of BS12, and BS13: high fat diet plus 100 mg/kg/day of BS13. Values are expressed as mean ± SEM ($n = 7$). $^{++}p < 0.01$ and $^{+++}p < 0.001$ (compared with ND) and $^{*}p < 0.05$, $^{**}p < 0.01$, and $^{***}p < 0.001$ (compared with HFD) express significant differences as determined by Duncan's multiple-range test.

(Figure 3(b)). BS treated groups seemed to have a tendency to upregulate serum adiponectin levels (Figure 3(c)). Among the five BS mixtures, BS21 appeared to have better effects on energy balancing metabolisms compared to the other BS groups (Figure 3).

3.4. Effects of BS Mixtures on Serum Toxicity Markers.
To evaluate both potential toxicity and protective effects of BS mixtures, serum toxicity markers for liver (ALT, AST) and kidney (creatinine) were assayed at the end of the experimental period. The levels of ALT and AST in serum were significantly increased in HFD control group compared to ND group (Figure 4(a)). Serum ALT level was significantly decreased in all BS groups while serum AST level was significantly decreased only in BS21 group (Figure 4(a)). There was no significant decrease in serum creatinine level in BS groups except BS21 group, which showed significant decrease in serum creatinine level (Figure 4(b)). On the whole, BS21

treatment seemed to cause no detectable adverse toxic effects and to protect to some extent the livers and kidneys of mice.

3.5. Effects of BS Mixtures on Fat Deposit (Weight of Adipose Tissues and Size of Adipocyte) and Histological Observations.
The weights of inguinal and epididymal adipose tissues were increased significantly in HFD control group compared to ND group (Figure 5(a)). The weights of inguinal and perirenal adipose tissues were decreased significantly in all BS groups compared to HFD control group.

Also BS21, BS12, and BS13 showed to decrease significantly the weight of epididymal adipose tissue compared to HFD control group. XNC group and BS21 group showed the most effective and statistically significant decreases ($p < 0.001$ for XNC and $p < 0.01$ for BS21) in the weights of inguinal, epididymal, and perirenal adipose tissues compared to HFD control (Figure 5(a)) while HCA group showed a little effect on reduction of fat deposit. The outcome of the other

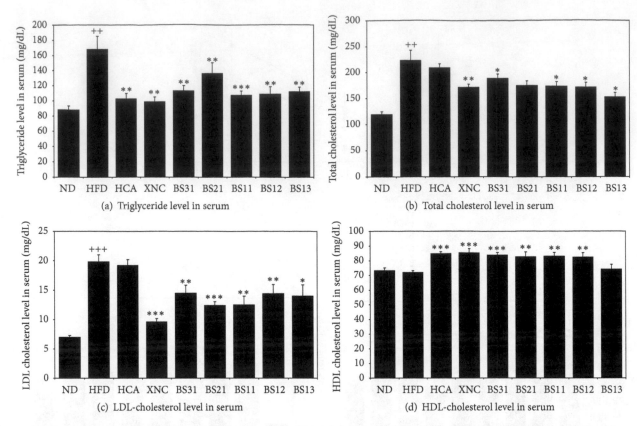

FIGURE 2: Effects of BS mixtures on the levels of (a) triglyceride, (b) total cholesterol, (c) LDL-cholesterol, and (d) HDL-cholesterol in serum. Values are expressed as mean ± SEM ($n = 7$). $^{++}p < 0.01$ and $^{+++}p < 0.001$ (compared with ND) and $^{*}p < 0.05$, $^{**}p < 0.01$, and $^{***}p < 0.001$ (compared with HFD) express significant differences as determined by Duncan's multiple-range test.

BS groups (BS31, BS11, BS12, and BS13) lay in between those of XNG/BS21 groups and HCA group.

To estimate the adipocyte size, the area comprising 20 adipocytes in H&E stained sections was measured. HFD control group showed significant increase in adipocyte area size compared to ND group (Figure 5(b)). All the positive control groups and BS groups showed significant decreases in adipocyte area size compared to HFD control group (Figure 5(b)). These results were supported by the histological observations that demonstrated clearly the difference in adipocyte size among the experimental groups (Figure 6). We presume in the consideration of these results that the decrease in body fat mass by BS treatment is partly due to the decrease in adipocyte size. We obtained no statistically significant results with respect to the weight of liver, kidney, and spleen (Figure 5(c)). The weight of liver appeared to show a tendency to be decreased in BS groups compared to HFD control group. However, BS groups showed no significant reduction in liver weight increment except BS11, which showed significant reduction (Figure 5(c)).

Our data from histochemistry showed that the liver of HFD control group showed more extensive lipid droplet accumulation compared to ND group in histological observations (Figure 7). The liver of HFD control group contained macrovesicular lipid droplets as well as numerous microlipid droplets demonstrating a typical fatty liver developed by high fat diet. BS groups showed less lipid droplet accumulation than HFD control group (Figure 7). In particular, the liver conditions of BS21 and BS12 groups appeared to be close to those of ND group.

3.6. Chromatographic Separation of BS21 to Identify Marker Compounds.

HPLC/PDA chromatograms of BS21, *Scutellaria* root extract, and bamboo leaf extract are shown in Figure 8. The two marker compounds of BS21 were determined from the major peaks of HPLC/PDA chromatogram in comparison to the retention times and UV spectra of commercially available standards. As shown in Figure 8, the high performance liquid chromatographic analysis of BS21 revealed two major compounds, isoorientin originated from bamboo leaf extract and baicalin originated from *Scutellaria* root extract at the retention times of approximately 22.4 min and 32.1 min, respectively. Quantitation of the two marker compounds, isoorientin and baicalin, was made by chromatographic comparison between BS21 and mixture of the two commercial standards of isoorientin and baicalin (Figure 8). The result revealed that BS21 contained 7.2 ± 0.5 mg/g of isoorientin and 64.7 ± 3.2 mg/g of baicalin.

4. Discussion

In this study, we found that BS mixtures prepared from mixing with different ratios of the two herbal extracts,

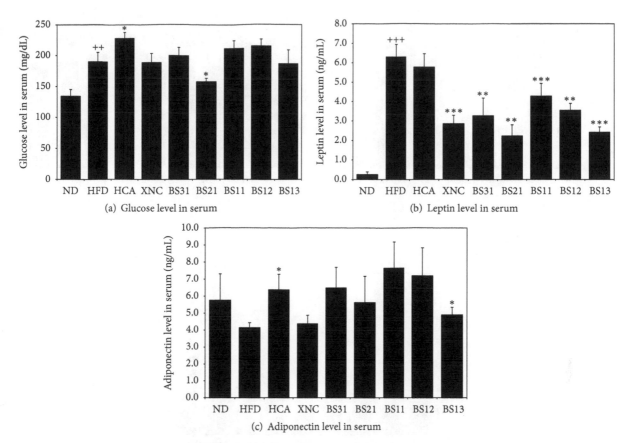

FIGURE 3: Effects of BS mixtures on the levels of (a) glucose, (b) leptin, and (c) adiponectin in serum. Values are expressed as mean ± SEM ($n = 7$). $^{++}p < 0.01$ and $^{+++}p < 0.001$ (compared with ND) and $^{*}p < 0.05$, $^{**}p < 0.01$, and $^{***}p < 0.001$ (compared with HFD) express significant differences as determined by Duncan's multiple-range test.

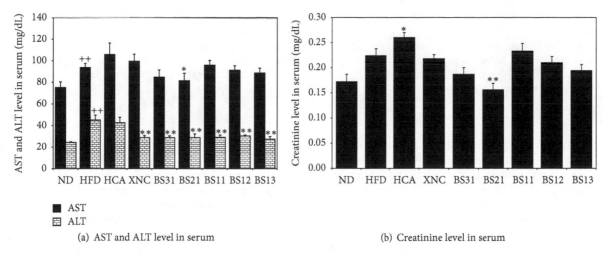

FIGURE 4: Effects of BS mixtures on the levels of ALT, AST, and creatinine in serum. Values are expressed as mean ± SEM ($n = 7$). $^{++}p < 0.01$ (compared with ND) and $^{*}p < 0.05$ and $^{**}p < 0.01$ (compared with HFD) express significant differences as determined by Duncan's multiple-range test.

Phyllostachys pubescens leaf and *Scutellaria baicalensis* root, decreased body weight gain of mice fed with a high fat diet. BS21 treatment appeared to be the most effective in decreasing body weight gain among the five BS mixtures. The inhibitory effect of BS21 on the body weight gain was similar to that of Xenical, a well known prescription drug. The data from the measurement of daily amount of food intake and food efficiency ratio also suggested that BS21 was the most effective in reduction of body weight gain among the five BS mixtures.

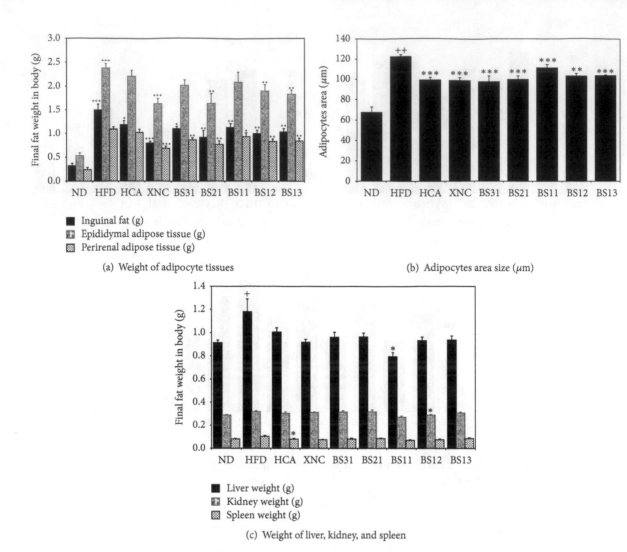

(a) Weight of adipocyte tissues

(b) Adipocytes area size (μm)

(c) Weight of liver, kidney, and spleen

FIGURE 5: Effects of BS mixtures on fat deposit: (a) the weight of inguinal, epididymal, and perirenal adipose tissues, (b) adipocyte area size, and (c) the weight of liver, kidney, and spleen. Values are expressed as mean ± SEM ($n = 7$). $^+p < 0.05$, $^{++}p < 0.01$, and $^{+++}p < 0.001$ (compared with ND) and $^*p < 0.05$, $^{**}p < 0.01$, and $^{***}p < 0.001$ (compared with HFD) express significant differences as determined by Duncan's multiple-range test.

The treatment of BS mixtures showed significant reductions in the amount of inguinal, epididymal, and perirenal adipose tissues. In the estimation of adipocyte size by measuring the area comprising 20 adipocytes, BS groups showed significant decreases in adipocyte size. This result was supported by comparative microscopic observations, between BS groups and HFD control group, made on the adipocytes of the stained adipose tissue slices. BS21 treatment appeared to be most effective for the inhibition of fat accumulation and adipocyte size expansion in adipose tissues.

Considering the results of body weight gain and internal fat mass, we made an assumption that BS21 treatment had potency to tackle obesity and its associated disorders.

HFD control group showed to increase significantly the levels of triglyceride, total cholesterol, and LDL-cholesterol in serum compared to ND group, demonstrating the development of hyperlipidemia (hypercholesterolemia and hypertriglyceridemia). BS groups showed to decrease significantly

the levels of triglycerides, total cholesterol, and LDL-cholesterol in serum and to increase significantly HDL-cholesterol level in serum compared to HFD control group. The result suggested a possibility for the use of BS to help to prevent and/or relieve from adverse events caused by hyperlipidemia.

The increment of liver weight most probably by fat deposition seemed to reduce in BS groups compared to HFD control. In histological observations, the liver of HFD control group contained macrovesicular lipid droplets as well as numerous microlipid droplets, demonstrating a typical fatty liver developed by a high fat diet. BS groups showed less accumulation of lipid droplet in liver compared to HFD control group. We suggest in consideration of this result that BS treatment may help to prevent and/or relieve from fatty liver.

Adiponectin was known to modulate a number of metabolic processes, including glucose regulation and fatty acid oxidation [25]. Adiponectin was also reported to be inversely correlated with body fat percentage in adults and

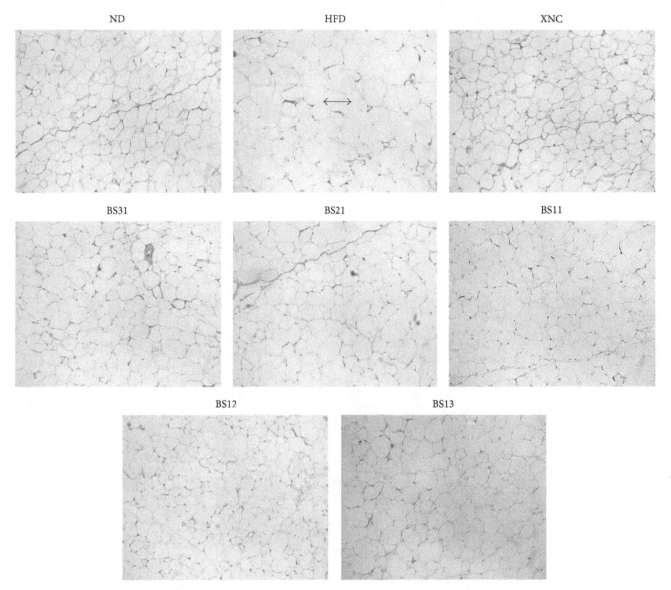

FIGURE 6: Effects of BS mixtures on adipocyte size. Histological observations of H&E stained adipose tissues of the experimental groups. Representative photographs of H&E stained epididymal adipose tissue (magnification: 400x). The arrow for the control group indicates the size of an adipocyte.

to mediate insulin-sensitizing effect to ameliorate hyperglycemia and hyperinsulinemia without inducing weight gain or even inducing weight loss [26]. The reduction of adiponectin level in serum was associated with insulin resistance, dyslipidemia, and atherosclerosis [27]. In obesity, a decreased sensitivity to leptin occurred, resulting in an inability to detect satiety despite the accumulation of high energy [28]. BS21 showed to lower the levels of glucose and leptin in serum and to elevate adiponectin level in serum.

Therefore, BS21 seemed to influence insulin sensitizing, fat mass reduction, and weight loss with the aids of numerous energy related processes mediated by reduced serum level of leptin and elevated serum level of adiponectin in obese conditions.

In the evaluation of the levels of ALT, AST, and creatinine in serum, BS treatment appeared to cause no detectable

adverse toxic effects and to protect to some extent the livers and kidneys.

For the standardization of BS21, we identified two marker compounds, isoorientin and baicalin, each of which is the highest content constituent of *Phyllostachys pubescens* leaf extract and *Scutellaria baicalensis* root extract, respectively. Both baicalin [29] and isoorientin [17] have been reported to work as antiadipogenic regulators of the adipogenesis pathway.

5. Conclusions

In this study, BS21 showed the most reliable antiobesity effects among the five BS mixtures.

We demonstrated that BS21 treatment significantly lowered body weight gain. This study also showed that BS21

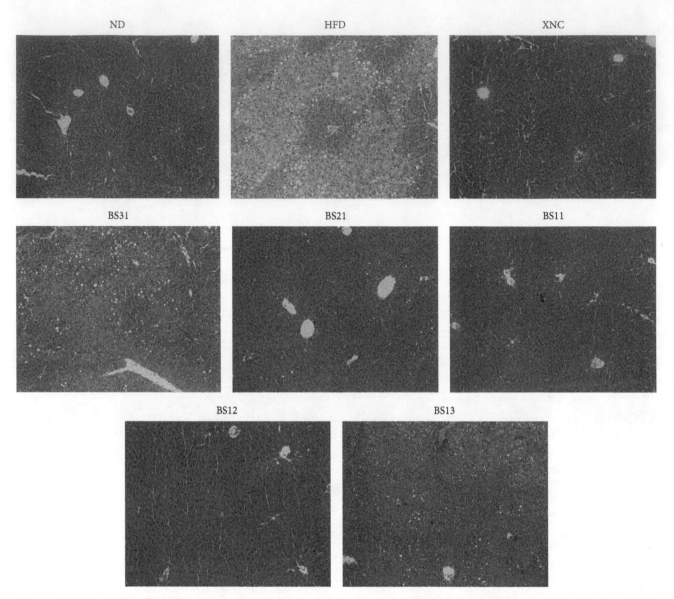

FIGURE 7: Histological profile of the representative H&E stained liver tissue section for the experimental groups (magnification, 200x).

treatment effectively reduced adipose tissue mass as well as adipocyte size and improved positively the serum lipid profile including triglycerides, total cholesterol, LDL-cholesterol, and HDL-cholesterol.

BS21 treatment showed remarkable reduction in lipid droplet accumulation in fatty liver induced by a high fat diet and reduction in the serum glucose level. BS21 treatment also lowered the serum leptin level and elevated serum adiponectin level.

We, therefore, suggest as an extension of this study to explore further the possibilities of BS21 to apply for preventing and/or relieving from obesity and from hyperlipidemia, fatty liver, and other adverse events that may occur concomitantly with obesity.

By chromatographic separation of BS21, the two maker compounds, isoorientin for *Phyllostachys pubescens* leaf extract and baicalin for *Scutellaria baicalensis* root extract,

were identified and quantified for the standardization of BS21. The two compounds, isoorientin and baicalin, were of extraordinarily high content in *Phyllostachys pubescens* leaf extract and *Scutellaria baicalensis* root extract, respectively. Therefore, isoorientin and baicalin were chosen as marker compounds considering profitability as quality control markers in comparison to the other constituents in trace level.

Competing Interests

The authors declare that there is no conflict of interests regarding the publication of this paper.

Acknowledgments

This work has been carried out with the government funded projects, "the Clinical Trial and Product Development of

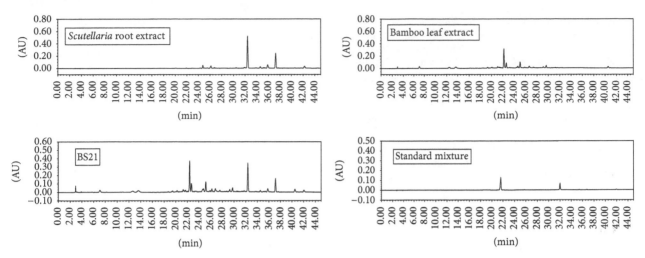

Figure 8: HPLC chromatograms of 80% (v/v) ethanol extracts of *Scutellaria* root and bamboo leaf, the mixture of two extracts (BS21), and the mixture of two reference standards, isoorientin (1) and baicalin (2). UV peaks were detected at 350 nm. Isoorientin and baicalin appeared at the retention times of approximately 22.4 min and 32.1 min, respectively.

Antiobesity Herbal Complex" (Project G14150) and "The Development of Korean Medicine Initiatives for Treating Gout" (Project K16030), granted to the Korea Institute of Oriental Medicine by the Ministry of Science, ICT & Future Planning, Republic of Korea.

References

[1] S. E. Kahn, R. L. Hull, and K. M. Utzschneider, "Mechanisms linking obesity to insulin resistance and type 2 diabetes," *Nature*, vol. 444, no. 7121, pp. 840–846, 2006.

[2] L. F. Van Gaal, I. L. Mertens, and C. E. De Block, "Mechanisms linking obesity with cardiovascular disease," *Nature*, vol. 444, no. 7121, pp. 875–880, 2006.

[3] S. M. Grundy, "Obesity, metabolic syndrome, and coronary atherosclerosis," *Circulation*, vol. 105, no. 23, pp. 2696–2698, 2002.

[4] D. Coggon, I. Reading, P. Croft et al., "Knee osteoarthritis and obesity," *International Journal of Obesity and Related Metabolic Disorders*, vol. 25, no. 5, pp. 622–627, 2001.

[5] I. Vucenik and J. P. Stains, "Obesity and cancer risk: evidence, mechanisms, and recommendations," *Annals of the New York Academy of Sciences*, vol. 1271, no. 1, pp. 37–43, 2012.

[6] F. Lei, X. N. Zhang, W. Wang et al., "Evidence of anti-obesity effects of the pomegranate leaf extract in high-fat diet induced obese mice," *International Journal of Obesity*, vol. 31, no. 6, pp. 1023–1029, 2007.

[7] M. A. Friedman and K. D. Brownell, "Psychological correlates of obesity: moving to the next research generation," *Psychological Bulletin*, vol. 117, no. 1, pp. 3–20, 1995.

[8] J. E. Rodríguez and K. M. Campbell, "Past, present, and future of pharmacologic therapy in obesity," *Primary Care: Clinics in Office Practice*, vol. 43, no. 1, pp. 61–67, 2016.

[9] A. R. Saltiel, "New therapeutic approaches for the treatment of obesity," *Science Translational Medicine*, vol. 8, no. 323, Article ID 323rv2, 2016.

[10] G. A. Bray, G. Frühbeck, D. H. Ryan, and J. P. H. Wilding, "Management of obesity," *The Lancet*, 2016.

[11] T. Shimada, T. Kudo, T. Akase, and M. Aburada, "Preventive effects of bofutsushosan on obesity and various metabolic disorders," *Biological and Pharmaceutical Bulletin*, vol. 31, no. 7, pp. 1362–1367, 2008.

[12] S. Akagiri, Y. Naito, H. Ichikawa et al., "Bofutsushosan, an oriental herbal medicine, attenuates the weight gain of white adipose tissue and the increased size of adipocytes associated with the increase in their expression of uncoupling protein 1 in high-fat diet-fed male KK/Ta mice," *Journal of Clinical Biochemistry and Nutrition*, vol. 42, no. 2, pp. 158–166, 2008.

[13] A. Khan, M. Safdar, M. M. Ali Khan, K. N. Khattak, and R. A. Anderson, "Cinnamon improves glucose and lipids of people with type 2 diabetes," *Diabetes Care*, vol. 26, no. 12, pp. 3215–3218, 2003.

[14] C. Hioki, K. Yoshimoto, and T. Yoshida, "Efficacy of bofu-tsusho-san, an oriental herbal medicine, in obese Japanese women with impaired glucose tolerance," *Clinical and Experimental Pharmacology and Physiology*, vol. 31, no. 9, pp. 614–619, 2004.

[15] E. Cho, S. Kim, I. Na, D. C. Kim, M. J. In, and H. J. Chae, "Antioxidant and anticoagulant activities of water and ethanol extracts of phyllostachys pubescence leaf produced in Geoje," *Journal of Applied Biological Chemistry*, vol. 53, no. 3, pp. 170–173, 2010.

[16] M. In, M. Park, S. Kim et al., "Composition analysis and antioxidative activity of maengjong-juk (*Phyllostachys pubescence*) leaves tea," *Journal of Applied Biological Chemistry*, vol. 53, no. 2, pp. 116–119, 2010.

[17] Y. M. Lee, B. Poudel, S. Nepali et al., "Flavonoids from *Triticum aestivum* inhibit adipogenesis in 3T3-L1 cells by upregulating the insig pathway," *Molecular Medicine Reports*, vol. 12, no. 2, pp. 3139–3145, 2015.

[18] H. J. Yoon and Y. S. Park, "Effects of *Scutellaria baicalensis* water extract on lipid metabolism and antioxidant defense system in rats fed high fat diet," *Journal of the Korean Society of Food Science and Nutrition*, vol. 39, no. 2, pp. 219–226, 2010.

[19] K. H. Song, S. H. Lee, B.-Y. Kim, A. Y. Park, and J. Y. Kim, "Extracts of *Scutellaria baicalensis* reduced body weight and blood triglyceride in db/db mice," *Phytotherapy Research*, vol. 27, no. 2, pp. 244–250, 2013.

[20] Y. M. Kang, S. Kim, Y. Lee, H. K. Kim, and D. Kim, "Synergistic combination effect of anti-obesity in the extracts of *Phyllostachys pubescence* Mael and *Scutellaria baicalensis* Georgi," *The Korea Journal of Herbology*, vol. 29, no. 6, pp. 7–13, 2014.

[21] H. Choi, H. Eo, K. Park et al., "A water-soluble extract from *Cucurbita moschata* shows anti-obesity effects by controlling lipid metabolism in a high fat diet-induced obesity mouse model," *Biochemical and Biophysical Research Communications*, vol. 359, no. 3, pp. 419–425, 2007.

[22] S. B. Heymsfield, D. B. Allison, J. R. Vasselli, A. Pietrobelli, D. Greenfield, and C. Nunez, "*Garcinia cambogia* (Hydroxycitric Acid) as a potential anti-obesity agent," *The Journal of the American Medical Association*, vol. 280, no. 18, pp. 1596–1600, 1998.

[23] J. S. Cheah, "Orlistat (Xenical) in the management of obesity," *Annals of the Academy of Medicine Singapore*, vol. 29, no. 4, pp. 419–420, 2000.

[24] D. Isler, C. Moeglen, N. Gains, and M. K. Meier, "Effect of the lipase inhibitor orlistat and of dietary lipid on the absorption of radiolabelled triolein, tri-γ-linolenin and tripalmitin in mice," *British Journal of Nutrition*, vol. 73, no. 6, pp. 851–862, 1995.

[25] J. J. Díez and P. Iglesias, "The role of the novel adipocyte-derived hormone adiponectin in human disease," *European Journal of Endocrinology*, vol. 148, no. 3, pp. 293–300, 2003.

[26] O. Ukkola and M. Santaniemi, "Adiponectin: a link between excess adiposity and associated comorbidities?" *Journal of Molecular Medicine*, vol. 80, no. 11, pp. 696–702, 2002.

[27] A. Yadav, M. A. Kataria, V. Saini, and A. Yadav, "Role of leptin and adiponectin in insulin resistance," *Clinica Chimica Acta*, vol. 417, pp. 80–84, 2013.

[28] H. Pan, J. Guo, and Z. Su, "Advances in understanding the interrelations between leptin resistance and obesity," *Physiology and Behavior*, vol. 130, pp. 157–169, 2014.

[29] H. Lee, R. Kang, Y. Hahn et al., "Antiobesity effect of baicalin involves the modulations of proadipogenic and antiadipogenic regulators of the adipogenesis pathway," *Phytotherapy Research*, vol. 23, no. 11, pp. 1615–1623, 2009.

Therapeutic Effects of Traditional Chinese Medicine on Spinal Cord Injury: A Promising Supplementary Treatment in Future

Qian Zhang,[1] **Hao Yang,**[1] **Jing An,**[1] **Rui Zhang,**[1] **Bo Chen,**[1] **and Ding-Jun Hao**[2]

[1] *Translational Medicine Center, Hong Hui Hospital, Xi'an Jiaotong University College of Medicine, Xi'an 710054, China*
[2] *Department of Spine Surgery, Hong Hui Hospital, Xi'an Jiaotong University College of Medicine, Xi'an, China*

Correspondence should be addressed to Qian Zhang; zq-melody@163.com

Academic Editor: Khalid Rahman

Objective. Spinal cord injury (SCI) is a devastating neurological disorder caused by trauma. Pathophysiological events occurring after SCI include acute, subacute, and chronic phases, while complex mechanisms are comprised. As an abundant source of natural drugs, Traditional Chinese Medicine (TCM) attracts much attention in SCI treatment recently. Hence, this review provides an overview of pathophysiology of SCI and TCM application in its therapy. *Methods.* Information was collected from articles published in peer-reviewed journals via electronic search (PubMed, SciFinder, Google Scholar, Web of Science, and CNKI), as well as from master's dissertations, doctoral dissertations, and Chinese Pharmacopoeia. *Results.* Both active ingredients and herbs could exert prevention and treatment against SCI, which is linked to antioxidant, anti-inflammatory, neuroprotective, or antiapoptosis effects. The detailed information of six active natural ingredients (i.e., curcumin, resveratrol, epigallocatechin gallate, ligustrazine, quercitrin, and puerarin) and five commonly used herbs (i.e., Danshen, Ginkgo, Ginseng, Notoginseng, and Astragali Radix) was elucidated and summarized. *Conclusions.* As an important supplementary treatment, TCM may provide benefits in repair of injured spinal cord. With a general consensus that future clinical approaches will be diversified and a combination of multiple strategies, TCM is likely to attract greater attention in SCI treatment.

1. Introduction

Spinal cord injury (SCI) is a catastrophic event that can profoundly affect a patient's life, with far-reaching social and economic effects. The estimated annual global incidence of SCI is approximately 15–40 cases per million and is increasing with the development of modern society [1]. Thus, the treatment of SCI is currently a significant challenge in clinic and in research around the world. With ongoing advances in neurobiology, materials science, pharmacology, and other related sciences, great progress has been made in the prevention and treatment of SCI. Considerable advances have been made to relieve the symptoms of SCI and the suffering of patients, which are achieved by preventing injury progression, managing deafferentation pain syndromes, implementing bowel and bladder training regimens, and teaching patients to cope with their disabilities [2].

Today, the routine therapy employed in the early stage of SCI mainly involves surgical procedures combined with high-dose methylprednisolone (MP). The surgical procedures might stabilize and decompress spinal cord, while MP can inhibit lipid peroxidation, maintain the blood-spinal cord barrier, enhance spinal cord blow flow, inhibit endorphin release, and limit the inflammatory response. However, the question of optimal timing of surgical interventions (or even the intervention itself) has generated considerable debate and remains unanswered. Moreover, MP is also highly controversial due to a lack of consensus with regard to its true beneficial effects [3, 4]. Thus, various other novel strategies for SCI repair have emerged and received considerable research focus, including cell therapy (e.g., transplantation of neural stem cells, mesenchymal stem cells, olfactory ensheathing cells, Schwann cells, activated macrophages, and embryonic stem cells), molecular therapy (e.g., neurotrophin, anti-Nogo antibody, and interleukin-10), and tissue engineering (e.g., construction of a 3D scaffold including hydrogels, sponges, guidance tubes, and nanofibrous scaffolds) [2]. However, more related research needs to be carried out before these novel strategies are widely applied in clinic.

As an abundant source of natural drugs, Traditional Chinese Medicine (TCM) has many thousands of years of history in clinical applications in China and other Asian countries. TCM comprises hundreds of commonly used herbs, which is mostly used in intervention therapy as a form of compound prescription in clinic. Each herb contains numerous chemical constituents which belong to different categories, and the active ingredients exert therapeutic action in the treatment of some disease. In recent years, TCM has attracted much attention in the field of SCI treatment. Both active ingredients and herbs [5–8], and even compound prescriptions [9–12], have shown effectiveness in the prevention and treatment of SCI. Although it could not replace regular surgical procedures, as a complementary and alternative treatment, intervention of TCM plays an important role in preoperative prevention and postoperative recovery. Meanwhile, combined application of multiple therapeutic approaches would benefit the functional recovery of spinal cord, for example, TCM combined with cell therapy, molecular therapy, or tissue engineering. Thus, application of TCM would be an important focus of future research in the field of SCI treatment.

This review intends to provide an overview of TCM applications in the field of SCI. It will provide the readers with the detailed prevention and treatment effects of six active natural ingredients (i.e., curcumin, resveratrol, epigallocatechin gallate, ligustrazine, quercitrin, and puerarin) and five commonly used herbs (i.e., Danshen, Ginkgo, Ginseng, Notoginseng, and Astragali Radix), on the basis of the pathophysiology and therapeutic mechanisms of SCI.

2. Pathophysiology of SCI

In the past 30–40 years, much research has focused on elucidating the mechanisms and complex pathophysiologic processes of SCI. Pathophysiological events occurring after SCI include acute, subacute, and chronic phases.

The acute phase refers to the immediate postinjury period, when the spinal cord is lacerated or macerated by a sharp penetrating force, contused or compressed by a blunt force (most common), or infarcted by a vascular insult [13]. This stage is also called "primary injury," and the processes cannot be reversed. The extent of injury is hard to control, which depends on the violence severity, compression time of spinal cord, fracture-dislocation situation of spine, and acceleration of impact force, as well as absorption circumstances of impact energy by surrounding tissues.

The subacute phase occurs over the time course of minutes to weeks following SCI and leads to further damage that is described as "secondary injury." The secondary stage consists of the following events. (1) Vascular changes: it includes hemorrhage, thrombosis, vasospasm, loss of autoregulation, breakdown of blood brain barrier, and infiltration of inflammatory cells. This leads to edema, necrosis, and ischemia [14]. (2) Free radical formation and lipid peroxidation: SCI results in a rapid and extensive oxidative stress reaction, which causes oxidative death of the spinal cord neurons and reduces spinal cord blood flow that leads to edema and an inflammatory response [15]. (3) Disruption of an ionic balance of K^+, Na^+, and Ca^{2+}: it leads to depolarization of cell membranes, ATPase failure, and increase of intracellular Ca^{2+}. (4) Glutamate excitotoxicity: it is an increased release of extracellular glutamate after SCI that induces excessive activation of glutamate receptors leading to further neuronal cell death. (5) Apoptosis: it is a form of programmed cell death seen in populations of neurons, oligodendrocytes, microglia, and, perhaps, astrocytes after SCI [16]. The death of oligodendrocytes in white matter tracts continues for many weeks after injury and may contribute to postinjury demyelination [17]. (6) Inflammatory response: resident microglia are activated after SCI, along with proinflammatory cytokines that are produced by infiltrating neutrophils and macrophages, which induce higher extravasation of leukocytes and further tissue damage of the surrounding original injury site [18]. Nevertheless, some studies have demonstrated that inflammation also plays an important role in neural tissue repair [19].

Finally, the chronic phase of SCI occurs days to even years after injury and comprises many events, such as white matter demyelination, gray matter dissolution, connective tissue deposition, and reactive gliosis, that lead to glial scar formation. Microglia and astrocytes become activated, undergo proliferation, increase in size, activate astrogliosis, and produce a glial scar, which subsequently inhibits regeneration of neurons. Increased glial fibrillary acidic protein (GFAP) expression is a hallmark of reactive astrocytes, and this cytoskeletal protein contributes to the barrier effect [20]. A cystic cavity is surrounded by glial scar that progressively expands and leads to a condition called syringomyelia in approximately 25% of SCI patients. Finally, in many cases, SCI leads to neurological impairments in both orthograde and retrograde directions, including brain regions, as well as the development of pain syndromes and mood disorders such as depression [21].

3. Pharmacological Intervention with Natural Compounds

3.1. Curcumin. Curcumin is a natural polyphenolic compound extracted from Curcumae Longae Rhizoma, the dried rhizome of *Curcuma longa* L. in Zingiberaceae [22], which is prevalent in tropical and subtropical regions including India, China, and Southeast Asia. Structure of curcumin is shown in Figure 1(a), and studies indicate that it has potent anticancer, antiarthritic, and antidiabetic activities [23].

In recent years, curcumin has emerged as a potential therapeutic drug in SCI treatment. Behavioral scores, including tilt board test and Basso, Beattie, and Bresnahan (BBB) scores, have confirmed improvement in rat hindlimb motor functions ($P < 0.01$) [24, 25]. Wet/dry weight ratio assay showed that administration of curcumin (100 mg/kg, i.p.) could significantly alleviate edema of the injured spinal cord ($P < 0.01$) [26]. Many studies have indicated that curcumin exerts a treatment effect in SCI by protecting neurons, inhibiting oxidant and inflammatory reactions.

3.1.1. Antioxidant and Anti-Inflammatory Effects. The antioxidant and anti-inflammatory effects of curcumin have been demonstrated by many studies [27]; thus it is reasonable that curcumin is used in SCI treatment. In the group receiving

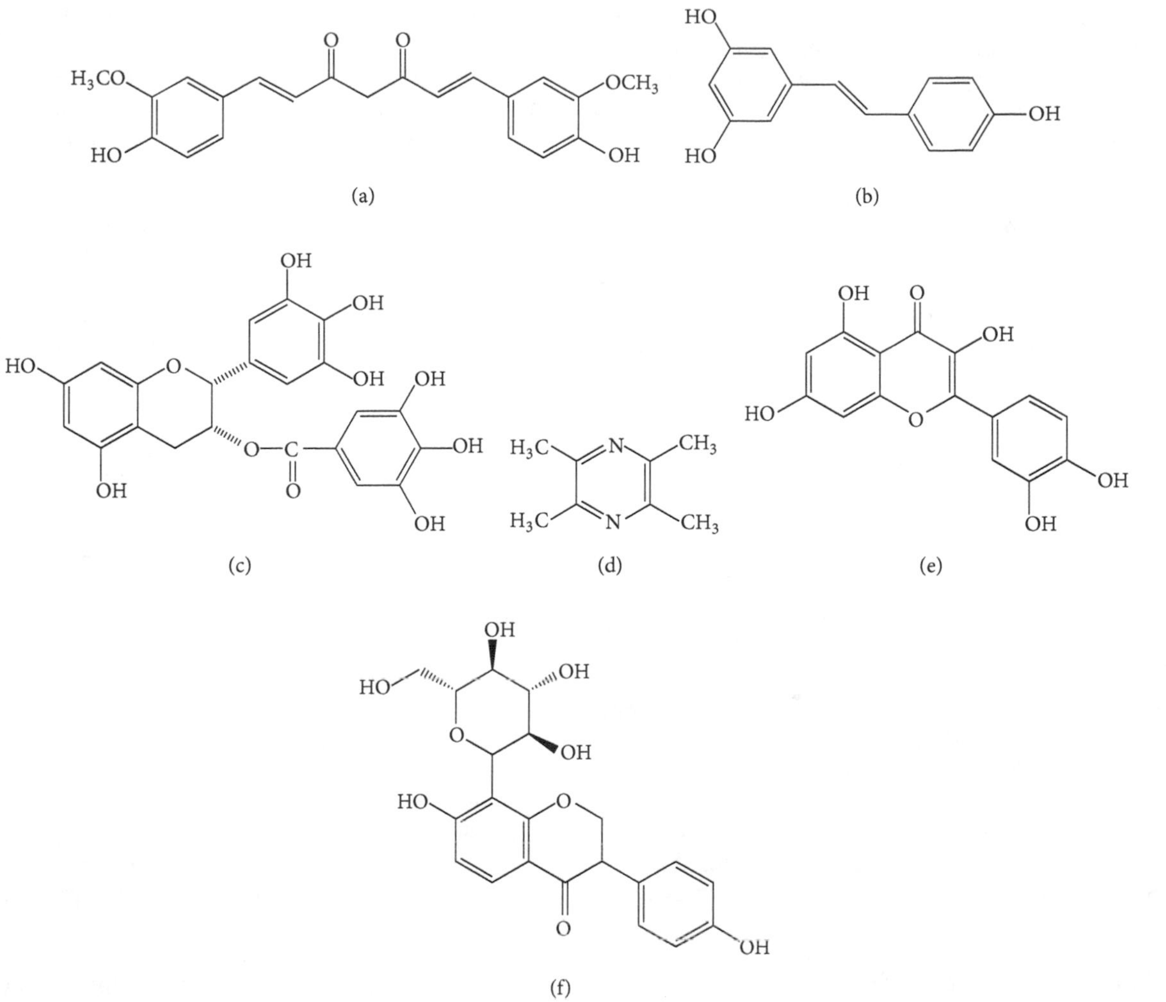

FIGURE 1: Structures of natural compounds ((a) curcumin; (b) resveratrol; (c) epigallocatechin gallate (EGCG); (d) ligustrazine; (e) quercitrin; (f) puerarin).

curcumin (200 mg/kg/d, p.o.), serum superoxide dismutase (SOD) level was significantly increased ($P < 0.01$), while the malondialdehyde (MDA) level significantly decreased ($P < 0.05$) compared with the control group and MP group [28]. As an important measure of oxidative stress, glutathione (GSH) level, glutathione/oxidized-glutathione ratio (GSH/GSSH), and glutathione peroxidase (GSH-PX) level all increased, while catalase (CAT) level decreased significantly *in vitro* (SK-N-SH cells) and *in vivo* (SCI mice) [24, 29].

In the context of anti-inflammatory pathways, inflammatory cytokines network is believed to be central to the pathophysiology of inflammatory processes. After SCI, the inflammatory related factors including NF-κB and proinflammatory cytokines (e.g., TNF-α, IL-1β, IL-6, and RANTES) in the injured spinal cord were significantly upregulated following SCI and could be suppressed when treated with curcumin (100 mg/kg, i.p.) [26, 30]. In the antioxidant Nrf2/ARE pathway, which regulates the expression of inflammatory cytokines, the activity of pleiotropic transcription factor Nrf2 was significantly activated following SCI and could be further induced when treated with curcumin. Induction of Nrf2

activity by curcumin markedly decreased NF-κB activation and reduced expression of TNF-α and IL-1β [26].

3.1.2. Neuroprotective and Antiapoptosis Effects. As a hallmark of reactive astrocytes, increased GFAP expression indicates the production of glial scar and inhibition of axonal extension. After treatment with curcumin (1 μM) for 7 d, GFAP mRNA isolated from reactivated astrocytes was significantly downregulated ($P < 0.001$), and a reduction of GFAP protein expression was observed following immunofluorescent staining of primary cultured astrocytes *in vitro* [25]. Western immunoblotting signals showed that level of neuron-specific enolase (NSE) was significantly increased in curcumin posttreatment groups (1 μM, 24 h), indicating protection and preservation of the neuronal phenotype [29]. As the key intracellular cysteine protease of the cascade of events associated with apoptosis, both caspase-3 and caspase-7 were activated and significantly upregulated after neural injury. Administration of curcumin significantly and dose-dependently inhibited caspase-3 and caspase-7 levels and exerted antiapoptosis effects [29, 31, 32].

3.2. Resveratrol. Resveratrol (Figure 1(b)) is a natural polyphenol antioxidant and the active constituent of *Polygonum cuspidatum* (Japanese knotweed, 0.524 mg/g), red wine (0.1–14.3 mg/L), red grape skins (50–100 μg/g), and berries such as blueberries, as well as peanuts and other nuts [33]. As early as 1970, it was noticed that there was a positive relationship between wine consumption and the incidence of heart disease [34]. Through modern pharmacological research, resveratrol has been widely used in preventing or slowing the progression of a wide variety of diseases, including cardiovascular disease, cancer, ischemic injury, and Alzheimer's disease [33, 35].

In recent years, the potential therapeutic effect of resveratrol in SCI treatment has been confirmed by behavioral scores (i.e., BBB scores, Rivlin, and Tator's angle board test) and histopathological changes [36, 37]. Hematoxylin and eosin (HE) staining showed that administration of resveratrol (100 mg/kg or 200 mg/kg, i.p.) could alleviate hemorrhage and edema in both gray and white matter as well as reversing the tissue necrosis, liquefaction, pyknosis, and dissolution of nucleus, and appearance of apoptotic bodies 3 d after SCI. Nissl staining showed that, with resveratrol intervention, neurons displayed partially restored functions, especially in cellular nutrient supply and energy biosynthesis [38]. According to previous reports, resveratrol protects the injured spinal cord mainly by inhibiting oxidant formation and apoptosis.

3.2.1. Antioxidant Effects. Many studies have shown the effectiveness of resveratrol on oxidative stress caused by SCI. In an SCI model, resveratrol (100 μg/kg or 10 mg/kg, i.v.; 50 mg/kg or 100 mg/kg, i.p.) reduced the expression and level of MDA in injured spinal cord tissues ($P < 0.05$) [36, 37, 39, 40]. Additionally, the increase of xanthine oxidase (XO) and NO levels, as well as the decrease of SOD activity and GSH level in rat injured spinal cord tissues, could be reversed ($P < 0.01$) by administration of resveratrol after SCI (100 mg/kg or 200 mg/kg, i.p.) [36, 38].

3.2.2. Antiapoptosis Effects. Firstly, electron microscopic (EM) identification and TUNEL staining clearly showed that the number of TUNEL-positive cells distributed dramatically decreased after resveratrol treatment in both the white and the gray matter of spinal cord in an SCI rat model ($P < 0.01$). By contrast, the apoptosis index significantly declined ($P < 0.01$). Resveratrol (200 mg/kg, i.p.) could significantly improve abnormal morphology, including neuronal shrinking, breaking, or disappearance of mitochondrial ridges, cytoplasm vacuolization, and marked enlarging of the endoplasmic reticulum [38]. Secondly, resveratrol intervention obviously inhibited the upregulation of protein expression of the proapoptosis factor Bax and the terminal executing enzyme for substrate cleavage of caspase-3 ($P < 0.01$). In addition, resveratrol inhibited the downregulation in the protein expression of the antiapoptosis factor Bcl-2 ($P < 0.01$) that was induced by SCI [38]. Finally, several studies have revealed that resveratrol (20 mg/kg or 60 mg/kg, i.p.) could activate the PI3K/Akt pathway, prevent neuronal apoptosis [41], and attenuate activation of the mitogen-activated protein kinases (MAPKs) signaling pathways [42].

3.3. Epigallocatechin Gallate (EGCG). The natural product (–)-epigallocatechin-3-gallate (EGCG, Figure 1(c)) is the major polyphenolic constituent found in green tea (dried fresh leaves of the plant *Camellia sinensis* L. Ktze. in Theaceae) [43]. As the second most consumed beverage globally, numerous epidemiological studies have reported an inverse association between tea consumption and cardiovascular events. Moreover, ingestion of green teas significantly increased anticarcinogenic, anti-inflammatory, antioxidant, antithrombotic, and antimutagenic capacity. A number of scientific researches have suggested that EGCG is responsible for the majority of the potential health benefits attributed to green tea consumption [44].

In recent years, research has focused on the therapeutic effect of EGCG in SCI that is attributed to its potent antioxidant, anti-inflammatory, antiapoptotic, and neuroprotective activities [45]. After administration of EGCG (10 mg/kg or 20 mg/kg, i.p.) for 1 w after SCI, behavioral scores (i.e., BBB scores and tilt board test) have confirmed an improvement of rat locomotor functional recovery ($P < 0.05$). LFB staining indicated that EGCG administration decreased the cavity area, while increasing the myelin sheath area as compared with the SCI group [46, 47].

3.3.1. Antioxidant and Anti-Inflammatory Effects. The study of Deng et al. indicated that EGCG (50 mg/kg or 100 mg/kg, i.p.) could significantly upregulate the levels of O^{2-} and SOD, while significantly downregulating the activity of MDA 24 h following SCI ($P < 0.01$). Meanwhile, EGCG (50 mg/kg or 100 mg/kg, i.p.) significantly reduced the production of IL-1β, TNF-α, and ICAM-1 in SCI rat serum ($P < 0.01$). In particular, the antioxidant and anti-inflammatory effects of 100 mg/kg EGCG were similar to MP in the treatment of SCI ($P > 0.05$) [48, 49].

3.3.2. Antiapoptosis and Neuroprotective Effects. The level of Bcl-2 was depressed, while Bax level and the Bcl-2/Bax ratio were increased in spinal cord tissues 24 h after SCI ($P < 0.01$). EGCG (50 or 100 mg/kg, i.p.) treatment significantly increased Bcl-2 level, and the Bcl-2/Bax ratio, while decreasing Bax level [48].

EGCG enhanced the expression of endogenous neurotrophic factors like neurotrophin-3 (NT-3) and brain-derived neurotrophic factor (BDNF) in SCI rats and protected spinal motor neurons from death after SCI [48]. In the study of Ge et al., both IHC and Western blot assays showed that aquaporin-4 (AQP4) and GFAP expression were significantly increased from 24 to 72 h after SCI, while EGCG treatment (100 mg/kg, i.p.) obviously decreased its expression. Conceivably, the downregulation of AQP4 expression by EGCG (100 mg/kg, i.p.) treatment might be beneficial to reducing spinal cord edema in SCI rats [50].

3.4. Ligustrazine. Ligustrazine (tetramethylpyrazine, TMP, Figure 1(d)) is a natural alkaloid extracted from Chuanxiong Rhizoma, the dried rhizome of *Ligusticum chuanxiong* Hort. in Umbelliferae, which is chiefly found in China [51]. In TCM, Chuanxiong Rhizoma can treat neurovascular, cardiovascular, and brain and kidney diseases, while TMP has a diverse array of pharmacological functions, including dilation of blood vessels, inhibition of platelet aggregation, improvement of microcirculation, inhibition of cell apoptosis, elimination of oxygen free radicals, and exertion of a calcium antagonist action [52, 53].

In recent years, it has been revealed that TMP could protect injured spinal cord by suppressing inflammatory cytokines, inhibiting cell apoptosis, and scavenging oxygen free radicals. TMP (30 mg/kg, i.p.) could significantly increase behavioral scores (i.e., BBB scores) and improve rat hindlimb motor functions ($P < 0.01$) [54].

3.4.1. Anti-Inflammatory and Antioxidant Effects. Systemic administration of TMP (30 mg/kg, i.p.) exerted potent neuroprotective effects against spinal cord injury by reducing the expression of proinflammatory cytokines (i.e., IL-1β and TNF-α), upregulating the expression of anti-inflammatory cytokine IL-10, and inhibiting NF-κB activation ($P < 0.01$) [54]. Several studies suggested that TMP effectively protects the central nervous system by scavenging reactive oxygen species and regulating nitric oxide production, and consequently preventing peroxynitrite formation [52]. SCI significantly decreased SOD level and increased MDA level in spinal cord as compared with the sham group ($P < 0.05$). In addition, TMP treatment (30 mg/kg, i.p.) significantly reversed the changes in SOD and MDA activities ($P < 0.01$) [55], while significantly suppressing oxidative stress and preventing excitotoxic cell damage in neuronal cultures [56].

3.4.2. Antiapoptosis Effects. Western blot analysis showed that spinal cord injury obviously reduced Bcl-2 expression and increased Bax expression as compared with the sham group ($P < 0.01$), while treatment with TMP (30 mg/kg, i.p.) was associated with greater Bcl-2 and attenuated Bax expression relative to the vehicle control group ($P < 0.01$) [55]. TMP could also reduce caspase-3 activity, activate the PI3K/Akt pathway, inhibit neuronal apoptosis, and prevent neuronal loss [57, 58].

3.5. Quercitrin. Quercetin (Figure 1(e)) is a typical flavonol-type flavonoid that is ubiquitously present in many fruits and vegetables, such as apples, onions, citrus fruits, berries, red grapes, red wine, and broccoli. As a flavonol essential in many plants, quercetin is rich mainly in its sugar derivatives [59]. Quercetin exhibits antioxidative, anti-inflammatory, and vasodilating activity and has been proposed as a potential approach in the prevention and therapy of cardiovascular diseases and cancer. Recently, quercetin has been marketed in the United States primarily as a dietary supplement [60, 61].

Recently, quercetin has emerged as a potential therapeutic drug in the treatment of SCI. Quercetin could significantly increase BBB scores and inclined plane test score in SCI rats, which is similar to the positive control drug MP [62]. Many studies have indicated that SCI treatment of quercetin is attributed to its antioxidant, anti-inflammatory, and antiapoptosis activities.

3.5.1. Antioxidant and Anti-Inflammatory Effects. Quercetin treatment (20 mg/kg twice daily, i.p.) could reverse the

upregulation of MDA level ($P < 0.05$), NO level ($P < 0.001$), and MPO activity ($P < 0.001$) and the downregulation of GSH level ($P < 0.001$) and SOD activities ($P < 0.05$) after SCI, thus reducing oxidative damage in tissues [63]. Immunohistochemistry results also showed that the rate of iNOS-positive cells was significantly higher from days 1 to 7 postoperatively ($P < 0.05$), while being significantly lower in the injured spinal cord after administration of quercetin (0.2 mg/kg/d, i.p.) ($P < 0.05$) [62].

Enzyme-linked immunosorbent assay (ELISA) showed that plasma TNF-α, IL-1β, and IL-6 levels were significantly increased in the vehicle-treated SCI group ($P < 0.01$–$P < 0.001$), whereas treatment with quercetin suppressed any increases of these proinflammatory cytokines ($P < 0.05$–$P < 0.001$) [63].

3.5.2. Antiapoptosis Effects. There was no statistically significant difference between the quercetin and p38MAPK inhibitor (SB203580) treatment groups ($P > 0.05$), which indicated that the potential mechanism of action of quercetin is through inhibiting the activation of the p38MAPK signaling pathway [62]. Moreover, semiquantitative Western blot analysis revealed that increased caspase-3 protein expression in bladder tissues of SCI rats was attenuated following quercetin treatment (0.2 mg/kg/d, i.p.) ($P < 0.01$) [63].

3.6. Puerarin. Puerarin (Figure 1(f)) is the most important phytoestrogen extracted from the dried root of *Pueraria lobata* (Willd.) Ohwi in Leguminosae, which is a commonly used traditional Chinese medicine. Researchers have concentrated on the pharmacological activities of puerarin, which displays a series of beneficial activities on hangover, cardiovascular disease, osteoporosis, neurological dysfunction, fever, and liver injury in clinical treatment and experimental research [64].

In recent years, several studies have shown that puerarin was effective in treating SCI. Administration of puerarin (50 mg/kg/d, i.p.) for 3 d significantly improved motor function (neurological deficit score 48 h after SCI, $P < 0.05$) and reduced spinal infarction volume ($P < 0.05$), while the optimal time of treatment with puerarin was within 4 h after SCI [65]. The therapeutic effect of puerarin on SCI was mainly attributed to its neuroprotective activity.

Puerarin exhibits a neuroprotective action in SCI and is associated with several aspects. Firstly, following SCI, the expression of p35 was downregulated, while p25 was upregulated in a mechanism dependent on cleaving p35. The enhanced expression of p25 resulted in a hyperactivation of Cdk5. The pretreatment with puerarin significantly depressed the upregulation of p25 and inhibited the downregulation of p35 ($P < 0.05$), by way of a roscovitine-like function [66]. Secondly, it is well-known that release of a high amount of glutamate and activation of metabotropic glutamate receptors lead to spinal tissue injury following SCI. The excitotoxicity of glutamate to spinal cells is mediated via glutamate receptors of the spinal cord. Intraperitoneal injection with puerarin (50 mg/kg), at 1 h, 2 h, 4 h, and 6 h after SCI, significantly decreased glutamate release ($P < 0.05$) and inhibited mGluR mRNA expression ($P < 0.05$) [67]. Thirdly, puerarin

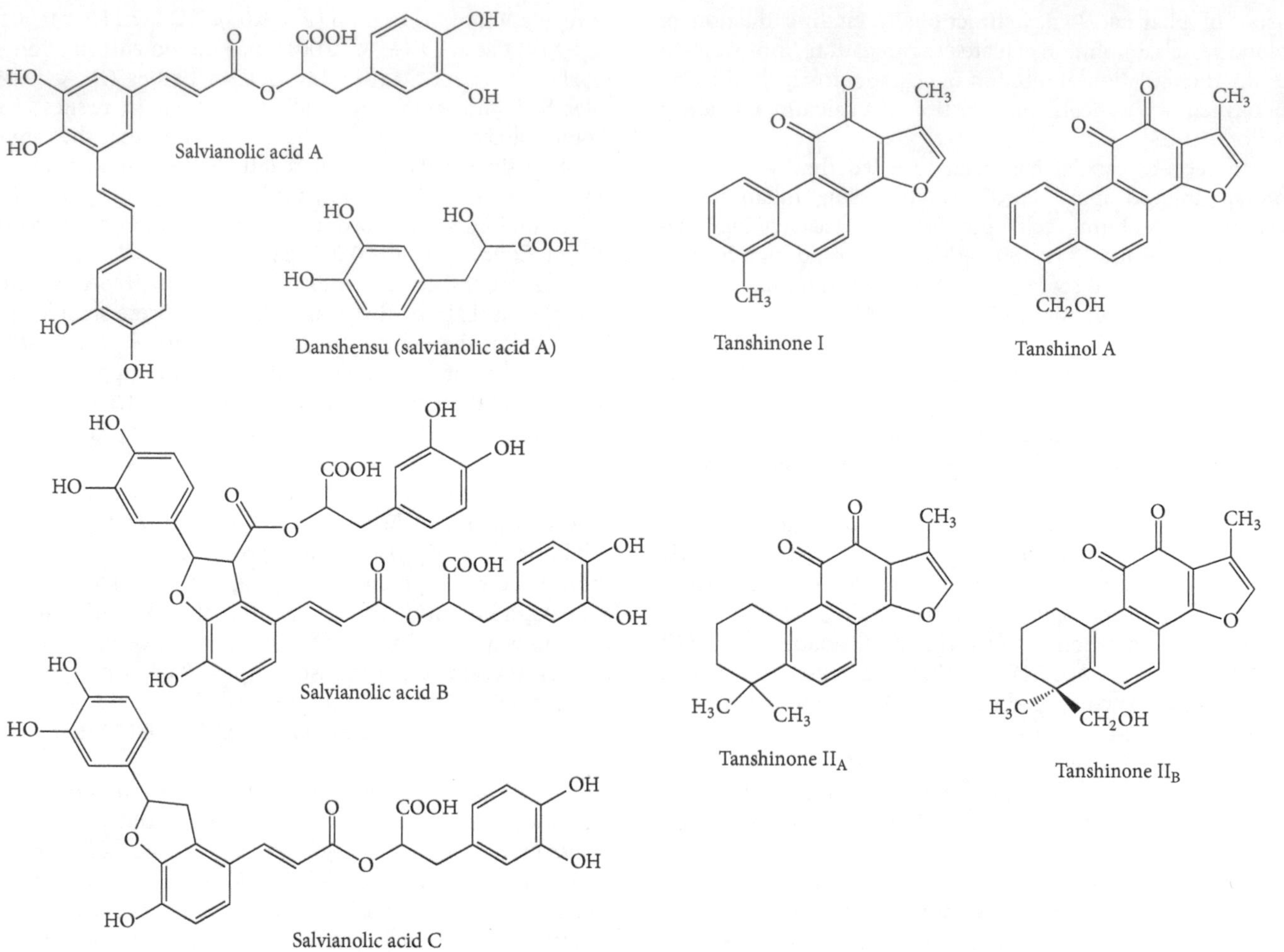

FIGURE 2: Structures of major constituents in Danshen (danshensu, salvianolic acids B and C; tanshinones I, II$_A$, and II$_B$, and tanshinol A).

treatment significantly reversed the decrease in Trx-1 and Trx-2 mRNA expression after SCI ($P < 0.05$) and elevated number of apoptotic cells in the spinal cord ($P = 0.01$) [65].

3.7. Summary. The sources, structures, doses, and mechanisms of all six natural compounds in SCI treatment are summarized in Table 1. Besides the six natural compounds mentioned above, there are also some other compounds that have been reported in the treatment of SCI, including hydroxysafflor yellow A [68], tetrandrine [69], and piperine [70]. However, there are insufficient studies describing SCI treatment of these compounds, and more related research is required before these compounds are considered as potential therapeutic agents in treating SCI.

4. Pharmacological Intervention with Chinese Herbs

4.1. Danshen

4.1.1. Source, Chemical Constituents, and Pharmacology of Danshen.
Danshen (Salviae Miltiorrhizae Radix et Rhizoma) is the dried root and rhizome of *Salvia miltiorrhiza* Bge. in genus *Salvia* of mint family [22]. As one of the best-known

Chinese traditional herbs, it has been clinically used for more than 2000 years and is mainly produced in Anhui, Shanxi, Hebei, and Jiangsu provinces in China.

Until now, more than 70 compounds have been isolated and structurally identified from Danshen with various concentrations. The major components reported from Danshen are hydrophilic depside derivatives (e.g., danshensu, salvianolic acids A–C, E–G, caffeic acid, and ferulic acid) and lipophilic diterpenoids (e.g., tanshinones I, II$_A$, and II$_B$, tanshinol A, and tanshindiols A and B). Some of the structures are given in Figure 2 [71].

In TCM, Danshen is characterized as a common hemorheological drug with the following functions: (1) to promote blood flow in menstruation, (2) to remove blood stasis, (3) to reduce pain, (4) to resolve mental uneasiness and restlessness, (5) to nourish the blood, and (6) to tranquilize the mind. Based on modern investigations, the most important and frequent clinical application of Danshen is in the treatment of coronary heart disease, like angina pectoris, coronary artery spasm, myocardial infarction, and other conditions [72]. In addition, Danshen is used to treat cerebrovascular disease, hepatitis, hepatocirrhosis, hypertension dysmenorrhea, and osteoporosis [73].

TABLE 1: Sources, structures, doses, and mechanisms of six natural compounds in SCI treatment.

Name	Source	Structure	Dose	Mechanism
Curcumin	Dried rhizome of *Curcuma longa* L. in Zingiberaceae; Curcumae Longae Rhizoma	H$_3$CO, OCH$_3$, OH, HO	(1) *In vivo:* 100 mg/kg, i.p.; 200 mg/kg/day, p.o. (2) *In vitro:* 1 μM for 24 h or 7 days	(1) Antioxidant (SOD, MDA, GSH/GSSH, GSH-PX, and CAT) (2) Anti-inflammatory (NF-κB, TNF-α, IL-1β, IL-6, RANTES, and Nrf2/ARE pathway) (3) Neuroprotective effect (GFAP, NSE) (4) Antiapoptosis effect (caspase-3 and caspase-7)
Resveratrol	*Polygonum cuspidatum*, red wine, red grape skins, berries such as blueberries, peanuts, and other nuts	HO, OH, HO	*In vivo:* 100 μg/kg, i.v.; 10 mg/kg, i.v. (New Zealand white rabbit); 20 mg/kg, i.p.; 50 mg/kg, i.p.; 60 mg/kg, i.p.; 100 mg/kg, i.p.; 200 mg/kg, i.p.	(1) Antioxidant (MDA, SOD, XO, NO, and GSH) (2) Antiapoptosis (Bax, Bcl-2, caspase-3, PI3K/Akt pathway, and MAPKs signaling pathways)
EGCG	Dried fresh leaves of the plant *Camellia sinensis* L. Ktze. in Theaceae	OH, OH, OH, OH, OH, HO, OH	*In vivo:* 50 mg/kg, i.p.; 100 mg/kg, i.p.	(1) Antioxidant (O^{2-}, SOD, and MDA) (2) Anti-inflammatory (IL-1β, TNF-α, and ICAM-1) (3) Antiapoptosis (Bax, Bcl-2, and Bcl-2/Bax ratio) (4) Neuroprotective effect (NT-3, BDNF, AQP4, and GFAP)
Ligustrazine	Dried rhizome of *Ligusticum chuanxiong* Hort. in Umbelliferae	H$_3$C, CH$_3$, N, N, CH$_3$, H$_3$C	*In vivo:* 30 mg/kg, i.p.	(1) Anti-inflammatory (IL-1β, TNF-α, IL-10, and NF-κB) (2) Antioxidant (MDA, SOD) (3) Antiapoptosis (Bcl-2, Bax, caspase-3, and PI3K/Akt pathway)

TABLE 1: Continued.

Name	Source	Structure	Dose	Mechanism
Quercetin	Apples, onions, citrus fruits, berries, red grapes, red wine, and broccoli		*In vivo:* 0.2 mg/kg/d, i.p; 20 mg/kg twice daily, i.p.	(1) Antioxidant (MDA, SOD, GSH, NO, and MPO) (2) Anti-inflammatory (TNF-α, IL-1β, and IL-6) (3) Antiapoptosis (caspase-3, p38MAPK signaling pathway)
Puerarin	Dried root of *Pueraria lobata* (Willd.) Ohwi in Leguminosae		50 mg/kg, i.p.	Neuroprotective activity (p35, p25, glutamate, Trx-1, and Trx-2)

Animals used in experiments are rats without special explanation.

4.1.2. Danshen for SCI Treatment. In recent years, Danshen has attracted increased attention in SCI treatment and is mostly employed as an intervention approach in the form of herbal extract or Chinese medicine injection. Behavioral scores (i.e., tilt board test) and histopathological changes confirmed the improvement in rat motor functions ($P < 0.01$), while bleeding and edema in the damage zone were significantly reduced after administration of Danshen (2.67 g/kg/d, i.p.) for 7 and 14 days, respectively [74].

(1) Hemorheology Changes. Considering the properties of promoting blood circulation and relieving blood stasis, it was reasonable that Danshen could improve microcirculation and increase blood flow of the injured spinal cord tissues, inhibit platelet aggregation, and reduce release of TXA_2. The upregulation of hemodynamic indices of ηb, Fib, and RAI induced by SCI was significantly reversed by administration of Danshen (6.0 g/kg, i.p., $P < 0.01$) [75].

(2) Antioxidant and Anti-Inflammatory Effects. Administration of Danshen injection (3 mg/kg) reversed the increase of MDA and decrease of SOD levels in white tissue of spinal cord after acute SCI ($P < 0.01$). By contrast, Danshen downregulated the increase of NO level in serum and spinal cord tissues ($P < 0.05$) [76].

Both immunohistochemistry and Western blot assays demonstrated that the increase of NF-κB expression induced by SCI was ameliorated by Danshen injection (9 g/kg, twice per day, $P < 0.05$) [77].

(3) Neuroprotective Effects. Danshen injection (2.67 g/kg/d) could significantly increase glial cell line-derived neurotrophic factor (GDNF) (1 d after SCI), choline acetyltransferase (ChAT) (3 d after SCI), synaptophysin (7 d after SCI), synapsin I (7 d after SCI), and synaptic adhesion protein I (syt I) (7 d after SCI) in gray matter of spinal cord after acute SCI ($P < 0.01$) [74]. Therefore, the mechanisms of Danshen on SCI treatment could be attributed to increasing the activity of ChAT in attempt to restore the motor function of spinal cord gray matter and increase the activity of associated proteins in the synapse to promote the transfer of nerve impulses.

The mRNA expression and level of myelin basic protein (MBP) in the cytoplasm of oligodendroglia were also continuously upregulated following multiple administration of Danshen injection (50 mg/kg, twice per day) after SCI. This was important in promoting the regeneration of myelin and the recovery of neurological function [78].

4.2. Ginkgo

4.2.1. Source, Chemical Constituents, and Pharmacology of Ginkgo. Ginkgo biloba L. is well-known globally although grown mainly in China and Japan. In China, the dried leaf of *Ginkgo biloba* L. is used as a medicine and is named as Ginkgo Folium [22]. In Western countries, medical interest in Ginkgo has grown dramatically since the 1980s, and extracts from *Ginkgo biloba* leaves (EGb) are one of the most commonly used herbal medicinal products in Europe and in the US today [79]. The extract taken most is the standardized extract EGb761® [80].

EGb has been well investigated chemically for various classes of constituents. It is reported to contain a number of secondary metabolites including terpenoids, flavonoids, polyphenols, allyl phenols, organic acids, carbohydrates, fatty acids and lipids, inorganic salts, and amino acids. However terpene trilactones (e.g., ginkgolides A, B, C, and J and bilobalide) (Figure 3(a)) and flavonoid glycosides (e.g., quercetin, kaempferol, and isorhamnetin) are considered the main bioactive constituents [81].

The therapeutic indications of EGb include chest impediment, heart pain, stroke, hemiplegia, and dysphasia due to blockage of the meridians by stagnated blood and angina pectoris of the stable type in coronary heart disease and cerebral infarction with the above noted symptoms [22]. Nowadays, EGb is widely used for diseases like cerebral ischemia, cardiovascular disease, Alzheimer's disease, dementia, and memory loss [82].

4.2.2. EGb for SCI Treatment. Although EGb is not regularly used to treat SCI in Western countries and China, behavioral scores (i.e., tilt board test and BBB scores) and histopathological changes have confirmed the improvement in rat hindlimb motor functions ($P < 0.01$) [83]. HE staining results showed that rats given EGb (17.5 mg/kg/d or 25 mg/kg/d) had fewer incidences of hemorrhage, edema, necrosis, axonal demyelination, swelling of nerve cells, infiltration of inflammatory cells, and astroglial responses in spinal cord as compared with that of the control group [84, 85]. In addition, several studies suggested antioxidant and antiapoptosis effects *in vivo*, providing a possible alternative mechanism for improvement of SCI symptoms [86].

(1) Antioxidant Effects. Intraperitoneal injection of EGb (100 mg/kg/d) could significantly upregulate SOD levels, while downregulating MDA and NO levels ($P < 0.05$) in the injured spinal cord after SCI [87, 88].

(2) Antiapoptosis Effects. The presence of apoptotic cells, Bcl-2 and Bax expression, caspase-3 and caspase-9 expression, and iNOS were upregulated after SCI in the injured spinal cord ($P < 0.01$). EGb (17.5 mg/kg/d) treatment significantly increased the ratio of apoptosis cells, Bcl-2 expression, caspase-3, caspase-9, and iNOS levels ($P < 0.05$), while it decreased Bax expression ($P < 0.01$) in anterior horn motor neurons of the spinal cord [84, 85, 89].

4.2.3. Active Constituents in Ginkgo for SCI Treatment. In recent years, investigators have focused attention from EGb to terpene trilactones in the field of SCI treatment, and ginkgolides A and B are two active constituents that have attracted the most attention.

The combined behavioral and BBB scores have confirmed an improvement to the recovery of muscular function and limb coherence after intraperitoneal injection of ginkgolide A (10 mg/kg/d) and ginkgolide B (2 mg/kg/d or 4 mg/kg/d), respectively [90, 91]. Ginkgolide B (2 mg/kg/d) could also improve hemorrhage, edema, necrosis, and inflammatory cell infiltrates in injured spinal cord [92].

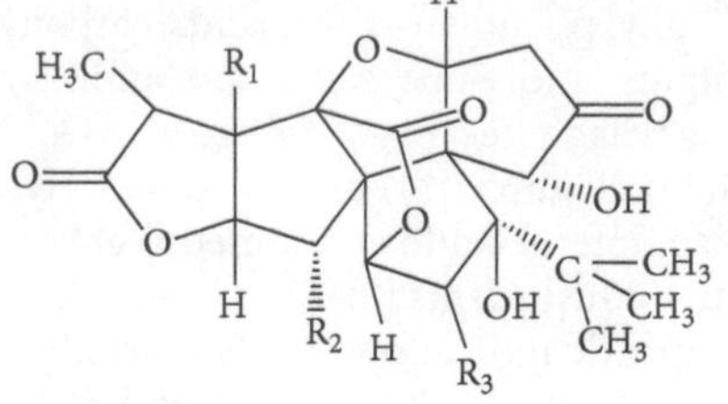

Ginkgolide A: R_1 = OH, R_2 = H, R_3 = H

Ginkgolide B: R_1 = OH, R_2 = OH, R_3 = H

Ginkgolide C: R_1 = OH, R_2 = OH, R_3 = OH

Ginkgolide J: R_1 = H, R_2 = OH, R_3 = OH

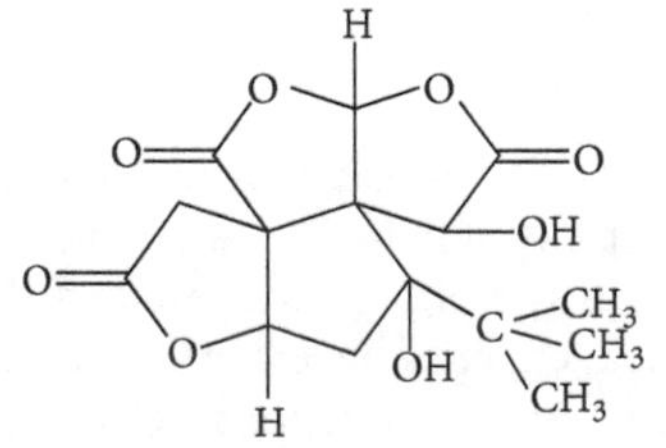

Bilobalide

(a)

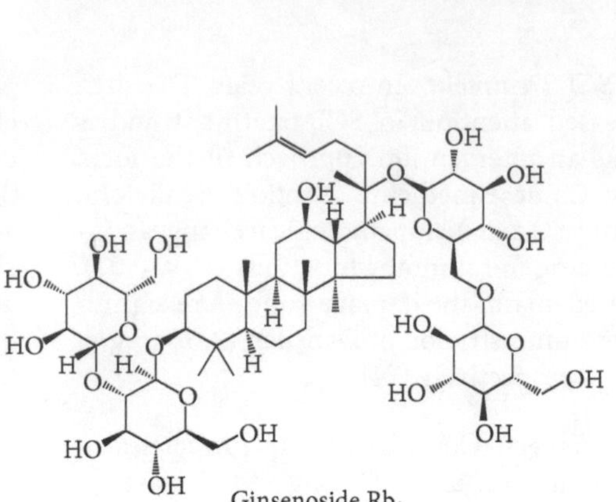

Ginsenoside Rb_1

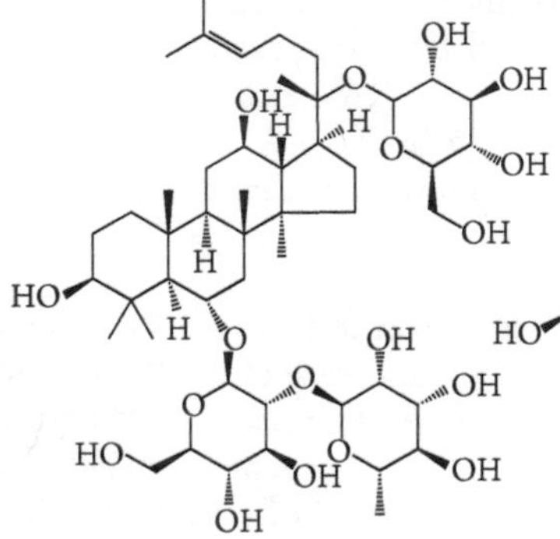

Ginsenoside Re

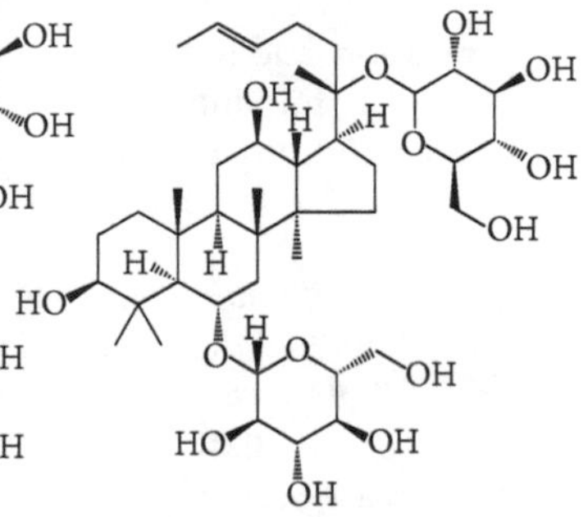

Ginsenoside Rg_1

(b)

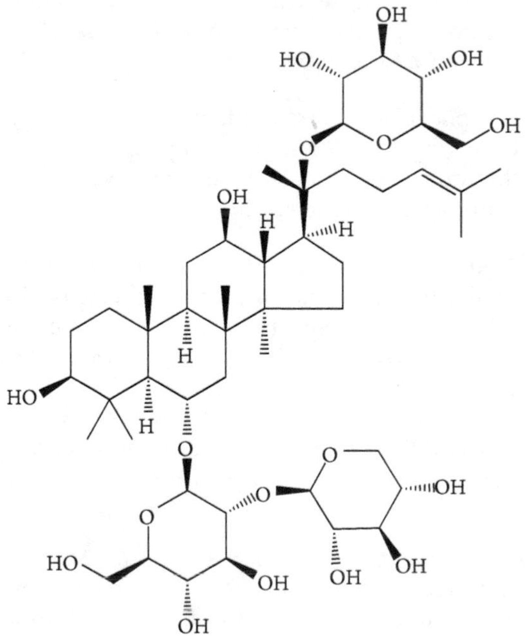

Notoginsenoside R_1

(c)

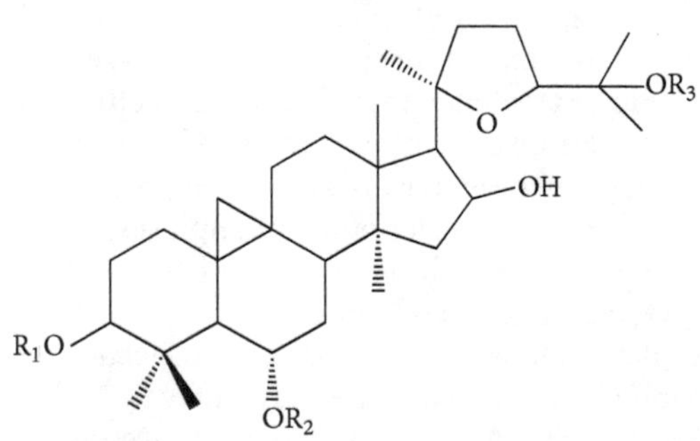

	R_1	R_2	R_3
Astragalosides I	β-D-xylp(2′,3′-di-OAc)	β-D-glcp	H
Astragalosides II	β-D-xylp(2′-OAc)	β-D-glcp	H
Astragalosides III	β-D-xylp(2′-β-D-glcp)	H	H
Astragalosides IV	β-D-xylp	β-D-glcp	H

(d)

FIGURE 3: Structures of major constituents in Ginkgo, Ginseng, Notoginseng, and Astragali Radix ((a) structures of ginkgolides A, B, C, and J and bilobalide in Ginkgo; (b) structures of ginsenosides Rb_1, Re, and Rg_1 in Ginseng; (c) structures of notoginsenoside R_1 in Notoginseng; (d) structures of astragalosides I–IV in Astragali Radix).

(1) Antiapoptosis Effects. Ginkgolide B (2 mg/kg/d) could significantly reverse the increase of apoptosis rates ($P < 0.05$), caspase-3 expression in injured spinal cord nerve cells ($P < 0.01$), and caspase-3 p20 immunostaining positive cells in the penumbra areas ($P < 0.01$) at 3, 7, and 14 days after acute SCI [92]. Another report indicated that the underlying mechanism of Ginkgolide B (4 mg/kg/d) protection of rats against acute SCI may be related to inhibition of the JAK/STAT signaling pathway ($P < 0.05$), improvement of the Bcl-2/Bax ratio ($P < 0.05$), and decreases of caspase-3 gene and protein expression ($P < 0.05$) [91].

(2) Neuroprotective Effects. SP immunostaining indicated that continuous intraperitoneal injection of ginkgolide B (2 mg/kg/d) could significantly reverse the upregulation of ED-1 positive cells, S100β-positive cells, and GFAP-positive cells numbers 3 d after SCI ($P < 0.01$). Meanwhile, the downregulation of MBP-positive cells in the injured spinal cord region ($P < 0.01$) was also reversed by continuous administration of ginkgolide B (2 mg/kg/d) for 3 d after SCI. These results indicated that ginkgolide B could efficiently decrease hyperplasia and overgrowth of astrocytes, prevent the formation of glial scar, and decrease the accumulation of macrophages and activation of microglia, as well as preventing demyelination of axons and promoting regeneration of axons to some extent [93].

4.3. Ginseng

4.3.1. Source, Chemical Constituents, and Pharmacology of Ginseng. Ginseng is the dried root and rhizome of *Panax ginseng* C. A. Mey. in genus *Panax* of Araliaceae family and is also known as Ginseng Radix et Rhizoma [22]. Although it is a traditional herbal medicine in oriental countries, especially China, Korea, and Japan, Ginseng has been widely used all over the world. For its promising healing and restorative properties, it has occupied a prominent position in the list of best-selling natural products in the world.

Since the first isolation of six ginsenosides derived from Ginseng in the 1960s [94], many ginsenosides have been isolated and identified. Among various ginsenosides, Rb_1, Rg_1, Rg_3, Re, and Rd are the most frequently studied variants, and the structures of some typical constituents are given in Figure 3(b). Many pharmacological activities of Ginseng extracts have been discovered since the 1950s, and most of them are attributed to ginsenosides, which include antioxidant, anti-inflammatory, antidiabetic, anticancer, anti-ischemic, antiarrhythmic, antihypertensive, inhibiting platelet aggregation, adjusting lipid profiles, and improving aging [95].

4.3.2. Ginsenoside for SCI Treatment. Although ginsenosides are not used to treat SCI regularly, its potential therapeutic effect in SCI treatment has been confirmed by behavioral scores (i.e., CBS scores) and histopathological changes. Both EM and HE staining showed that administration of ginsenosides (3 g/kg/d or 100 mg/kg/d) could improve the hemorrhage and edema seen in the injured spinal cord, as well as tissue necrosis, vacuolar degeneration of neurons, pyknosis

and dissolution of the nucleus, disappearance of the Nissl body in the gray matter, infiltration of inflammatory cells, nerve fiber fractures, and axonal demyelination in the white matter [96, 97]. Ginsenosides protect spinal cord neurons from both oxidative stress and apoptosis *in vivo* and *in vitro*, which may be two of the major mechanisms of SCI.

(1) Antioxidant Effects. Intraperitoneal injection of ginsenosides (3 g/kg/d) could significantly upregulate SOD and GSH levels ($P < 0.05$), while downregulating MDA level ($P < 0.05$) and Ca^{2+} influx ($P < 0.01$) in the injured spinal cord after SCI [96].

In the oxidative stress model, spinal cord neurons were treated with 30 mM H_2O_2 for 24 h. Rb_1 ($\geq$20 mM) and Rg_1 ($\geq$20 mM) could significantly reduce neuronal death by approximately 52–57% ($P < 0.01$), although the protective ability against oxidative damage was limited.

In the excitotoxic model, spinal cord neurons were treated with 500 mM glutamate for 1 h (or 100 mM kainic acid for 24 h). A 20 mM concentration of Rb_1 and 40 mM Rg_1 appeared to be sufficient to provide full protection, as measured by both direct cell counts and neuron-specific enolase (NSE) ELISA ($P < 0.01$) [98].

(2) Antiapoptosis Effects. Intraperitoneal injection of ginsenosides (100 mg/kg/d) upregulated the expression of Bcl-2 protein and the ratio of Bcl-2/Bax, while downregulating the expression of Bax, caspase-3 protein, and apoptotic cell numbers ($P < 0.01$), as measured by TUNEL, immunohistochemistry, and Western blot assays [97, 99].

4.4. Notoginseng

4.4.1. Source, Chemical Constituents, and Pharmacology of Notoginseng. *Panax notoginseng* (Burk.) F. H. Chen (Araliaceae) is a Chinese medicinal herb, distributed throughout the southwest of China, Burma, and Nepal. According to the Chinese Pharmacopoeia (2010 edition), the dried root and rhizome of *Panax notoginseng* are used as medicines, which are given the name Notoginseng Radix et Rhizoma [22].

There are various chemical constituents in Notoginseng, including ginsenosides, notoginsenosides, flavonoids, volatile oils, amino acids, and polysaccharides. Extensive chemical studies on this herb have shown that dammarane-type saponins are the main bioactive components [100]. The *Panax notoginseng* Saponins (PNS) contain protopanaxadiol glucosides (e.g., ginsenosides Rb_1 and Rd), protopanaxatriol glucosides (e.g., ginsenosides Rg_1 and Re), and notoginsenosides (e.g., notoginsenoside R_1) (Figure 3(c)), which account for 12% of the root [101].

In addition, Notoginseng has various pharmacological actions and is traditionally used in the treatment of cardiovascular diseases, inflammation, trauma, and hemorrhage. It is also reported to have antihypertensive, antithrombotic, antiatherosclerotic, hemostatic, antitumour, neuroprotective, immunological adjuvant, and hypoglycaemic activities [102].

4.4.2. PNS for SCI Treatment. As the similarity in chemical constituents between Ginseng and Notoginseng, it is reasonable to suspect that PNS is used in SCI treatment. Behavioral scores (i.e., tilt board test and BBB scores) have confirmed improvement in rat hindlimb motor functions ($P < 0.01$). EM showed that neurons shrank and exhibited abnormal morphology. Following the treatment of PNS (30 mg/kg/d), the ultrastructure of the neurons demonstrated a much clearer morphology, including an evenly distributed chromatin, integrative nuclear membranes with decreased introcession, and intact granular ER and mitochondria [103].

(1) Anti-Inflammatory and Neuroprotective Effects. Both immunohistochemical and Western blot assays indicated that PNS (30 mg/kg/d) could exert anti-inflammatory effects against SCI by reducing the expression of IL-1β and TNF-α, as well as increasing the expression of IL-10 ($P < 0.01$) [103]. Besides, AQP4 in the central ependymal cells and the gliocytes that surround the blood vessels, as well as GFAP expression in the gray matter, was significantly increased after SCI ($P < 0.01$). After PNS treatment (30 mg/kg/d or 20 mg/kg/d), AQP4 and GFAP staining was significantly reduced ($P < 0.01$), which was similar to the effect of MP therapy (30 mg/kg/d) in the positive control group ($P > 0.05$) [103, 104].

(2) Antiapoptosis Effects. Intraperitoneal injection of PNS (30 mg/kg/d) downregulated the increase of expression of two apoptosis-related proteins Fas and FasL in the injured spinal cord after acute SCI, as quantified by immunohistochemical and Western blot assays [103, 105].

4.5. Astragali Radix

4.5.1. Source, Chemical Constituents, and Pharmacology of Astragali Radix. Astragali Radix is a perennial herbaceous plant of the Leguminosae family, which is widely distributed throughout the temperate regions of the world. It is derived from the dried root of *Astragalus membranaceus* (Fisch.) Bge. var. *mongholicus* (Bge.) Hsiao or *Astragalus membranaceus* (Fisch.) Bge. [22] and is one of the most popular health-promoting herbal medicines commonly used in China.

The compounds contained in Astragali Radix have been isolated and identified as polysaccharides (APS), triterpene saponins (e.g., astragalosides I–IV, AST I–IV), flavonoids, amino acids, alkaloids, and trace elements [106]. Up to now, various biological activities of these compounds or Astragali Radix extract have been investigated and reported, such as immunomodulatory, antioxidant, anti-inflammatory, antitumour, antidiabetic, antiviral, cardioprotective, antihyperglycemic, antiatherosclerotic, and hepatoprotective effects [107].

The polysaccharides and triterpene saponins have been identified as the major active ingredients responsible for the bioactivities. The structures of AST I–IV are given in Figure 3(d).

4.5.2. Astragali Radix for SCI Treatment. In recent years, Astragali Radix has emerged as a potential therapeutic drug in the treatment of SCI and is mostly used as a form of herbal extract or Chinese medicine injection.

Behavioral scores (i.e., BBB scores, CBS scores, and tilt board test) and changes in somatosensory evoked potentials (SEP) have confirmed the improvement to rat motor functions ($P < 0.01$). HE staining showed that bleeding and edema were significantly reduced in the damage zone, with the necrotic area decreasing ($P < 0.01$), after intraperitoneal injection of Astragali Radix for 21 d (4 g/kg/d or 8 g/kg/d) [108, 109].

Several studies have indicated that Astragali Radix has both antioxidant and neuroprotective effects *in vivo*, providing a possible mechanism for SCI symptoms improvement. Intraperitoneal injection of Astragali Radix (8 g/kg/d or 4 g/kg/d) could significantly increase the downregulation of SOD, while decreasing any enhanced levels of MDA and GFAP expression ($P < 0.01$) in the injured spinal cord of SCI rats [110].

4.6. Summary. The pharmacological intervention mechanism of all five Chinese herbs in SCI treatment is summarized in Table 2. Besides the five herbs mentioned above, there are also some classic compound prescriptions currently used in SCI treatment, which are mainly Buyang Huanwu decoction and Zibu Piyin recipe [111–113]. It is worth noting that most of the related references of herbs and compound prescriptions are published in Chinese Journal. It indicates that researches of these herbs and compound prescriptions in prevention and treatment of SCI are still in a preliminary stage, and more systematic and thorough researches need to be done.

Compared with natural compounds used in the treatment of SCI, Chinese herbs have their own inherent advantages and disadvantages. On the one hand, similar "Drug-Drug Interaction" (DDI) would occur between the numerous compounds in the herb. Because of the enormous quantity and differential chemical properties of these compounds, it is too complicated to attempt clarification of the adverse reactions resulting from DDI, not to mention predicting and preventing such effects. On the other hand, multiconstituents of Chinese herbs have the superiority of synergistic effect and multitarget action, which can only be achieved by coadministration of several compounds in Western medicine. However, in order to give full play to superiority of Chinese herbs, more work needs to be done to explore their possible therapeutic mechanism.

5. Final Remarks

Spinal cord injury remains a frequent and devastating problem in modern society. Although there are no fully restorative treatments, in part because of the extremely complicated pathophysiologic mechanisms involved in SCI, various tissue engineering and cellular and molecular therapies have been tested in animal models. Many of these have reached, or are approaching, the clinical trials phase. However, none of them has been proven successfully in treating SCI patients to date. As an important supplementary treatment for SCI, TCM may provide benefits in the therapy or repair of the injured spinal cord, which has potential to replace the use of nonsteroidal anti-inflammatory drugs, neurotrophic factors, or even MP.

It is now of general consensus that successful functional recovery will not simply rely on a single therapeutic approach.

TABLE 2: Sources, major components, dosage form, and mechanisms of five Chinese herbs in SCI treatment.

Name	Picture	Source	Major components	Dosage form	Mechanism
Danshen (Salviae Miltiorrhizae Radix et Rhizoma)		Dried root and rhizome of *Salvia miltiorrhiza* Bge. in genus *Salvia* of mint family	Hydrophilic depsides derivatives (danshensu, salvianolic acids A–C, E–G, caffeic acid, ferulic acid, etc.) and lipophilic diterpenoids (tanshinones I, II_A, and II_B, tanshinol A, tanshindiols A, B, etc.)	(1) Herb extract (2) Chinese medicine injection	(1) Hemorheology change (blood flow, platelet aggregation, TXA_2, ηb, Fib, and RAI) (2) Antioxidant (MDA, SOD, and NO) (3) Anti-inflammatory (NF-κB) (4) Neuroprotective effect (GDNF, ChAT, synapsin I, syt I, and MBP) (5) Antiapoptosis (apoptotic cell index, iNOS expression)
Ginkgo (Ginkgo Folium)		Leaves of *Ginkgo biloba* L. in Ginkgoaceae	Terpenoids trilactones (ginkgolides A, B, C, and J and bilobalide), flavonoid glycosides (quercetin, kaempferol, and isorhamnetin), polyphenols, allyl phenols, organic acids, carbohydrates, fatty acids and lipids, inorganic salts, and amino acids	(1) Extracts from *Ginkgo biloba* leaves (EGb) (2) Active constituents: ginkgolides A and B	*EGb:* (1) Antioxidant (SOD, MDA, and NO) (2) Antiapoptosis (iNOS, ratio of apoptotic cells, caspase-3, Bcl-2, and Bax) *Ginkgolides A and B:* (1) Antiapoptosis (Bcl-2/Bax ratio, caspase-3, and JAK/STAT signaling pathway) (2) Neuroprotective effect (ED-1 positive cells, S100β-positive cells, GFAP-positive cells, and MBP-positive cells)
Ginseng (Ginseng Radix et Rhizoma)		Dried root and rhizome of *Panax ginseng* C. A. Mey. in genus *Panax* of Araliaceae family	Ginsenosides (Rb_1, Rg_1, Rg_3, Re, Rd, etc.)	(1) Herb extract (2) Chinese medicine injection	(1) Antioxidant (SOD, GSH, MDA, Ca^{2+} influx, and NSE) (2) Antiapoptosis (apoptotic cells numbers, Bcl-2, Bax, and caspase-3)

TABLE 2: Continued.

Name	Picture	Source	Major components	Dosage form	Mechanism
Notoginseng (Notoginseng Radix et Rhizoma)		Dried root and rhizome of *Panax notoginseng* (Burk.) F. H. Chen in Araliaceae	Ginsenosides (ginsenosides Rb₁, Rd, Rg₁, and Re), notoginsenosides (notoginsenoside R₁), flavonoids, volatile oils, amino acids, and polysaccharide	Herb extract: *Panax notoginseng* Saponins (PNS)	(1) Anti-inflammatory (IL-1β, TNF-α, and IL-10) (2) Neuroprotective effect (AQP4, GFAP) (3) Antiapoptosis (Fas, FasL)
Astragali Radix		Dried root of *Astragalus membranaceus* (Fisch.) Bge. var. *mongholicus* (Bge.) Hsiao or *Astragalus membranaceus* (Fisch.) Bge.	Polysaccharides (APS), triterpene saponins (astragalosides I–IV, AST I–IV), flavonoids, amino acids, alkaloids, and trace elements	Astragali Radix injection	(1) Antioxidant (SOD, MDA) (2) Neuroprotective effect (GFAP)

Future clinical approaches will become increasingly diversified and multimodal and will likely include a combination of multiple strategies. In this context, TCM is bound to attract increased attention in the field of SCI treatment.

Competing Interests

All authors declare that they have no competing interests.

Acknowledgments

The authors would like to acknowledge the support provided by a grant from the National Natural Science Foundation of China (Grant no. 81403278).

References

[1] L. H. S. Sekhon and M. G. Fehlings, "Epidemiology, demographics, and pathophysiology of acute spinal cord injury," *Spine*, vol. 26, no. 24, pp. S2–S12, 2001.

[2] N. A. Silva, N. Sousa, R. L. Reis, and A. J. Salgado, "From basics to clinical: a comprehensive review on spinal cord injury," *Progress in Neurobiology*, vol. 114, pp. 25–57, 2014.

[3] J. P. White and P. Thumbikat, "Acute spinal cord injury," *Surgery*, vol. 30, no. 7, pp. 326–332, 2012.

[4] B. Suberviola, A. González-Castro, J. Llorca, F. Ortiz-Melón, and E. Miñambres, "Early complications of high-dose methylprednisolone in acute spinal cord injury patients," *Injury*, vol. 39, no. 7, pp. 748–752, 2008.

[5] C. Zhang, J. Ma, L. Fan et al., "Neuroprotective effects of safranal in a rat model of traumatic injury to the spinal cord by anti-apoptotic, anti-inflammatory and edema-attenuating," *Tissue and Cell*, vol. 47, no. 3, pp. 291–300, 2015.

[6] C. Wang, P. Wang, W. Zeng, and W. Li, "Tetramethylpyrazine improves the recovery of spinal cord injury via Akt/Nrf2/HO-1 pathway," *Bioorganic & Medicinal Chemistry Letters*, vol. 26, no. 4, pp. 1287–1291, 2016.

[7] J. H. Song, M. Liu, W. L. Lei, J. Lu, D. Q. Wang, and Y. M. Yang, "Effect of extracts from leaves of ginkgo bilobe on hindlimbs locomator after spinal cord injury in rats," *Journal of Xi'an Jiaotong University (Medical Sciences)*, vol. 26, no. 2, pp. 166–168, 2005.

[8] T. B. Ng, "Pharmacological activity of sanchi ginseng (*Panax notoginseng*)," *The Journal of Pharmacy and Pharmacology*, vol. 58, no. 8, pp. 1007–1019, 2006.

[9] H. M. Ye, M. X. Yang, and Y. B. Gao, "Empirical study on Fangjifangqi decoction in treating hemitransected spinal cord injury in rats," *Zhejiang Journal of Integrated Traditional Chinese and Western Medicine*, vol. 18, no. 1, pp. 9–11, 2008.

[10] L. Wang and D.-M. Jiang, "Neuroprotective effect of Buyang Huanwu Decoction on spinal ischemia-reperfusion injury in rats is linked with inhibition of cyclin-dependent kinase 5," *BMC Complementary and Alternative Medicine*, vol. 13, article 309, 2013.

[11] A. Chen, H. Wang, J. Zhang et al., "BYHWD rescues axotomized neurons and promotes functional recovery after spinal cord injury in rats," *Journal of Ethnopharmacology*, vol. 117, no. 3, pp. 451–456, 2008.

[12] L. Wang and D.-M. Jiang, "Neuroprotective effect of Buyang Huanwu Decoction on spinal ischemia/reperfusion injury in

rats," *Journal of Ethnopharmacology*, vol. 124, no. 2, pp. 219–223, 2009.

[13] M. J. DeVivo, B. K. Go, and A. B. Jackson, "Overview of the national spinal cord injury statistical center database," *Journal of Spinal Cord Medicine*, vol. 25, no. 4, pp. 335–338, 2002.

[14] F. M. Bareyre and M. E. Schwab, "Inflammation, degeneration and regeneration in the injured spinal cord: insights from DNA microarrays," *Trends in Neurosciences*, vol. 26, no. 10, pp. 555–563, 2003.

[15] M. Toborek, A. Malecki, R. Garrido, M. P. Mattson, B. Hennig, and B. Young, "Arachidonic acid-induced oxidative injury to cultured spinal cord neurons," *Journal of Neurochemistry*, vol. 73, no. 2, pp. 684–692, 1999.

[16] M. S. Beattie, A. A. Farooqui, and J. C. Bresnahan, "Review of current evidence for apoptosis after spinal cord injury," *Journal of Neurotrauma*, vol. 17, no. 10, pp. 915–925, 2000.

[17] M. J. Crowe, J. C. Bresnahan, S. L. Shuman, J. N. Masters, and M. S. Beattie, "Apoptosis and delayed degeneration after spinal cord injury in rats and monkeys," *Nature Medicine*, vol. 3, no. 1, pp. 73–76, 1997.

[18] L. Yang, N. R. Jones, P. C. Blumbergs et al., "Severity-dependent expression of pro-inflammatory cytokines in traumatic spinal cord injury in the rat," *Journal of Clinical Neuroscience*, vol. 12, no. 3, pp. 276–284, 2005.

[19] D. J. Donnelly and P. G. Popovich, "Inflammation and its role in neuroprotection, axonal regeneration and functional recovery after spinal cord injury," *Experimental Neurology*, vol. 209, no. 2, pp. 378–388, 2008.

[20] T. Morino, T. Ogata, H. Horiuchi et al., "Delayed neuronal damage related to microglia proliferation after mild spinal cord compression injury," *Neuroscience Research*, vol. 46, no. 3, pp. 309–318, 2003.

[21] G. Yiu and Z. He, "Glial inhibition of CNS axon regeneration," *Nature Reviews Neuroscience*, vol. 7, no. 8, pp. 617–627, 2006.

[22] Chinese Pharmacopoeia: Part 1, pp. 264–265, 2015.

[23] L. Shen and H.-F. Ji, "The pharmacology of curcumin: is it the degradation products?" *Trends in Molecular Medicine*, vol. 18, no. 3, pp. 138–144, 2012.

[24] B. Cemil, K. Topuz, M. N. Demircan et al., "Curcumin improves early functional results after experimental spinal cord injury," *Acta Neurochirurgica*, vol. 152, no. 9, pp. 1583–1590, 2010.

[25] M.-S. Lin, Y.-H. Lee, W.-T. Chiu, and K.-S. Hung, "Curcumin provides neuroprotection after spinal cord injury," *Journal of Surgical Research*, vol. 166, no. 2, pp. 280–289, 2011.

[26] W. Jin, J. Wang, T. Zhu et al., "Anti-inflammatory effects of curcumin in experimental spinal cord injury in rats," *Inflammation Research*, vol. 63, no. 5, pp. 381–387, 2014.

[27] V. P. Menon and A. R. Sudheer, "Antioxidant and anti-inflammatory properties of curcumin," *Advances in Experimental Medicine and Biology*, vol. 595, pp. 105–125, 2007.

[28] H. Ş. Kavakli, C. Koca, and Ö. Alici, "Antioxidant effects of curcumin in spinal cord injury in rats," *Ulusal Travma ve Acil Cerrahi Dergisi*, vol. 17, no. 1, pp. 14–18, 2011.

[29] B. Ray, S. Bisht, A. Maitra, A. Maitra, and D. K. Lahiri, "Neuroprotective and neurorescue effects of a novel polymeric nanoparticle formulation of curcumin (NanoCurc™) in the neuronal cell culture and animal model: implications for Alzheimer's disease," *Journal of Alzheimer's Disease*, vol. 23, no. 1, pp. 61–77, 2011.

[30] J. K. Alexander and P. G. Popovich, "Neuroinflammation in spinal cord injury: therapeutic targets for neuroprotection and

regeneration," *Progress in Brain Research*, vol. 175, pp. 125–137, 2009.

[31] M. Bishnoi, K. Chopra, L. Rongzhu, and S. K. Kulkarni, "Protective effect of curcumin and its combination with piperine (bioavailability enhancer) against haloperidol-associated neurotoxicity: cellular and neurochemical evidence," *Neurotoxicity Research*, vol. 20, no. 3, pp. 215–225, 2011.

[32] P. Kumar, Y. E. Choonara, G. Modi, D. Naidoo, and V. Pillay, "Cur(Que)min: a neuroactive permutation of curcumin and quercetin for treating spinal cord injury," *Medical Hypotheses*, vol. 82, no. 4, pp. 437–441, 2014.

[33] J. A. Baur and D. A. Sinclair, "Therapeutic potential of resveratrol: the in vivo evidence," *Nature Reviews Drug Discovery*, vol. 5, no. 6, pp. 493–506, 2006.

[34] G. J. Soleas, E. P. Diamandis, and D. M. Goldberg, "Wine as a biological fluid: history, production, and role in disease prevention," *Journal of Clinical Laboratory Analysis*, vol. 11, no. 5, pp. 287–313, 1997.

[35] E.-J. Park and J. M. Pezzuto, "The pharmacology of resveratrol in animals and humans," *Biochimica et Biophysica Acta*, vol. 1852, no. 6, pp. 1071–1113, 2015.

[36] O. Ates, S. Cayli, E. Altinoz et al., "Effects of resveratrol and methylprednisolone on biochemical, neurobehavioral and histopathological recovery after experimental spinal cord injury," *Acta Pharmacologica Sinica*, vol. 27, no. 10, pp. 1317–1325, 2006.

[37] Y.-B. Yang and Y.-J. Piao, "Effects of resveratrol on secondary damages after acute spinal cord injury in rats," *Acta Pharmacologica Sinica*, vol. 24, no. 7, pp. 703–710, 2003.

[38] C. J. Liu, Z. B. Shi, L. H. Fan, C. Zhang, K. Z. Wang, and B. Wang, "Resveratrol improves neuron protection and functional recovery in rat model of spinal cord injury," *Brain Research*, vol. 1374, pp. 100–109, 2011.

[39] U. Kiziltepe, N. N. D. Turan, U. Han, A. T. Ulus, and F. Akar, "Resveratrol, a red wine polyphenol, protects spinal cord from ischemia-reperfusion injury," *Journal of Vascular Surgery*, vol. 40, no. 1, pp. 138–145, 2004.

[40] S. Kaplan, G. Bisleri, J. A. Morgan, F. H. Cheema, and M. C. Oz, "Resveratrol, a natural red wine polyphenol, reduces ischemia-reperfusion- induced spinal cord injury," *Annals of Thoracic Surgery*, vol. 80, no. 6, pp. 2242–2249, 2005.

[41] X.-M. Zhou, M.-L. Zhou, X.-S. Zhang et al., "Resveratrol prevents neuronal apoptosis in an early brain injury model," *Journal of Surgical Research*, vol. 189, no. 1, pp. 159–165, 2014.

[42] F. Zhang, J. Liu, and J.-S. Shi, "Anti-inflammatory activities of resveratrol in the brain: role of resveratrol in microglial activation," *European Journal of Pharmacology*, vol. 636, no. 1–3, pp. 1–7, 2010.

[43] D. G. Nagle, D. Ferreira, and Y.-D. Zhou, "Epigallocatechin-3-gallate (EGCG): chemical and biomedical perspectives," *Phytochemistry*, vol. 67, no. 17, pp. 1849–1855, 2006.

[44] E. G. de Mejia, M. V. Ramirez-Mares, and S. Puangpraphant, "Bioactive components of tea: cancer, inflammation and behavior," *Brain, Behavior, and Immunity*, vol. 23, no. 6, pp. 721–731, 2009.

[45] I. Paterniti, T. Genovese, C. Crisafulli et al., "Treatment with green tea extract attenuates secondary inflammatory response in an experimental model of spinal cord trauma," *Naunyn-Schmiedeberg's Archives of Pharmacology*, vol. 380, no. 2, pp. 179–192, 2009.

[46] X. G. Han, W. Tian, and B. Liu, "The therapeutic effect of epigallocatechin gallate on the neurological recovery after spinal cord injury in rat," *Chinese Journal of Spine and Spinal Cord*, vol. 23, no. 11, pp. 998–1005, 2013.

[47] W. M. Renno, G. Al-Khaledi, A. Mousa, S. M. Karam, H. Abul, and S. Asfar, "(-)-Epigallocatechin-3-gallate (EGCG) modulates neurological function when intravenously infused in acute and, chronically injured spinal cord of adult rats," *Neuropharmacology*, vol. 77, pp. 100–119, 2014.

[48] F. Deng, R. Li, Y. Yang, D. Zhou, Q. Wang, and J. Xu, "Neuroprotective effect of epigallocatechin-3-gallate on hemisection-induced spinal cord injury in rats," *Neural Regeneration Research*, vol. 6, no. 6, pp. 405–411, 2011.

[49] A. R. Khalatbary and H. Ahmadvand, "Anti-inflammatory effect of the epigallocatechin gallate following spinal cord trauma in rat," *Iranian Biomedical Journal*, vol. 15, no. 1-2, pp. 31–37, 2011.

[50] R. Ge, Y. Zhu, Y. Diao, L. Tao, W. Yuan, and X.-C. Xiong, "Anti-edema effect of epigallocatechin gallate on spinal cord injury in rats," *Brain Research*, vol. 1527, pp. 40–46, 2013.

[51] Y. Q. Jin, Y. L. Hong, J. R. Li, X. Li, X. X. Wang, and L. G. Hua, "Advancements in the chemical constituents and pharmacological effects of Chuanxiong," *Pharmacy and Clinics of Chinese Materia Medica*, vol. 4, no. 3, pp. 44–48, 2013.

[52] Z. Zhang, T. Wei, J. Hou, G. Li, S. Yu, and W. Xin, "Tetramethylpyrazine scavenges superoxide anion and decreases nitric oxide production in human polymorphonuclear leukocytes," *Life Sciences*, vol. 72, no. 22, pp. 2465–2472, 2003.

[53] C.-C. Wu, W.-F. Chiou, and M.-H. Yen, "A possible mechanism of action of tetramethylpyrazine on vascular smooth muscle in rat aorta," *European Journal of Pharmacology*, vol. 169, no. 2-3, pp. 189–195, 1989.

[54] L. Fan, K. Wang, Z. Shi, J. Die, C. Wang, and X. Dang, "Tetramethylpyrazine protects spinal cord and reduces inflammation in a rat model of spinal cord ischemia-reperfusion injury," *Journal of Vascular Surgery*, vol. 54, no. 1, pp. 192–200, 2011.

[55] L.-H. Fan, K.-Z. Wang, B. Cheng, C.-S. Wang, and X.-Q. Dang, "Anti-apoptotic and neuroprotective effects of Tetramethylpyrazine following spinal cord ischemia in rabbits," *BMC Neuroscience*, vol. 7, pp. 48–56, 2006.

[56] Y.-H. Shih, S.-L. Wu, W.-F. Chiou, H.-H. Ku, T.-L. Ko, and Y.-S. Fu, "Protective effects of tetramethylpyrazine on kainate-induced excitotoxicity in hippocampal culture," *NeuroReport*, vol. 13, no. 4, pp. 515–519, 2002.

[57] L. Lv, S.-S. Jiang, J. Xu, J.-B. Gong, and Y. Cheng, "Protective effect of ligustrazine against myocardial ischaemia reperfusion in rats: the role of endothelial nitric oxide synthase," *Clinical and Experimental Pharmacology and Physiology*, vol. 39, no. 1, pp. 20–27, 2012.

[58] X. Xiao, Y. Liu, C. Qi et al., "Neuroprotection and enhanced neurogenesis by tetramethylpyrazine in adult rat brain after focal ischemia," *Neurological Research*, vol. 32, no. 5, pp. 547–555, 2010.

[59] M. Russo, C. Spagnuolo, I. Tedesco, S. Bilotto, and G. L. Russo, "The flavonoid quercetin in disease prevention and therapy: facts and fancies," *Biochemical Pharmacology*, vol. 83, no. 1, pp. 6–15, 2012.

[60] Nutrient Data Laboratory, Food Composition Laboratory, Beltsville Human Nutrition Research Center, and Agricultural Research Service, *USDA Database for the Flavonoid Content of Selected Foods*, U.S. Department of Agriculture, Baltimore, Md, USA, 2007, http://www.ars.usda.gov/nutrientdata.

[61] M. Harwood, B. Danielewska-Nikiel, J. F. Borzelleca, G. W. Flamm, G. M. Williams, and T. C. Lines, "A critical review of the data related to the safety of quercetin and lack of evidence of in vivo toxicity, including lack of genotoxic/carcinogenic properties," *Food and Chemical Toxicology*, vol. 45, no. 11, pp. 2179–2205, 2007.

[62] Y. Song, J. Liu, F. Zhang, J. Zhang, T. Shi, and Z. Zeng, "Antioxidant effect of quercetin against acute spinal cord injury in rats and its correlation with the p38MAPK/iNOS signaling pathway," *Life Sciences*, vol. 92, no. 24–26, pp. 1215–1221, 2013.

[63] Ö. Çevik, M. Erşahin, T. E. Şener et al., "Beneficial effects of quercetin on rat urinary bladder after spinal cord injury," *Journal of Surgical Research*, vol. 183, no. 2, pp. 695–703, 2013.

[64] S.-Y. Wei, Y. Chen, and X.-Y. Xu, "Progress on the pharmacological research of puerarin: a review," *Chinese Journal of Natural Medicines*, vol. 12, no. 6, pp. 407–414, 2014.

[65] F. Tian, L.-H. Xu, W. Zhao, L.-J. Tian, and X.-L. Ji, "The optimal therapeutic timing and mechanism of puerarin treatment of spinal cord ischemia-reperfusion injury in rats," *Journal of Ethnopharmacology*, vol. 134, no. 3, pp. 892–896, 2011.

[66] F. Tian, L.-H. Xu, B. Wang, L.-J. Tian, and X.-L. Ji, "The neuroprotective mechanism of puerarin in the treatment of acute spinal ischemia-reperfusion injury is linked to cyclin-dependent kinase 5," *Neuroscience Letters*, vol. 584, pp. 50–55, 2015.

[67] F. Tian, L.-H. Xu, W. Zhao, L.-J. Tian, and X.-L. Ji, "The neuroprotective mechanism of puerarin treatment of acute spinal cord injury in rats," *Neuroscience Letters*, vol. 543, pp. 64–68, 2013.

[68] L.-Q. Shan, S. Ma, X.-C. Qiu et al., "Hydroxysafflor yellow A protects spinal cords from ischemia/reperfusion injury in rabbits," *BMC Neuroscience*, vol. 11, article 98, 2010.

[69] L. Wang and X. Tian, "Effects of Tetrandrine on the nerve cells' apoptosis and the expression of Bcl-2 and Bax after spinal cord injury," *Bone*, vol. 44, supplement 1, pp. S116–S117, 2009.

[70] Z.-H. Zhao, *Experimental study on neuroprotective effect and mechanism of piperine for spinal cord injury in rats [Master of Medicine thesis]*, Hebei Medical University, 2012.

[71] Y.-G. Li, L. Song, M. Liu, Z. B. Hu, and Z.-T. Wang, "Advancement in analysis of Salviae miltiorrhizae Radix et Rhizoma (Danshen)," *Journal of Chromatography A*, vol. 1216, no. 11, pp. 1941–1953, 2009.

[72] T. O. Cheng, "Danshen: a versatile Chinese herbal drug for the treatment of coronary heart disease," *International Journal of Cardiology*, vol. 113, no. 3, pp. 437–438, 2006.

[73] L. Zhou, Z. Zuo, and M. S. S. Chow, "Danshen: an overview of its chemistry, pharmacology, pharmacokinetics, and clinical use," *Journal of Clinical Pharmacology*, vol. 45, no. 12, pp. 1345–1359, 2005.

[74] L. Wei, *Effect of Salvia miltiorrhiza on motor function in gray matter of acute spinal cord injury in rat and its mechanism [Doctor of Medicine thesis]*, Fujian University of Traditional Chinese Medicine, 2013.

[75] G. Wang, S. Liu, W. Zheng, and Y. Hu, "Effect of Danshen on spinal cord blood flow and hemorrheological indexes after spinal cord injury in rabbits," *Chinese Journal of Microcirculation*, vol. 13, no. 4, pp. 11–12, 2003.

[76] D. Q. Guo, L. Yang, D. P. Wang, X. Chen, H. Guan, and J. D. Xiao, "Experimental study on how Salvia miltiorrhiza works on changes of free radical at early stage of spinal cord injury," *Journal of Chinese Microcirculation*, vol. 9, no. 1, pp. 38–40, 2005.

[77] J. Wang, K. Kong, W. Qi et al., "Effects of Salvia miltiorrhiza on nuclear factor-κB activity in rats with acute traumatic spinal cord injury," *Chinese Journal of Bone and Joint Injury*, vol. 22, no. 4, pp. 307–309, 2007.

[78] L. Wang and Y. H. Liu, "Effects of Salvia Miltiorrhiza on the myelin basic protein after the spinal cord injury of rats," *Chinese Archives of Traditional Chinese Medicine*, vol. 24, no. 8, pp. 1537–1539, 2006.

[79] European Medicines Agency and Committee on Herbal Medicinal Products, "Assessment report on Ginkgo biloba L., folium," Tech. Rep., European Medicines Agency, London, UK, 2014, http://www.ema.europa.eu/ema/.

[80] T. Heinonen and W. Gaus, "Cross matching observations on toxicological and clinical data for the assessment of tolerability and safety of Ginkgo biloba leaf extract," *Toxicology*, vol. 327, pp. 95–115, 2015.

[81] T. A. van Beek, "Chemical analysis of Ginkgo biloba leaves and extracts," *Journal of Chromatography A*, vol. 967, no. 1, pp. 21–55, 2002.

[82] H. Herrschaft, A. Nacu, S. Likhachev, I. Sholomov, R. Hoerr, and S. Schlaefke, "Ginkgo biloba extract EGb 761⁵ in dementia with neuropsychiatric features: a randomised, placebo-controlled trial to confirm the efficacy and safety of a daily dose of 240 mg," *Journal of Psychiatric Research*, vol. 46, no. 6, pp. 716–723, 2012.

[83] H. J. Song, M. Liu, W. L. Lei, J. Lu, D. Q. Wang, and Y. M. Yang, "Effect of extracts from leaves of ginkgo bilobe on hindlimbs locomotor after spinal cord injury in rats," *Journal of Xi'an Jiaotong University (Medical Sciences)*, vol. 26, no. 2, pp. 166–168, 2005.

[84] F. Zhang, W. W. Feng, and H. T. Zhou, "The function of the extracts of Ginkgo biloba on rats spinal cord injury and its mechanism," *Chinese Journal of Spine and Spinal Cord*, vol. 17, no. 9, pp. 675–679, 2007.

[85] J. F. Jiang, F. Zhang, and A. C. Wei, "Experimental study on neuroprotective effect of EGb after spinal cord injury in rats," *Modern Journal of Integrated Traditional Chinese and Western Medicine*, vol. 21, no. 18, pp. 1958–1960, 2012.

[86] R. K. Koç, H. Akdemir, A. Kurtsoy et al., "Lipid peroxidation in experimental spinal cord injury," *Research in Experimental Medicine*, vol. 195, no. 1, pp. 117–123, 1995.

[87] J. J. Jiao, J. N. Jiang, B. Du, Y. Mo, M. Zhou, and H. Q. Zhang, "Effect of Ginkgo biloba extract EGb761 on healing of nerve injury after spinal cord injury in rats," *Journal of Clinical Medicine in Practice*, vol. 14, no. 15, pp. 5–8, 2010.

[88] J. J. Jiao, J. N. Jiang, B. Du, Y. Mo, M. Zhou, and H. Q. Zhang, "Neuro-protective effect of Ginkgo biloba extract EGb761 on spinal cord injury in rats," *Anhui Medical and Pharmaceutical Journal*, vol. 14, no. 10, pp. 1138–1140, 2010.

[89] B. Cheng, W. Wang, L. Lin, F. Li, and X. Wang, "The change of the spinal cord ischemia–reperfusion injury in mitochondrial passway and the effect of the Ginkgo biloba extract's preconditioning intervention," *Cellular and Molecular Neurobiology*, vol. 31, no. 3, pp. 415–420, 2011.

[90] X. S. Wang, R. S. Xu, Y. W. Sun, J. Xue, and J. S. Wu, "Effect of ginkgolide A on the repairing of nerve fibers after acute spinal cord injury in rats," *Jiangsu Medical Journal*, vol. 39, no. 19, pp. 2236–2238, 2013.

[91] Y. Song, Z. Zeng, C. Jin, J. Zhang, B. Ding, and F. Zhang, "Protective effect of ginkgolide B against acute spinal cord injury in rats and its correlation with the JAK/STAT signaling

pathway," *Neurochemical Research*, vol. 38, no. 3, pp. 610–619, 2013.

[92] H. Yu, *Study of the ginkgolide B improve motor capaeity and inhabit apoptosis after spinal cord injury in rats [M.S. thesis]*, 2006.

[93] M. Li, *The effect of ginkgolides B on glial cells after spinal cord injury in rats [Master of Medicine]*, 2006.

[94] G. B. Elyakov, L. I. Strigina, N. I. Uvarova, V. E. Vaskovsky, A. K. Dzizenko, and N. K. Kochetkov, "Glycosides from ginseng roots," *Tetrahedron Letters*, vol. 5, no. 48, pp. 3591–3597, 1964.

[95] C. H. Lee and J.-H. Kim, "A review on the medicinal potentials of ginseng and ginsenosides on cardiovascular diseases," *Journal of Ginseng Research*, vol. 38, no. 3, pp. 161–166, 2014.

[96] J. C. Liu, F. Yin, G. Zhao, and S. H. Yuan, "Spinal cord injury treated by Gen-seng saponin—an experiment study," *Chinese Journal of Gerontology*, vol. 5, pp. 303–305, 2000.

[97] J. W. Shang, *Effects of ginsenoside on apoptosis of neurons and expressions of Bcl-2 and Caspase-3 in rats with spinal cord injury [Master of Medicine]*, 2003.

[98] B. Liao, H. Newmark, and R. Zhou, "Neuroprotective effects of ginseng total saponin and ginsenosides Rb1 and Rg1 on spinal cord neurons *in vitro*," *Experimental Neurology*, vol. 173, no. 2, pp. 224–234, 2002.

[99] Y. X. Song, C. Y. Jin, Z. Y. Zeng, B. Wang, and J. Q. Zhang, "Study on the mechanism underlying neuroprotective effect of Ginsenosides in rats after spinal cord injury," *Hainan Medical Journal*, vol. 20, no. 5, pp. 6–9, 2009.

[100] H. Sun, Z. Yang, and Y. Ye, "Structure and biological activity of protopanaxatriol-type saponins from the roots of *Panax notoginseng*," *International Immunopharmacology*, vol. 6, no. 1, pp. 14–25, 2006.

[101] W.-Z. Yang, Y. Hu, W.-Y. Wu, M. Ye, and D.-A. Guo, "Saponins in the genus *Panax* L. (Araliaceae): a systematic review of their chemical diversity," *Phytochemistry*, vol. 106, pp. 7–24, 2014.

[102] T. B. Ng, "Pharmacological activity of sanchi ginseng (*Panax notoginseng*)," *Journal of Pharmacy and Pharmacology*, vol. 58, no. 8, pp. 1007–1019, 2006.

[103] N. Ning, X. Dang, C. Bai, C. Zhang, and K. Wang, "Panax notoginsenoside produces neuroprotective effects in rat model of acute spinal cord ischemia-reperfusion injury," *Journal of Ethnopharmacology*, vol. 139, no. 2, pp. 504–512, 2012.

[104] H. Li, Z. J. Zhao, D. Pan et al., "Protective effect of TSPN on spinal cord injury and its GFAP relative mechanism," *Progress in Modern Biomedicine*, vol. 10, no. 10, pp. 1825–1827, 2010.

[105] W.-Q. Yuan, H. Wang, Y.-X. Zhao, and Y.-J. Li, "Effect of panax notoginseng saponin on behavior changes and apoptosis in rats with spinal cord injury," *Chinese Journal of Clinical Rehabilitation*, vol. 10, no. 15, pp. 62–64, 2006.

[106] C. Chu, L.-W. Qi, E.-H. Liu, B. Li, W. Gao, and P. Li, "Radix astragali (Astragalus): latest advancements and trends in chemistry, analysis, pharmacology and pharmacokinetics," *Current Organic Chemistry*, vol. 14, no. 16, pp. 1792–1807, 2010.

[107] M. Jin, K. Zhao, Q. Huang, and P. Shang, "Structural features and biological activities of the polysaccharides from *Astragalus membranaceus*," *International Journal of Biological Macromolecules*, vol. 64, pp. 257–266, 2014.

[108] J. M. Zhang and K. M. Tang, "Neuroprotective function of astragalus injection on treatment of rats with acute spinal cord injury," *Journal of Clinical Medicine in Practice*, vol. 18, no. 24, pp. 7–10, 2014.

[109] S. Q. Liu, Y. G. Ma, H. Peng, and A. L. Wei, "Neuroprotective effects of Astragalus root on experimentally spinal cord injury in rats," *China Journal of Orthopaedics and Traumatology*, vol. 16, no. 8, pp. 463–465, 2003.

[110] X.-S. Ren, X.-Y. Leng, Y.-G. Yang, and X.-X. Xu, "Neuroprotective effect of astragalus root on experimental injury of spinal cord in rats," *Chinese Journal of Clinical Rehabilitation*, vol. 10, no. 7, pp. 31–33, 2006.

[111] G. F. Zhang and H. M. Wang, "Effect of Buyang-Huanwu decoction for treatment of spinal cord injury by mesenchymal stem cells transplantation in rats," *China Journal of Orthopaedics and Traumatology*, vol. 19, no. 8, pp. 452–454, 2006.

[112] J. P. Zhang, Z. B. Wang, A. H. Lin, S. G. Li, F. N. Wen, and H. Yao, "Influence of Buyang Huanwu Decoction on the ultrastructure of spinal cord tissue in rats with spinal cord injury," *Traditional Chinese Drug Research & Clinical Pharmacology*, vol. 22, no. 2, pp. 153–157, 2011.

[113] Y. Liu and Y. C. Miao, "Influence of zibu piyin recipe on expression of brain-derived neurotrophic factor after spinal cord injury in rats," *Journal of Shandong University (Health Sciences)*, vol. 50, no. 10, pp. 33–36, 2012.

Untargeted Metabolomics Reveals Intervention Effects of Total Turmeric Extract in a Rat Model of Nonalcoholic Fatty Liver Disease

Ya Wang,[1,2] Ming Niu,[2] Ge-liu-chang Jia,[2] Rui-sheng Li,[3] Ya-ming Zhang,[2] Cong-en Zhang,[2] Ya-kun Meng,[2] He-rong Cui,[2] Zhi-jie Ma,[4] Dong-hui Li,[1] Jia-bo Wang,[2] and Xiao-he Xiao[2]

[1]*Pharmacy College, Jinzhou Medical University, Jinzhou 121000, China*
[2]*China Military Institute of Chinese Medicine, 302 Military Hospital, Beijing 100039, China*
[3]*Animal Laboratory Center, 302 Hospital of PLA, Beijing 100039, China*
[4]*Beijing Friendship Hospital, Capital Medical University, Beijing 100050, China*

Correspondence should be addressed to Dong-hui Li; lidonghuilx@sina.com, Jia-bo Wang; pharm_sci@126.com, and Xiao-he Xiao; pharmacy302xxh@126.com

Academic Editor: Qihe Xu

Nonalcoholic fatty liver disease (NAFLD) is one of the most common forms of chronic liver disease. Currently, there are no recognized medical therapies effective for NAFLD. Previous studies have demonstrated the effects of total turmeric extract on rats with NAFLD induced by high-fat diet. In this study, serum metabolomics was employed using UHPLC-Q-TOF-MS to elucidate the underlying mechanisms of HFD-induced NAFLD and the therapeutic effects of TE. Supervised orthogonal partial least-squares-discriminant analysis was used to discover differentiating metabolites, and pathway enrichment analysis suggested that TE had powerful combined effects of regulating lipid metabolism by affecting glycerophospholipid metabolism, glycerolipid metabolism, and steroid hormone biosynthesis signaling pathways. In addition, the significant changes in glycerophospholipid metabolism proteins also indicated that glycerophospholipid metabolism might be involved in the therapeutic effect of TE on NAFLD. Our findings not only supply systematic insight into the mechanisms of NAFLD but also provide a theoretical basis for the prevention or treatment of NAFLD.

1. Introduction

As a chronic disease, nonalcoholic fatty liver disease is acknowledged to be the hepatic manifestation of obesity and metabolic syndrome [1], presenting an increasing incidence worldwide. NAFLD severity encompasses a wide spectrum, ranging from simple steatosis to more severe nonalcoholic steatohepatitis, involving inflammation and apoptosis with or without fibrosis and cirrhosis. To date, conventional and modern drugs used to treat NAFLD are sometimes insufficient and can have serious side effects [2, 3]. Therefore, there is no effective and safe medical therapy available for NAFLD. Continuous effort to develop a promising pharmacological therapy for the treatment of NAFLD is still urgently needed.

Traditional Chinese medicine has been practiced in China for centuries and its application in the prevention of a variety of chronic diseases [4, 5]. The perennial herb Curcuma longa *L.*, commonly known as Java turmeric, is a popular dietary spice used for food in Asia, especially Indonesia and India. In addition, it has been used as a traditional medicinal plant to reduce the sensitivity of the liver to lipid peroxidation, as well as therapeutic properties against cancer, abnormally reduced fatty acid levels, and inflammatory disorders in adipose tissue [6–8]. TE has also been proven to be effective in NAFLD treatment. In modern research, growing evidence indicates that TE markedly affects liver diseases, such as acute liver injury, hepatic steatosis, and oxidative stress and inflammation in liver which is associated

TABLE 1: Scoring of morphological changes.

	n	Macrovesicular steatosis	Microvesicular steatosis	Lobular inflammation	Portal inflammation
Control	6	0.0 ± 0.0	0.17 ± 0.41	0.33 ± 0.52	0.17 ± 0.41
Model (HFD)	6	$1.67 \pm 0.82^{**}$	$2.17 \pm 0.75^{**}$	$1.33 \pm 0.52^{**}$	$1.17 \pm 0.41^{**}$
Positive (CMCB)	6	$0.33 \pm 0.52^{\#\#}$	$1.00 \pm 0.63^{\#}$	$0.67 \pm 0.52^{\#}$	$0.33 \pm 0.52^{\#}$
LD-TE	6	0.83 ± 0.75	1.33 ± 0.82	1.33 ± 0.82	0.67 ± 0.52
MD-TE	6	$0.33 \pm 0.52^{\#\#}$	$1.17 \pm 0.75^{\#}$	0.83 ± 0.41	$0.50 \pm 0.55^{\#}$
HD-TE	6	$0.17 \pm 0.41^{\#\#}$	$0.67 \pm 0.52^{\#\#}$	$0.50 \pm 0.55^{\#}$	$0.33 \pm 0.52^{\#}$

$^{**}P < 0.01$ compared with the control group; $^{\#\#}P < 0.01$, $^{\#}P < 0.05$ compared with the model group.

with NAFLD [9, 10]. However, compared with studies of its clinical application and pharmacological effect, there is inadequate detailed information on the mechanism involved in the therapeutic effects of TE.

As a crucial component of systems biology, metabolomics offers a noninvasive platform and holistic insight into the whole metabolic profile by detecting 1000s of molecules in various biological fluids, such as the urine, saliva, and blood [11]. By analyzing specific early biomarkers during disease or drug treatment, metabolomics has shown great potential in understanding disease mechanisms, identifying diagnostic biomarkers or drug targets, and the relationship between a substance and metabolic pathways. Moreover, metabolomics reflects the terminal symptoms of metabolic network of biological systems in holistic context [12]. This trait is well coincident with the integrity and systemic feature of TCM, indicating it is a comprehensive analytical approach to clarify the underlying efficacies and therapeutic mechanisms of TCM [13, 14].

In this study, metabolic profiling with UHPLC-Q-TOF-MS was performed to obtain a systematic view of the mechanism of TE as an effective treatment for NAFLD. In addition, to provide a deep understanding of the mechanism, specific biomarkers and unique biochemical pathways were applied, coupled with multivariate data analysis techniques. Our findings might also provide guidance in the improvement of TCM therapy strategies in the future.

2. Materials and Methods

2.1. Chemicals and Reagents. Acetonitrile (HPLC grade) and formic acid (HPLC grade) were obtained from Sigma-Aldrich (St. Louis, MO, USA). Distilled water was purified using a Milli-Q ultrapure water system (Millipore, Billerica, MA). All other reagents were of analytical grade. The total turmeric extract was an ethanol extract of the dried root of Curcuma longa *L* supplied by Shenwei pharmaceutical group (Hebei, China).

2.2. Animal Handling and Sample Preparation

2.2.1. Animal Handling. Male Sprague-Dawley rats (200 ± 20 g) were supplied by the laboratory animal center of the Military Medical Science Academy of the PLA (permission number SCXK-(A) 2012-0004). The room temperature was regulated at 24 ± 2°C and a humidity of 50 ± 5%. The

research was conducted in accordance with the NIH policy. All efforts were made to alleviate the suffering of animals. After acclimatization, animals were randomized into control group, model group (fed with HFD), positive control group (Compound Methionine and Choline Bitartrate Tablets [15, 16], 162 mg/kg), LD-TE group (50 mg/kg), MD-TE group (100 mg/kg), and HD-TE group (200 mg/kg), 10 rats per group. All rats were fed a HFD ad libitum (control group was fed a regular diet) for 8 weeks. The TE doses were given after rats developed NAFLD. Besides, four rats in each group were sacrificed randomly, the livers were collected, and pathological changes in the liver tissues were observed by H&E staining and oil O staining. Histological changes were assessed by a modification of the scoring system for grading and staging for NASH described by Brunt et al. [17]. The histological evaluation of the liver sections was performed blindly. Scoring of morphological changes was shown in Table 1. The drugs were dissolved in 0.5% sodium carboxymethyl cellulose solution and orally administered for 6 weeks after rats developed NAFLD. Rats in the control group were intragastrically administered an equivalent volume of solvent. The rats were fasted for 12 h before the experiments, but tap water was provided ad libitum.

2.2.2. Sample Preparation. Animals were euthanized on the last day. Blood samples were collected and centrifuged at 3000 ×g for 10 min at 4°C. The supernatants were separated and stored at −80°C for metabolomics analysis. An Olympus AU5400 (Olympus, Tokyo, Japan) automated clinical biochemistry analyzer was employed to measure the serum ALT, AST, TC, TG, HDL-c, and LDL-c. Portions of liver tissues were excised, fixed in 4% paraformaldehyde solution, and stained with hematoxylin and eosin.

2.2.3. Western Blotting. Liver tissue (0.1 g) was homogenized and subsequently lysed in ice-cold lysis buffer containing 1 mM phenylmethylsulfonyl fluoride and a protease inhibitor mixture. The sample was centrifuged at 8000 ×g and 4°C for 10 min to remove any debris. After centrifugation, the supernatant was aliquoted and stored at −80°C for the western blotting assay to detect PEMT, PSD, and PLA2G4. Fifty micrograms of total liver protein was separated by 12% SDS-polyacrylamide gel electrophoresis and transferred to a nitrocellulose membrane. Immunodetection was performed using rabbit anti-PEMT antibody (1:1000), anti-PSD antibody (1:1000), anti-PLA2G4 antibody (1:1000), and anti-β

actin antibody (1 : 1000) in a solution of 5% milk in Tris-buffered saline and 0.05% Tween-20. After incubation with the appropriate secondary peroxidase-conjugated antibody, the membrane was washed in TBST for 60 min, and the immunoreactive bands were visualized with chemilumines-cence.

2.3. Handling of Serum Samples.
Six rats per group were analyzed. A total of 250 μL thawed serum samples and 750 μL prechilled acetonitrile were transferred to 1.5 mL polypropylene tubes, and the mixture was vortexed for 30 s and allowed to stand for 20 min at 4°C before use. The samples were centrifuged at 10,000 rpm for 10 min at 4°C, and the supernatant was transferred into new tubes.

2.4. Metabolic Profiling and Metabolite Analysis

2.4.1. Chromatography and Mass Spectrometry. An Agilent 6550 UHPLC-Q-TOF/MS system was used for analysis. A ZORBAX RRHD 300 SB-C18 column (2.1 × 100 mm, 1.8 μm, Agilent, USA) was performed to separate the serum constituents. Samples were maintained at 4°C and the column temperature was set at 30°C. The injection volume was set at 4 μL. The mobile phases were comprised of 0.1% formic acid in acetonitrile (solvent A) and 0.1% formic acid in water (solvent B). The gradient was operated at a flow rate of 0.30 mL/min employing a linear gradient of 95% A at 0.0–1.0 min, 95–60% A at 1.0–9.0 min, 60–10% A at 9.0–19.0 min, 10–0% A at 19.0–20.0 min, and 0% A at 20.0–25.0 min. A QC sample mixed with 10 μL in each sample was injected as a blank after every 5 samples were injected.

Electrospray capillary voltage was 3.0 kV in negative ionization mode and 4.0 kV in positive ionization mode. The gas temperature was 225°C in the ESI+ and 200°C in the ESI– mode. Gas flow was 11 L/min. Sheath gas temperature was 350°C and sheath gas flow was 12 L/min. Nozzle voltage was 500 V in both the negative and positive modes. The mass data were collected from m/z 80 to 1000 Da.

2.4.2. Statistical Analysis. Sample data were extracted by MassHunter Profinder software (Agilent, California, USA). Data were presented as mean ± SD and scaled to Pareto variance. The SPSS 20.0 software program (IBM, SPSS, Chicago, IL, USA) was used for the statistical analysis. The statistical significance between the groups was analyzed by ANOVA followed by Tukey's post hoc test, with $P < 0.05$ set as the confidence level of statistical significance (highly significant at $P < 0.01$).

2.4.3. Multivariate Data Analysis. The data were imported to SIMCA-P+ 13.0 software (Umetrics AB, Umea, Sweden) prior to modeling, and Pareto scaling and column centering were used for every variable. Then, multivariate statistical analyses, including PCA and PLS-DA were applied. These variables with a higher VIP value (VIP ≥ 1.0) and |p(corr)| ≥ 0.58 in OPLS-DA were further evaluated. Only the variables ($P < 0.05$ in ANOVA and above 2-fold changes) were selected as candidates and subjected to further identification.

2.4.4. Biomarkers Identification and Pathway Enrichment Analysis. Compounds with significant changes between groups (P value < 0.05 and fold-change > 2) were selected as biomarkers. The potential biomarkers were identified by Agilent MassHunter PCDL Manager software. 20 potential biomarkers and KEGG numbers were subjected to Metaboanalyst [18] (http://www.metaboanalyst.ca/) for further pathway enrichment analysis.

3. Results

3.1. Histopathological Observations and Biochemical Analysis.
Histological evaluations provided visual evidence for the injury of HFD-induced NAFLD and the protective efficacy of TE on NAFLD. As demonstrated in Figure 1, oil red O staining showed that HFD rats developed severe macrosteatosis (Figure 1(a1)) and H&E staining showed an increase in ballooning degeneration and inflammation in the liver of HFD groups, whereas no such change was observed in the control group (Figure 1(a2)). These changes were more prominent in the model group than in other groups. The generally required histopathologic observations for NAFLD diagnosis are macrosteatosis, lobular inflammation, and hepatocyte ballooning. These three features were all observed in the HFD rats. After being treated with TE doses, macrosteatosis, lobular inflammation, and hepatocyte ballooning were ameliorated.

Morphological changes were assessed and the scoring of morphological changes was shown in Table 1. The livers of the control group had no signs of macrovesicular steatosis. Minimal microvesicular steatosis and minimal lobular and portal inflammatory changes were present. The livers of the HFD rats showed evidence of mild to moderate deposition of macrovesicular and microvesicular steatosis. After being treated with TE doses, macrovesicular and microvesicular steatosis and portal inflammation were significantly reduced in HD-TE and MD-TE livers.

To evaluate the therapeutic effects of TE, the levels of ALT, AST, TG, TC, HDL, and LDL in serum were compared with those of control groups. As shown in Figure 1(b), HFD-induced liver injuries in the model group rats were significantly different compared with the control group. The results showed that AST and TG were significantly elevated in HFD-induced liver injuries, but serum AST and TG levels showed no significant change in administered groups compared with the model group. However, the serum level of ALT was significantly reduced after being treated with HD, MD, and LD-TE groups, respectively. In addition, the other biochemical indices, including serum TC, HDL, and LDL, were decreased significantly in rats treated with 3 doses (Figures 1(b)–1(g)).

3.2. Multivariate Statistical Analysis and Potential Biomarkers.
PCA was initially used as an unsupervised statistical method to study the metabolomic differences between control, model, positive control, and TE dose groups. A score plot provided a direct image of observational clusters. As shown in Figures 2(a) and 2(b), the clustering significantly differed between the control group, model group, and HD-TE group. However,

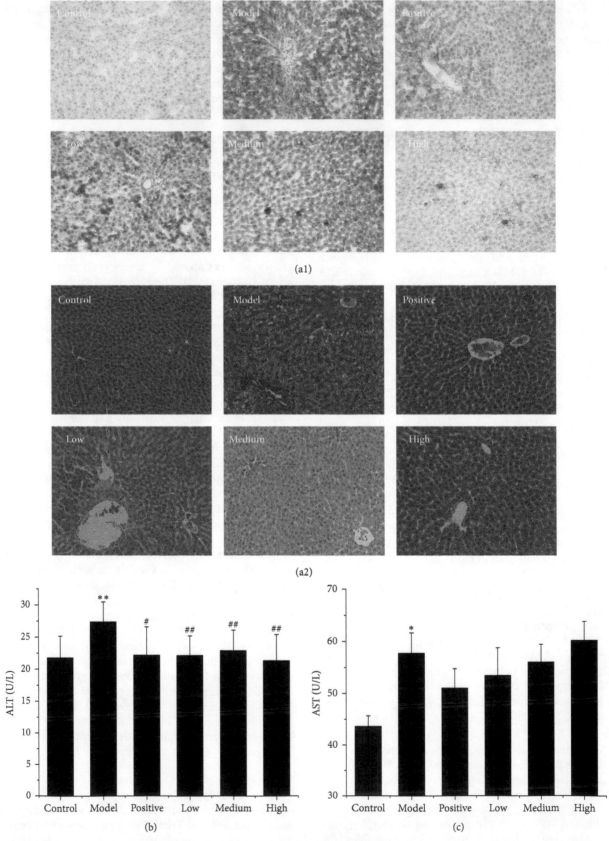

FIGURE 1: Continued.

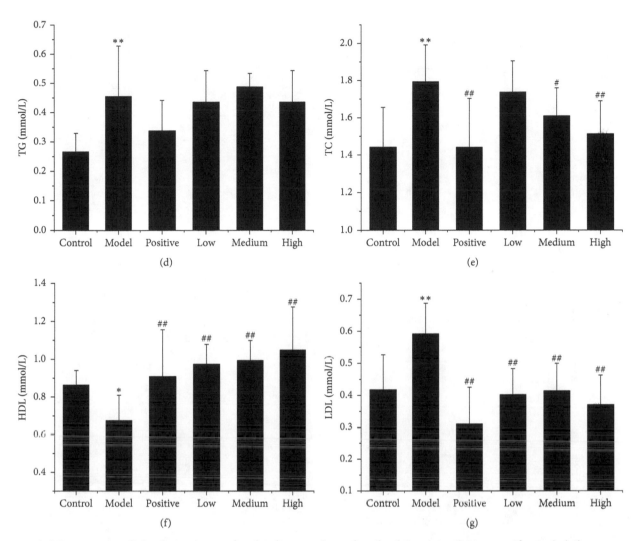

FIGURE 1: (a1) Representative light photomicrographs of rat liver specimens for oil red O staining (200x magnification); (a2) representative light photomicrographs of rat liver specimens for H&E analysis (200x magnification); (b–g) the serum levels of liver function indexes were assayed. (b) ALT; (c) AST; (d) TG; (e) TC; (f) HDL-c; (g) LDL-c. Data are expressed as the mean ± SD; control: control group; model: HFD group; positive: positive control group (CMCB); low: LD-TE; medium: MD-TE; high: HD-TE. $^{**}P < 0.01$, $^{*}P < 0.05$ compared with the control group; $^{##}P < 0.01$, $^{#}P < 0.05$ compared with the model group.

the clustering did not distinguish the model group, LD-TE group, and MD-TE group well in PCA. The results of the PCA indicated that the model of NAFLD induced by HFD was successfully reproduced, and HD-TE had a better effect on NAFLD. Further multivariate statistical analysis was necessary to discern the relationship among control, model, and HD-TE groups.

Supervised OPLS-DA is a powerful method to pick out discriminating ions that are contributing to the classification of samples and remove noncorrelated variations contained within spectra. Thus, OPLS-DA was applied to investigate potential biomarkers between the control group, model group, and HD-TE group. As shown in OPLS-DA score plot (Figures 2(c) and 2(d)), there was a distinguished classification among the clustering of the normal, model, and HD-TE groups in the ESI+ mode and ESI− mode, suggesting that metabolic profiles significantly changed in 3 groups. Commonly, the R^2Y and Q^2Y provide an estimate of predictive ability in OPLS-DA model. In the ESI+ model, the parameters for classification from the software were $R^2Y = 0.937$ and $Q^2Y = 0.819$, and, in the ESI− model, $R^2Y = 0.930$ and $Q^2Y = 0.722$, respectively, indicating that the OPLS-DA model was well established. To further demonstrate that the responsibility of each ion is more intuitive in these variations, an S-plot was employed (Figures 2(e) and 2(f)). The more away a red triangle is from the origin, the more influence it would have on the separation of samples. Thus, the further metabolite ions from the origin exhibiting a higher VIP and $|p(\text{corr})|$ were potential biomarkers, which are responsible for the difference between 3 groups. In this work, VIP ≥ 1.0 and $|p(\text{corr})| ≥ 0.58$ were used as a screening standard to select potential metabolites. We marked the variables with red triangles according to their VIP value and $|p(\text{corr})|$ in ESI+ mode and ESI− mode.

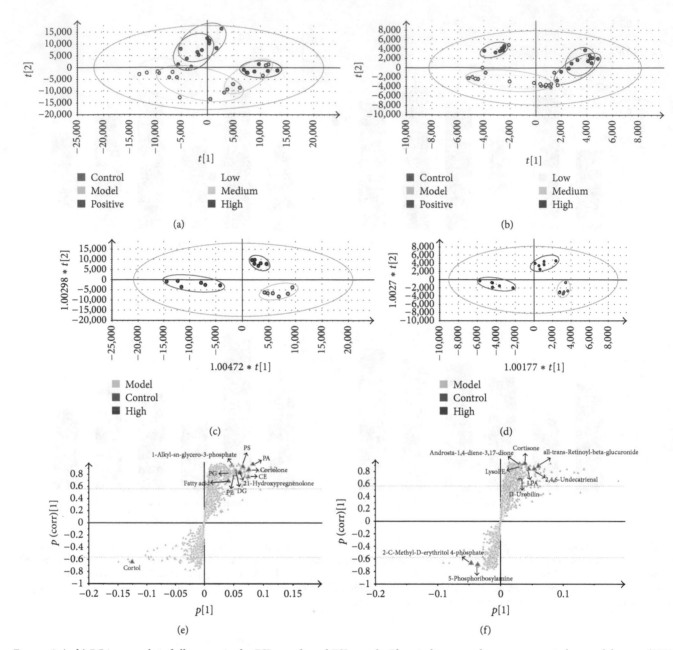

Figure 2: (a, b) PCA score plot of all groups in the ESI+ mode and ESI− mode. Blue circles: control group; green circles: model group (HFD group); violet circles: positive control group (CMCB); yellow circles: LD-TE group; cyan circles: MD-TE group; red circles: HD-TE group. (c, d) OPLS-DA score plot of the control group, model group, and HD-TE group in ESI+ mode and ESI− mode. (e, f) S-plot of the control group, model group, and HD-TE group in ESI+ mode and ESI− mode.

3.3. Identification of Potential Metabolites.

620 variables were selected as the candidates according to a threshold of VIP ≥ 1.0, and $|p(\text{corr})| \geq 0.58$ in OPLS-DA among the 2000 peaks. Then, candidates that differed among the groups with a significant P value below 0.05 and a fold-change greater than 2 times were identified with the PCDL database. Finally, 20 potential biomarkers showed significant differences among the three groups. The corresponding retention time, m/z, formula of the biomarkers, and variation trends in the different groups are listed in Table 1. The detailed changes

of potential biomarkers were also identified among the two respective groups.

3.4. Changes in Potential Metabolites in NAFLD with Different Doses of TE Treatment.

To further evaluate the reversed condition of the potential biomarkers by administration of TE doses more intuitively, we analyzed changes in 20 potential metabolites. The relative peak intensities of the 20 metabolites identified in different groups were shown in Figure 3. Compared with the control group, metabolites 13 and 16 were

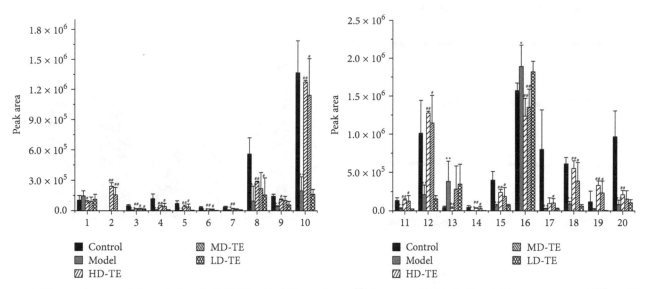

FIGURE 3: Changes in potential metabolites in NAFLD with different doses of TE treatment. Metabolites 1–20 were shown in Table 2. $^{**}P <$ 0.01, $^{*}P < 0.05$ compared with the control group; $^{##}P < 0.01$, $^{#}P < 0.05$ compared with the model group.

TABLE 2: List and change trends of differential metabolites.

Number	RT (min)	Mass (m/z)	Metabolites	Formula	Model trend[a]	HD-TE trend[b]
1	0.95	206.0419	2-C-Methyl-D-erythritol 4-phosphate	$C_5H_{13}O_7P$	↑	↓[#]
2	5.12	229.0371	5-Phosphoribosylamine	$C_5H_{12}NO_7P$	—	↑[##]
3	14.46	360.1873	Cortisone	$C_{20}H_{28}O_5$	↓[**]	↑[##]
4	15.24	284.1776	Androsta-1,4-diene-3,17-dione	$C_{19}H_{24}O_2$	↓[**]	↑[##]
5	15.95	476.2441	all-trans-Retinoyl-beta-glucuronide	$C_{26}H_{36}O_8$	↓[**]	↑[##]
6	16.17	535.3668	1-Acyl-sn-glycero-3-phosphoethanolamine (LysoPE)	$C_{27}H_{54}NO_7P$	↓[**]	↑
7	16.34	434.2463	1-Acyl-sn-glycerol-3-phosphate [LPA(18:2(9Z,12Z)/0:0)]	$C_{20}H_{39}O_7P$	↓[**]	↑[##]
8	17.19	757.5842	Phosphatidylethanolamine [PE(15:0/22:2(13Z,16Z))]	$C_{42}H_{80}NO_8P$	↓[**]	↑[#]
9	17.20	164.1220	2,4,6-Undecatrienal	$C_{11}H_{16}O$	↓[**]	↑[##]
10	17.42	368.2563	Cortol	$C_{20}H_{36}O_5$	↓[**]	↑[##]
11	17.45	332.2351	21-Hydroxypregnenolone	$C_{20}H_{32}O_3$	↓[**]	↑[##]
12	17.46	366.2473	Cortolone	$C_{20}H_{34}O_5$	↓[**]	↑[##]
13	18.49	408.3038	4Z,7Z,10Z,13Z,16Z,19Z,22Z,25Z-Octacosaoctaenoic acid (fatty acid)	$C_{28}H_{40}O_2$	↑[**]	↓[##]
14	19.31	588.2944	D-Urobilin	$C_{33}H_{40}N_4O_6$	↓[**]	↑[##]
15	20.48	424.3008	1-Alkyl-sn-glycero-3-phosphate (1-octadecyl lysophosphatidic acid)	$C_{20}H_{45}O_6P$	↓[**]	↑[##]
16	22.63	428.3684	Cholesteryl ester (CE(12:0))	$C_{29}H_{48}O_2$	↑[*]	↓[##]
17	22.74	686.4913	1,2-Diacyl-sn-glycerol	$C_{45}H_{66}O_5$	↓[**]	↑[#]
18	22.76	720.4941	Phosphatidylglycerol [PG(14:0/18:1(9Z))]	$C_{38}H_{73}O_{10}P$	↑[*]	↓[##]
19	22.93	727.4572	Phosphatidyl-L-serine [PS(14:1(9Z)/18:3(9Z,12Z,15Z))]	$C_{38}H_{66}NO_{10}P$	↓	↑[##]
20	23.04	660.5034	1,2-Diacyl-sn-glycerol 3-phosphate PA(P-20:0/14:0)	$C_{37}H_{73}O_7P$	↓[**]	↑[##]

[a]Compared to the normal group. [b]Compared to the model group. The significantly changed biomarkers were flagged with (↓) downregulated, (↑) upregulated, and (—) invalid data; $^{*,#}P < 0.05$, $^{**,##}P < 0.01$.

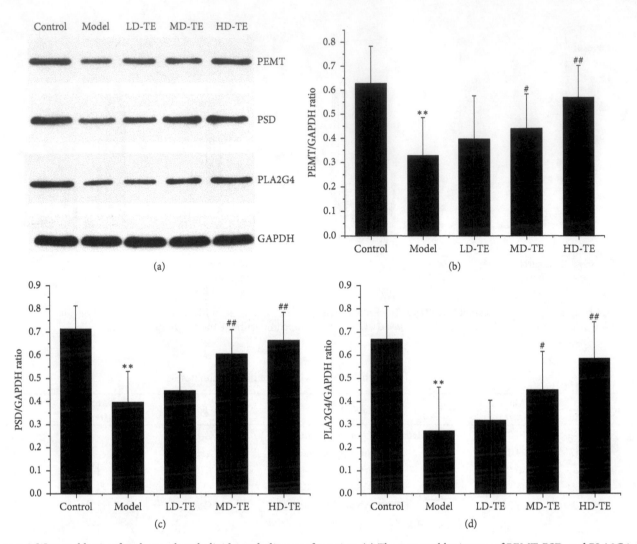

FIGURE 4: Western blotting for glycerophospholipid metabolism confirmation. (a) The western blot images of PEMT, PSD, and PLA2G4; (b) PEMT protein level in liver tissue; (c) PSD protein level in liver tissue; (d) PLA2G4 protein level in liver tissue. $^{**}P < 0.01$, compared with the control group; $^{##}P < 0.01$, $^{#}P < 0.05$ compared with the model group; control: control group; model: HFD group.

both significantly upregulated; meanwhile the significantly downregulated 4, 5, 6, 7, 9, 14, 8, 10, 11, 12, 15, 17, 18, and 20 were both identified in NAFLD group. The significantly perturbed metabolite was most pronounced in response to the distinction between NAFLD and healthy states. Additionally, compared to the NAFLD group, biomarkers 1, 2, 4, 5, 7, 8, 9, 10, 11, 12, 13, 14, 15, 16, 17, 18, 19, and 20 were significantly reversed in the TE-treated group, and the other metabolites were also reversed to different degrees.

3.5. Western Blotting for Bile Acid Metabolism Confirmation. To ensure that TE primarily exerts its effect by regulating glycerophospholipid metabolism, we further explored the protein expressions of several zymoproteins such as PEMT, PSD, and PLA2G4. The results showed that the expression of PEMT, PSD, and PLA2G4 was markedly decreased in NAFLD rats compared with the control. Furthermore, treatment with HD-TE significantly increased the low expression levels of

PEMT, PSD, and PLA2G4 in rats. However, these increases were limited in response to MD-TE and LD-TE (shown as in Figure 4).

4. Discussion

With the rapid growth of prevalence, NAFLD has become a common cause of chronic liver disease with a complex molecular pathogenesis. As reported previously, many pharmacological actions have been employed in NAFLD treatment [19, 20]. However, there are no widely accepted effective and safe medical therapy strategies for the treatment of NAFLD. Given this condition, the literature has reported the therapeutic effects of traditional Chinese medicine on NAFLD [4, 21, 22]. And *C. longa* was widely used for the treatment of NAFLD for many years [23].

In this study, the NAFLD model in rats was successfully reproduced, and TE was performed to treat NAFLD. Further,

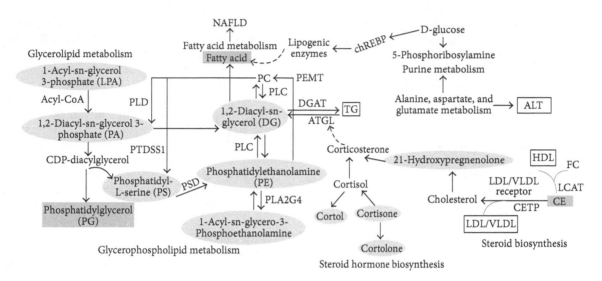

FIGURE 5: Schematic diagram of the disturbed metabolic pathway related to NAFLD and HD-TE treatment. The notations are as follows: yellow rectangle: metabolites increased in model group compared with control group; blue ovals: metabolites decreased in model group compared with control group; red metabolites: increased in HD-TE group compared with model group; and blue metabolites: decreased in HD-TE compared with model group; PEMT: phosphatidylethanolamine N-methyltransferase; PSD: phosphatidylserine decarboxylase; PLA2G4: phospholipase A2G4; ATGL: adipose triglyceride lipase; LCAT: lecithin cholesterol acyl transferase; CETP: cholesteryl ester transfer protein; PLC: phospholipase C.

metabolomics and multivariate statistical analysis were used to analyze serum samples. Here, potential biomarkers associated with NAFLD were further analyzed, and the networks correlated with the potential biomarkers, the main disturbed metabolic pathway related to NAFLD, and the possible metabolic mechanisms of HD-TE treatment are summarized in Figure 5.

As demonstrated in Figure 5, we found that most pathways of the potential biomarkers were related to glycerophospholipid metabolism, glycerolipid metabolism, and steroid hormone biosynthesis according to the KEGG pathway maps (01100, metabolic pathways). Several lipid mediators typically associated with lipotoxicity such as diacylglycerols (DGs), oxysterols, and fatty acids are commonly found in metabolic syndrome, insulin resistance, and type 2 diabetes [24], which are frequent comorbidities associated with NAFLD [25].

Fatty acids are common lipid mediators produced by fatty acid synthases from acetyl-CoA and malonyl-CoA precursors, by lipases in the degradation of glycerolipids, or by phospholipase in the breakdown of glycerophospholipids [26]. NAFLD results from imbalanced lipid homeostasis in the liver, which may be induced by HFD. In agreement with this, the elevation of fatty acid was detected in the serum. Despite the fundamental physiological importance, an oversupply of FAs is highly detrimental, leading to impaired membrane function, mitochondrial dysfunction, inflammation, and cell death [27]. In this study, the increased fatty acid provided the evidence of decreased DG and glycerophospholipids.

In this study, 6 biomarkers were related to glycerophospholipid metabolism, and 3 biomarkers were associated with glycerolipid metabolism. The levels of LPA, PA, PE, LysoPE, PS, and DG were elevated, indicating the glycerophospholipid and glycerolipid metabolism were inhibited. LPA, a lysophospholipid, the second product of reactions catalyzed by phospholipase A2, is rapidly acylated with acyl-CoA, resulting in the maintenance of the normal and essential neural membrane glycerophospholipid composition. However, under pathological situations (ischemia), the overstimulation of phospholipase A2 results in a rapid generation and accumulation of free fatty acids, resulting in inflammation, oxidative stress, and neurodegeneration [28]. It was reported that a 20% reduction in the hepatic PA content and 35% reduction in the PA/LPA ratio was observed in NAFLD rats with expression of PNPLA3, which were associated with a 50% reduction in hepatic DG content and increased hepatic insulin sensitivity [29]. In addition, all mammalian cell types synthesized hepatocytes PC is synthesized by the sequential methylation of PE, a reaction catalyzed by the enzyme PEMT. The conversion of PE to PC catalyzed by PEMT was impaired, which corroborates previous findings showing that the deficiency of the PEMT pathway led to hepatic TG accumulation [30]. Accordingly, the inhibition of glycerophospholipid and glycerolipid metabolism were closely associated with NAFLD. In HD-TE group, the downregulated PG and upregulated DG, PE, LysoPE, PS, and LPA were detected. As a result, concentration of FAs and TG was decreased. Therefore, HD-TE markedly regulated the levels of these bioactive lipid molecules in the serum, which suggested that the observed prevention mechanism is closely related to elevated lipid metabolism and fatty acid metabolism.

Glucocorticoids and hypercortisolemia caused elevation of circulating FFAs. The basis of this phenomenon had been linked to the effect of glucocorticoids enhancing the adipose lipolysis response to various hormones [31]. A recent study revealed that physiological hypercortisolemia may contribute to potent stimulus of lipolysis. In this study, the levels of several glucocorticoids and hypercortisolemia, such as cortisone, cortol, cortolone, and 21-hydroxypregnenolone, were significantly decreased in NAFLD rats, indicating adipose lipolysis was inhibited. Notably, the metabolites were relevant to corticosterone, which had direct effects on ATGL, supporting the notion that glucocorticoids increase lipolysis through glucocorticoid-induced increases of lipase expression in response to treatment with HD-TE compared with NAFLD [32]. Finally, the lipolytic action of glucocorticoids liberates excess TG efflux from adipocytes to the bloodstream in HD-TE rats.

Abnormal cholesterol metabolism is closely related to HDL and LDL levels. The main atheroprotective mechanism of HDL is reverse cholesterol transport, whereby excess cholesterol is transported from peripheral tissues to the liver for elimination [33]. In contrast, cholesterol is removed from the liver to surrounding tissues by LDL, and LDL levels are related to the risk of atherosclerosis [34]. As shown in this network, HDL converts FC to CE by the LCAT enzyme. In humans, CE would be transferred to other lipoproteins by CETP, promoting the removal of CE from HDL in exchange for TG derived primarily from VLDL. Finally, it is absorbed in the liver by the VLDL/LDL receptor. Therefore, the downregulated level of CE indicates the regulation of abnormal cholesterol metabolism, contributing to regulated levels of HDL and LDL.

Lipid metabolism is regulated by multiple signaling pathways and generates a variety of bioactive lipid molecules, such as fatty acid, eicosanoids, DGs, PA, LPA, sphingosine, phosphatidylinositol-3 phosphate, and cholesterol, which are involved in the activation or regulation of different signaling pathways [27]. In this study, glycerophospholipid metabolism, glycerolipid metabolism, and steroid hormone biosynthesis were recognized as the main signaling pathways in NAFLD and TE treatment. Impaired glycerophospholipid metabolism and glycerolipid metabolism lead to the lipidosis in the liver, causing hepatocyte steatosis and inflammation. The changed metabolites, such as LPA, PA, PS, PE, DG, PG, and LysoPE, constitute both the phenotype and cause of the progression of NAFLD. In our study, several proteins in hepatocytes are also specifically changed during NAFLD, including PEMT, PSD, and PLA2G4. PEMT catalyzes PC synthesis from PE. Studies have shown that the deficiency of either of the PEMT pathways led to hepatic TG accumulation. PSD and PLA2G4 are the enzymes that catalyze PS and PE metabolism. Our data indicated that the expressions of PEMT, PSD, and PLA2G4 were decreased in NAFLD rats. The lower expression of enzymes could cause accumulation of lipids. Treatment with HD-TE was able to significantly

increase the lower expression of PEMT, PSD, and PLA2G4 as well as bile acid such as LPA, PA, PS, PE, DG, PG, and LysoPE, indicating that the regulation of lipid metabolism effect of HD-TE on NAFLD was probably associated with the glycerophospholipid metabolism and glycerolipid metabolism signaling pathways. Furthermore, the in vitro effects of cortisol and cortisone on basal and stimulated lipolysis in human adipose tissue were studied in previous studies [35, 36]. Several glucocorticoids and hypercortisolemia, such as cortisone, cortol, cortolone, and 21-hydroxypregnenolone were detected in our study, and they may ultimately regulate lipolysis associated with the steroid hormone biosynthesis. In addition, the degradation of TG to DG was catalyzed by ATGL [37, 38], which catalyzed the initial step of lipolysis. As shown in schematic diagram, ATGL was affected by the upregulated 21-hydroxypregnenolone in the HD-TE group, and it was activated by downregulated CE associated with steroid biosynthesis. Therefore, the lipolytic effect of HD-TE was also probably relative to the steroid biosynthesis signaling pathways. Thus TE had powerful combined effects of regulating lipid metabolism by affecting glycerophospholipid metabolism, glycerolipid metabolism, and steroid hormone biosynthesis signaling pathways.

In this study, a UHPLC-Q-TOF-MS-based metabolomics approach was applied to investigate the biomarkers of NAFLD with the administration of TE. According to the metabolic pathways of these significantly changed metabolites, it is confirmed that TE had powerful combined effects of regulating lipid metabolism by affecting glycerophospholipid metabolism, glycerolipid metabolism, and steroid hormone biosynthesis signaling pathways. Moreover, the effects of glucocorticoids on adipose tissue metabolism are conflicting, and the contradictory effects of glucocorticoids on lipid metabolism occur through a number of different mechanisms, some of which are well defined and others remain to be elucidated. Our study can be applied in glucocorticoids on lipid metabolism research in the future.

5. Conclusion

A serum metabolomic study based on UHPLC-Q-TOF-MS was successfully performed to explore potential biomarkers in NAFLD and investigate the mechanism of TE treatment on NAFLD. With the help of serum biochemistry and histopathology, the HFD-induced NAFLD was confirmed. The control, model, and HD-TE groups were successfully discriminated by PCA and OPLS-DA. As a result, 20 significantly changed metabolites were identified as potential biomarkers associated with HD-TE of NAFLD. All the data yielded the conclusion that TE could reverse the pathological process of NAFLD through the powerful combined effects of regulating lipid metabolism by affecting glycerophospholipid metabolism, glycerolipid metabolism, and steroid hormone biosynthesis signaling pathways. The results implied that a UHPLC-Q-TOF-MS-based metabolomics approach could provide a systematic view of the characteristics of NAFLD. It also offered better guidance for the investigation of safe and effective herbal medicines for the prevention or treatment of NAFLD.

Abbreviations

NAFLD: Nonalcoholic fatty liver disease
TE: Total turmeric extract
HFD: High-fat diet
CMCB: Compound Methionine and Choline Bitartrate Tablets
TCM: Traditional Chinese medicine
HD-TE: High dose of total turmeric extract
MD-TE: Medium dose of total turmeric extract
LD-TE: Low dose of total turmeric extract
ALT: Alanine amino transferase
AST: Aspartate amino transferase
TG: Triglyceride
TC: Total cholesterol
HDL-c: High-density lipoprotein cholesterol
LDL-c: Low-density lipoprotein cholesterol
PCA: Principal component analysis
OPLS-DA: Orthogonal partial least squares
PA: 1,2-Diacyl-sn-glycerol 3-phosphate
PG: Phosphatidylglycerol
PS: Phosphatidyl-L-serine
PE: Phosphatidylethanolamine
PC: Phosphatidylcholine
CE: Cholesteryl ester
DG: Diglyceride
FC: Free cholesterol
LCAT: Lecithin cholesterol acyltransferase enzyme
CETP: CE transfer protein
VLDL: Very low-density lipoprotein
PEMT: Phosphatidylethanolamine N-methyltransferase
PSD: Phosphatidylserine decarboxylase
PLA2G4: Phospholipase A2G4
ATGL: Adipose triglyceride lipase
LCAT: Lecithin cholesterol acyl transferase
CETP: Cholesteryl ester transfer protein
PLC: Phospholipase C.

Competing Interests

The authors declare that they have no competing interests.

Authors' Contributions

Ya Wang, Ming Niu, and Ge-liu-chang Jia contributed equally to this work.

Acknowledgments

This work was supported by the Beijing Special Foundation of R&D in Ten Drugs for Ten Diseases (no. Z141100002204017).

References

[1] G. Marchesini, R. Marzocchi, F. Agostini, and E. Bugianesi, "Nonalcoholic fatty liver disease and the metabolic syndrome," Current Opinion in Lipidology, vol. 16, no. 4, pp. 421–427, 2005.

[2] K. D. Lindor, "Ursodeoxycholic acid for treatment of non-alcoholic steatohepatitis: results of a randomized, placebo-controlled trial," Gastroenterology, vol. 124, no. 4, pp. A708–A709, 2003.

[3] J. E. Lavine, J. B. Schwimmer, M. L. Van Natta et al., "Effect of vitamin e or metformin for treatment of nonalcoholic fatty liver disease in children and adolescents the tonic randomized controlled trial," The Journal of the American Medical Association, vol. 305, no. 16, pp. 1659–1668, 2011.

[4] H. Dong, F.-E. Lu, and L. Zhao, "Chinese herbal medicine in the treatment of nonalcoholic fatty liver disease," Chinese Journal of Integrative Medicine, vol. 18, no. 2, pp. 152–160, 2012.

[5] T. Y. C. Poon, K. L. Ong, and B. M. Y. Cheung, "Review of the effects of the traditional Chinese medicine Rehmannia Six Formula on diabetes mellitus and its complications," Journal of Diabetes, vol. 3, no. 3, pp. 184–200, 2011.

[6] A. M. Neyrinck, M. Alligier, P. B. Memvanga et al., "Curcuma longa extract associated with white pepper lessens high fat diet-induced inflammation in subcutaneous adipose tissue," PLoS ONE, vol. 8, no. 11, Article ID e81252, 2013.

[7] S. O. Nwozo, D. A. Osunmadewa, and B. E. Oyinloye, "Anti-fatty liver effects of oils from Zingiber officinale and Curcuma longa on ethanol-induced fatty liver in rats," Journal of Integrative Medicine, vol. 12, no. 1, pp. 59–65, 2014.

[8] S. Kaul and T. P. Krishnakantha, "Influence of retinol deficiency and curcumin/turmeric feeding on tissue microsomal membrane lipid peroxidation and fatty acids in rats," Molecular and Cellular Biochemistry, vol. 175, no. 1-2, pp. 43–48, 1997.

[9] R. K. Elahi, "Preventive effects of turmeric (Curcuma longa Linn.) powder on hepatic steatosis in the rats fed with high fat diet," Life Science Journal, vol. 9, no. 4, pp. 5462–5468, 2012.

[10] Y. Nishimura, Y. Kitagishi, H. Yoshida, N. Okumura, and S. Matsuda, "Ethanol extracts of black pepper or turmeric down-regulated SIRT1 protein expression in Daudi culture cells," Molecular Medicine Reports, vol. 4, no. 4, pp. 727–730, 2011.

[11] J. L. Griffin, "The Cinderella story of metabolic profiling: does metabolomics get to go to the functional genomics ball?" Philosophical Transactions of the Royal Society B: Biological Sciences, vol. 361, no. 1465, pp. 147–161, 2006.

[12] M. Wang, R.-J. A. N. Lamers, H. A. A. J. Korthout et al., "Metabolomics in the context of systems biology: bridging traditional Chinese medicine and molecular pharmacology," Phytotherapy Research, vol. 19, no. 3, pp. 173–182, 2005.

[13] X. Wang, H. Wang, A. Zhang et al., "Metabolomics study on the toxicity of aconite root and its processed products using ultraperformance liquid-chromatography/electrospray-ionization synapt high-definition mass spectrometry coupled with pattern recognition approach and ingenuity pathways analysis," Journal of Proteome Research, vol. 11, no. 2, pp. 1284–1301, 2012.

[14] H. Sun, A. Zhang, and X. Wang, "Potential role of metabolomic approaches for Chinese medicine syndromes and herbal medicine," Phytotherapy Research, vol. 26, no. 10, pp. 1466–1471, 2012.

[15] H. Zheng, J. Zhao, Y. Zheng et al., "Protective effects and mechanisms of total alkaloids of Rubus alceaefolius Poir on non-alcoholic fatty liver disease in rats," Molecular Medicine Reports, vol. 10, no. 4, pp. 1758–1764, 2014.

[16] W.-X. Zhao, X.-Y. Liu, and Y.-F. Shi, "Effect of Xiaozhi Hugan capsule on the pathologic changes and PPARα expression of rat models with non-alcoholic fatty liver disease," Journal of Traditional Chinese Medicine, vol. 11, article 33, 2007.

[17] E. M. Brunt, C. G. Janney, A. M. Di Bisceglie, B. A. Neuschwander-Tetri, and B. R. Bacon, "Nonalcoholic steatohepatitis: a proposal for grading and staging the histological lesions," *American Journal of Gastroenterology*, vol. 94, no. 9, pp. 2467–2474, 1999.

[18] J. Xia, N. Psychogios, N. Young, and D. S. Wishart, "MetaboAnalyst: a web server for metabolomic data analysis and interpretation," *Nucleic Acids Research*, vol. 37, supplement 2, pp. W652–W660, 2009.

[19] T. Foster, M. J. Budoff, S. Saab, N. Ahmadi, C. Gordon, and A. D. Guerci, "Atorvastatin and antioxidants for the treatment of nonalcoholic fatty liver disease: the St francis heart study randomized clinical trial," *American Journal of Gastroenterology*, vol. 106, no. 1, pp. 71–77, 2011.

[20] H. Tilg and A. Kaser, "Treatment strategies in nonalcoholic fatty liver disease," *Nature Clinical Practice Gastroenterology & Hepatology*, vol. 2, no. 3, pp. 148–155, 2005.

[21] J.-J. Li, J. Yang, W.-X. Cui et al., "Analysis of therapeutic effect of *Ilex hainanensis* Merr. extract on nonalcoholic fatty liver disease through urine metabolite profiling by ultraperformance liquid chromatography/quadrupole time of flight mass spectrometry," *Evidence-Based Complementary and Alternative Medicine*, vol. 2013, Article ID 451975, 12 pages, 2013.

[22] J. Pan, M. Wang, H. Song, L. Wang, and G. Ji, "The efficacy and safety of Traditional Chinese Medicine (Jiang Zhi Granule) for nonalcoholic fatty liver: a multicenter, randomized, placebo-controlled study," *Evidence-Based Complementary and Alternative Medicine*, vol. 2013, Article ID 965723, 8 pages, 2013.

[23] W.-F. Yiu, P.-L. Kwan, C.-Y. Wong et al., "Attenuation of fatty liver and prevention of hypercholesterolemia by extract of Curcuma longa through regulating the expression of CYP7A1, LDL-receptor, HO-1, and HMG-CoA reductase," *Journal of Food Science*, vol. 76, no. 3, pp. H80–H89, 2011.

[24] H. Malhi and G. J. Gores, "Molecular mechanisms of lipotoxicity in nonalcoholic fatty liver disease," in *Seminars in Liver Disease*, NIH Public Access, 2008.

[25] L. A. Adams, O. R. Waters, M. W. Knuiman, R. R. Elliott, and J. K. Olynyk, "NAFLD as a risk factor for the development of diabetes and the metabolic syndrome: an eleven-year follow-up study," *The American Journal of Gastroenterology*, vol. 104, no. 4, pp. 861–867, 2009.

[26] C. Huang and C. Freter, "Lipid metabolism, apoptosis and cancer therapy," *International Journal of Molecular Sciences*, vol. 16, no. 1, pp. 924–949, 2015.

[27] R. Zechner, R. Zimmermann, T. O. Eichmann et al., "FAT SIGNALS—lipases and lipolysis in lipid metabolism and signaling," *Cell Metabolism*, vol. 15, no. 3, pp. 279–291, 2012.

[28] A. A. Farooqui, L. A. Horrocks, and T. Farooqui, "Deacylation and reacylation of neural membrane glycerophospholipids: a matter of life and death," *Journal of Molecular Neuroscience*, vol. 14, no. 3, pp. 123–135, 2000.

[29] N. Kumashiro, T. Yoshimura, J. L. Cantley et al., "Role of patatin-like phospholipase domain-containing 3 on lipid-induced hepatic steatosis and insulin resistance in rats," *Hepatology*, vol. 57, no. 5, pp. 1763–1772, 2013.

[30] D. E. Vance, C. J. Walkey, and Z. Cui, "Phosphatidylethanolamine N-methyltransferase from liver," *Biochimica et Biophysica Acta—Lipids and Lipid Metabolism*, vol. 1348, no. 1-2, pp. 142–150, 1997.

[31] C. Xu, J. He, H. Jiang et al., "Direct effect of glucocorticoids on lipolysis in adipocytes," *Molecular Endocrinology*, vol. 23, no. 8, pp. 1161–1170, 2009.

[32] A. J. Peckett, D. C. Wright, and M. C. Riddell, "The effects of glucocorticoids on adipose tissue lipid metabolism," *Metabolism: Clinical and Experimental*, vol. 60, no. 11, pp. 1500–1510, 2011.

[33] E. J. Niesor and R. Benghozi, "Potential signal transduction regulation by HDL of the β2-adrenergic receptor pathway. implications in selected pathological situations," *Archives of Medical Research*, vol. 46, no. 5, pp. 361–371, 2015.

[34] K. M. Habegger, E. Grant, P. T. Pfluger et al., "Ghrelin receptor deficiency does not affect diet-induced atherosclerosis in low-density lipoprotein receptor-null mice," *Frontiers in Endocrinology*, vol. 2, article 67, 2011.

[35] M. Ottosson, P. Lönnroth, P. Björntorp, and S. Edèn, "Effects of cortisol and growth hormone on lipolysis in human adipose tissue," *Journal of Clinical Endocrinology and Metabolism*, vol. 85, no. 2, pp. 799–803, 2000.

[36] S. Werner and H. Low, "Stimulation of lipolysis and calcium accumulation by parathyroid hormone in rat adipose tissue in vitro after adrenalectomy and administration of high doses of cortisone acetate," *Hormone and Metabolic Research*, vol. 5, no. 4, pp. 292–296, 1973.

[37] J. Ling, T. Chaba, L.-F. Zhu, R. L. Jacobs, and D. E. Vance, "Hepatic ratio of phosphatidylcholine to phosphatidylethanolamine predicts survival after partial hepatectomy in mice," *Hepatology*, vol. 55, no. 4, pp. 1094–1102, 2012.

[38] B. M. Arendt, D. W. Ma, B. Simons et al., "Nonalcoholic fatty liver disease is associated with lower hepatic and erythrocyte ratios of phosphatidylcholine to phosphatidylethanolamine," *Applied Physiology, Nutrition, and Metabolism*, vol. 38, no. 3, pp. 334–340, 2013.

Identification of "Multiple Components-Multiple Targets-Multiple Pathways" Associated with Naoxintong Capsule in the Treatment of Heart Diseases Using UPLC/Q-TOF-MS and Network Pharmacology

Xianghui Ma,[1] **Bin Lv,**[1] **Pan Li,**[1] **Xiaoqing Jiang,**[1] **Qian Zhou,**[1] **Xiaoying Wang,**[1,2] **and Xiumei Gao**[1]

[1]*State Key Laboratory of Modern Chinese Medicine, Tianjin University of Traditional Chinese Medicine, Tianjin 300193, China*
[2]*College of Traditional Chinese Medicine, Tianjin University of Traditional Chinese Medicine, Tianjin 300193, China*

Correspondence should be addressed to Xiaoying Wang; wxy@tjutcm.edu.cn

Academic Editor: Carmen Mannucci

Naoxintong capsule (NXT) is a commercial medicinal product approved by the China Food and Drug Administration which is used in the treatment of stroke and coronary heart disease. However, the research on the composition and mechanism of NXT is still lacking. Our research aimed to identify the absorbable components, potential targets, and associated pathways of NXT with network pharmacology method. We explored the chemical compositions of NXT based on UPLC/Q-TOF-MS. Then, we used the five principles of drug absorption to identify absorbable ingredients. The databases of PharmMapper, Universal Protein, and the Molecule Annotation System were used to predict the main targets and related pathways. By the five principles of drug absorption as a judgment rule, we identified 63 compositions that could be absorbed in the blood in all 81 chemical compositions. Based on the constructed networks by the significant regulated 123 targets and 77 pathways, the main components that mediated the efficacy of NXT were organic acids, saponins, and tanshinones. Radix Astragali was the critical herbal medicine in NXT, which contained more active components than other herbs and regulated more targets and pathways. Our results showed that NXT had a therapeutic effect on heart diseases through the pattern "multiple components-multiple targets-multiple pathways."

1. Introduction

Naoxintong capsule (NXT) is a commercial medicinal product approved by the China Food and Drug Administration which is widely used in the treatment of stroke and coronary heart disease. NXT contains 16 Chinese herbal medicines (Table 1). NXT exerts significant therapeutic effects and has high safety for stroke recovery in the clinical setting [1]. Recent studies showed that NXT could reduce the infarct size of acute myocardial infarction (AMI) patients by improving vascular endothelial function [2]. Long-term administration of NXT was also reported to alleviate inflammation, reduce the recurrence of angina pectoris, and decrease the incidence of ACS attack in borderline lesion coronary heart disease patients [3]. Some studies investigated the mechanisms of NXT in vitro or in vivo. NXT was reported to protect against atherosclerosis through its lipid-lowering activity [4] and to reduce the expression of iNOS mRNA and the NO level in the vessel wall to benefit the treatment of atherosclerosis [5]. NXT also protected cardiomyoblasts against H_2O_2-induced oxidative injury [6]. Although some mechanisms of NXT have been reported, existing studies on unilateral factors and single targets could not demonstrate the complex mechanisms of NXT, a herbal prescription with 16 medicines which is prescribed for the treatment of complex diseases like cardiovascular and cerebrovascular diseases.

With the prominence of network pharmacology in system biology, this distinct and novel approach to the study of complicated analytical systems is becoming more widely known and more frequently used in the field of drug research.

TABLE 1: Sixteen Chinese traditional medical herbs of NXT.

Abbreviation	Medicinal herbs	Original plants	Content (g)*
RA	Radix Astragali	*Astragalus membranaceus* (Fisch.) Beg. var. *mongholicus* (Bge.) Hsiao or *A. membranaceus* (Fisch.) Bge.	66
RPR	Radix Paeoniae Rubra	*Paeonia lactiflora* Pall. or *P. veitchii* Lynch	27
RSM	Radix Salviae Miltiorrhizae	*Salvia miltiorrhiza* Bge.	27
RAS	Radix Angelicae Sinensis	*Angelica sinensis (Oliv) Diels.*	27
RCX	Rhizoma Chuanxiong	*Ligusticum chuanxiong* Hort.	27
SP	Semen Persicae	*Prunus persica* (L.) Batsch or *Prunusdavidiana* (Carr.) Franch.	27
FC	Flos Carthami	*Carthamus tinctorius* L.	13
FK	Frankincense	*Boswellia carterii Birdw.*	13
MRH	Myrrha	*Commiphora myrrha* Engl.	13
CS	Caulis Spatholobi	*Spatholobus suberectus* Dunn	20
RAB	Radix Achyranthis Bidentatae	*Achyranthes bidentata* Bl. or *Cyathula officinalis* Kuan	27
RC	Ramulus Cinnamomi	*Cinnamomum cassia* Presl	20
RM	Ramulus Mori	*Morus alba* L.	27
PT	Pheretima	*Pheretima aspergillum* (E. Perrier) or *Pheretima vulgaris* Chen. or *Pheretima guillelmi* (Michaelsen) or *Pheretima pectinifera* Michaelsen	27
SCP	Scorpio	*Buthus martensii* Karsch	13
HRD	Hirudo	*Whitmania pigra* Whitman or *Hirudo nipponica* Whitman or *Whitmania acranulata* Whitman	27

*Note. The content of 16 Chinese traditional medical herbs of NXT came from Chinese Pharmacopoeia 2015.

The functions of network pharmacology include uncovering the functions of traditional Chinese medicines (TCMs), providing deeper insights into and scientific evidence for TCMs, and identifying TCMs as scientifically proven. Here, we attempt to explore the mechanism of NXT using this method.

In the current study, based on the use of UPLC/Q-TOF-MS to investigate the involved components, we aimed to analyse the absorbable components of NXT, to identify potential targets and associated pathways using the network pharmacology method, and to systematically discuss the mechanism of NXT in the treatment of heart diseases.

2. Material and Methods

2.1. Prediction of Components

2.1.1. Sample Preparation. NXT was obtained from Heze-Buchang Pharmaceutical Co., Ltd. (Heze, China). Deionized water was prepared from aqua distillate using a Milli-Q system (Millipore, Bedford, MA, USA). Analytical grade methanol was purchased from Merck (Darmstadt, Germany). We dissolved 1 g of NXT powder in 10 mL of 75% analytical grade methanol and subjected the mixture to ultrasonic extraction for 30 min. We then brought the solution to room temperature and obtained the supernatant as a capture reagent. The sample was filtered using a 0.22 μm microporous membrane before UPLC analysis.

2.1.2. UPLC/Q-TOF-MS. We used a Waters Acquity UPLC System (Waters Co., USA) furnished with a photodiode array detector for the analysis. The sample was diluted on a Waters Acquity UPLC BEH C18 column (2.1 mm × 100 mm, 1.7 μm). UV detection was achieved at 190–400 nm. The system was controlled using the MassLynx version 4.1 software (Waters Co.). The gradient duration program for A (UPLC-grade acetonitrile) and B (water with 0.1% formic acid) was performed as follows: 2% A from 0 min to 3 min, 10% to 50% A from 3 min to 12 min, 50% to 63% A from 12 min to 18 min, 63% to 83% A from 18 min to 21 min, 83% to 84% A from 21 min to 22 min, 84% to 87% A from 22 min to 26 min, 87% to 90% A from 26 min to 28 min, 90% to 95% A from 28 min to 31 min, 95% to 100% A from 31 to 33 min, 100% to 100% A from 33 to 35 min, and 100% to 2% A from 35 min to 37 min. The flow rate was maintained at 0.4 mL/min, and the column temperature was maintained at 30°C.

The components of NXT were identified using a Waters Q-TOF Premier with an electrospray ionization (ESI) system (Waters MS Technologies, Manchester, UK). The ESI-MS spectra were acquired at both negative and positive ion voltages. The capillary voltage was set to 2.5 kV for the negative mode and to 3.0 kV for the positive mode. The sample cone voltage was set to 30 V, and the source temperature was 110°C. High-purity nitrogen was used as the nebulization and auxiliary gas. The nebulization gas was set to 600 L/h, the cone gas was set to 50 L/h, and the desolation temperature was 350°C. The Q-TOF Premier acquisition rate was 0.1 s, and there was a 0.02 s interscan delay. Argon, which was

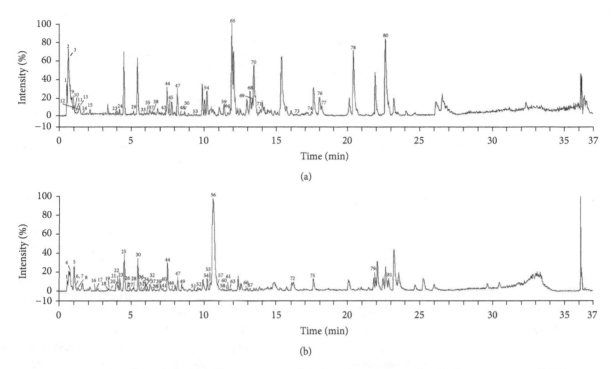

FIGURE 1: UPLC/Q-TOF-MS analysis of NXT. (a) Chromatograms of NXT in positive ion mode. (b) Chromatograms of NXT in negative ion mode.

used as the collision gas, was maintained at a pressure of 5.3×10^{-5} Torr. The instrument was operated with the first resolving quadruple in a wide pass mode (100 Da–1500 Da). Leucineen kephalinamide acetate was used as the lock mass ($[M - H]^{-} = 553.2775$, $[M + H]^{+} = 555.2931$).

2.2. Calculation and Prediction of Absorbable Components. First, we determined the structural formulas of the chemical components that were identified in compound NXT from the Chemical Book website and used the Chemdraw software to draw these formulas. Then, we imported these structural formulas into the Online SMILES Translator and Structure File Generator (http://cactus.nci.nih.gov/translate/) to obtain the smiles format. Finally, we input the smiles format of the chemical components into the Molispiration Smiles website (http://www.molinspiration.com/cgi-bin/properties) to calculate the prediction parameters of drug absorption. According to the five principles of drug absorption, if a component was subject to the following provisions of the corresponding parameters, it could be identified as an absorbable component: hydrogen bond donor (the number of hydrogen atoms attached to the O and N) $nOHNH \leq 5$; relative molecular mass MW ≤ 500; fat water partition coefficient miLog$P \leq 5$; and hydrogen bond acceptor (the number of O and N) $nON \leq 10$.

2.3. Prediction and Screening of Targets. Using the software of Chembio3D Ultrul2.0, we transformed the structure of the absorbed components into the sdf structure format. Then, to predict the possible targets, we imported the components into the public network server of the target database of the efficacy group PharmaMapper website

(http://59.78.96.61/pharmmapper/) to perform reverse docking. We selected the top 10 targets for subsequent study.

2.4. Prediction and Screening of Pathways. We imported the obtained targets into the Bio database (http://bioinfo.capitalbio.com/mas3/) and then screened for pathways that met the criterion of $P < 0.01$.

2.5. Construction of Network. According to the screening pathways with their corresponding targets and components, we created a component-target-pathway illustration using Cytoscape. Then, according to the main selected targets, we drew a target-composition diagram.

3. Results

3.1. UPLC/Q-TOF-MS Analysis. We analysed the chemical components of NXT using ultraperformance liquid chromatography combined with quadrupole time-of-flight mass spectrometry. Because different chemical components had better responses in different modes, MS data were obtained in both positive ion mode (Figure 1(a)) and negative ion mode (Figure 1(b)). MS data in (+/−) ESI modes and the identification results for the constituents in NXT were presented in Table 2. In all 16 herbs from NXT, no related component in Myrrha and Hirudo was found.

3.2. Absorption Parameters of Components. Using a computer prediction method to calculate the identified compounds of NXT, we obtained absorption parameters that could determine whether the chemical compositions could be absorbed.

TABLE 2: MS data in (+/−) ESI modes and the identification results for the constituents in NXT.

Peak number	RT (min)	Identification	Mode	MS (m/z)	Composition	Herbal source
1	0.647	Arginine	Pos/Neg	174.2024	$C_6H_{14}N_4O_2$	PT
2	0.702	Valine	Pos	117.1478	$C_5H_{11}NO_2$	PT
3	0.721	Proline	Pos	115.1331	$C_5H_9NO_2$	PT
4	0.776	Malic acid	Neg	134.0911	$C_4H_6O_5$	RA
5	1.053	Citric acid	Neg	192.1286	$C_6H_8O_7$	RA
6	1.201	D-5-oxoproline	Neg	129.1174	$C_5H_7NO_3$	RAS
7	1.201	L-5-oxoproline	Neg	129.1174	$C_5H_7NO_3$	RAS
8	1.275	Succinic acid	Neg	118.0910	$C_4H_6O_4$	RAS, RAB, PT
9	1.294	ρ-Coumaric acid	Pos	164.1601	$C_9H_8O_3$	RAS
10	1.310	o-Phthalic acid	Pos	166.1294	$C_8H_6O_4$	RAS
11	1.312	Adenosine	Pos	267.2403	$C_{10}H_{13}N_5O_4$	RAS, PT, RCX
12	1.331	Leucine	Pos	131.1688	$C_6H_{13}NO_2$	PT
13	1.460	Isoleucine	Pos	131.1688	$C_6H_{13}NO_2$	RAB
14	1.589	Gallic acid[a]	Neg	170.1207	$C_7H_6O_5$	RPR
15	2.199	Phenylalanine	Pos	165.1874	$C_9H_{11}NO_2$	FC
16	2.459	Danshensu	Neg	198.1701	$C_9H_{10}O_5$	RSM
17	2.606	Palmitic acid	Neg	256.3380	$C_{16}H_{32}O_2$	RAS, FC, RA, SCP
18	3.438	Senkyunolide B	Neg	204.2374	$C_{12}H_{12}O_3$	RCX
19	3.456	Senkyunolide C	Neg	204.2374	$C_{12}H_{12}O_3$	RCX
20	3.600	Protocatechuic aldehyde	Neg	138.1185	$C_7H_6O_3$	RSM, RC
21	3.974	Mulberroside A[a]	Neg	568.5277	$C_{26}H_{32}O_{14}$	RM
22	4.122	Gallicin	Neg	184.1453	$C_8H_8O_5$	RPR
23	4.230	Hydroxysafflor yellow A	Pos/Neg	612.5364	$C_{27}H_{32}O_{16}$	FC
24	4.232	7-Hydroxycoumarin	Pos	162.1457	$C_9H_6O_3$	RM
25	4.565	Vanillic acid	Neg	168.1459	$C_8H_8O_4$	RCX, RPR
26	4.694	Benzoic acid	Neg	122.1209	$C_7H_6O_2$	RPR
27	4.935	Epicatechin	Neg	290.2674	$C_{15}H_{14}O_6$	CS
28	5.157	Catechin	Neg	290.2674	$C_{15}H_{14}O_6$	RPR
29	5.212	Albiflorin	Pos	480.4653	$C_{23}H_{28}O_{11}$	RPR
30	5.730	Quercetin-7-O-glucoside	Neg	464.3754	$C_{21}H_{20}O_{12}$	FC
31	5.952	Rutin	Neg	610.5203	$C_{27}H_{30}O_{16}$	RA
32	5.970	Calycosin[a]	Neg	284.2679	$C_{16}H_{12}O_5$	RA
33	5.988	Calycosin-7-O-glucoside	Pos	446.4075	$C_{22}H_{22}O_{10}$	RA
34	5.989	Ferulic acid[a]	Neg	194.1815	$C_{10}H_{10}O_4$	RA, RCX, RAS, RAB
35	6.321	Paeoniflorin[a]	Pos	480.466	$C_{23}H_{28}O_{11}$	RPR
36	6.358	Pentagalloylglucose[a]	Neg	940.68	$C_{41}H_{32}O_{26}$	RPR
37	6.413	Kaempferol-3-O-rutinoside[a]	Pos/Neg	594.5179	$C_{27}H_{30}O_{15}$	FC
38	6.654	3,5-Di-O-caffeoylquinic acid[a]	Pos/Neg	516.4573	$C_{25}H_{24}O_{12}$	CS
39	6.987	Dicaffeoylquinic acid	Neg	516.1275	$C_{25}H_{24}O_{12}$	RCX
40	7.042	Z-Butylidenephthalide[a]	Neg	188.2259	$C_{12}H_{12}O_2$	RCX
41	7.210	Salvianolic acid A	Neg	494.4578	$C_{26}H_{22}O_{10}$	RSM
42	7.449	4-Hydroxyl-3-butylphthalide	Pos	206.2346	$C_{12}H_{14}O_3$	RCX
43	7.540	Salvianolic acid B	Neg	718.6220	$C_{36}H_{30}O_{16}$	RSM
44	7.688	Ononin	Pos	430.4107	$C_{22}H_{22}O_9$	CS
45	7.763	Senkyunolide F	Pos	206.1017	$C_{12}H_{14}O_3$	RCX, RAS
46	7.855	Salvianolic acid E	Neg	718.1512	$C_{36}H_{30}O_{16}$	RSM
47	8.243	Biochanin A	Pos/Neg	284.2689	$C_{16}H_{12}O_5$	CS
48	8.262	(6aR,11aR)-3-Hydroxy-9,10-dimethoxy pterocarpan	Pos	300.3107	$C_{17}H_{16}O_5$	RA
49	8.594	N1-N5-(Z)-N10-(E)-tri-p-coumaroylspermidine	Pos	583.2703	$C_{34}H_{37}N_3O_6$	FC

TABLE 2: Continued.

Peak number	RT (min)	Identification	Mode	MS (m/z)	Composition	Herbal source
50	8.740	Benzoylpaeoniflorin	Pos	584.5723	$C_{30}H_{32}O_{12}$	RPR
51	9.518	Pratensein	Neg	300.0679	$C_{16}H_{12}O_6$	RA
52	9.611	Hydroxyl calendic acid	Neg	294.4342	$C_{18}H_{30}O_3$	SP
53	9.648	Trans-oxyresveratrol	Pos	244.2435	$C_{14}H_{12}O_4$	RM
54	10.240	Formononetin[a]	Pos/Neg	268.2580	$C_{16}H_{12}O_4$	RA
55	10.405	Astragaloside IV	Neg	784.4633	$C_{41}H_{68}O_{14}$	RA
56	10.590	Senkyunolide H	Neg	220.2305	$C_{12}H_{12}O_4$	RCX
57	10.978	Astragaloside II	Neg	826.4701	$C_{43}H_{70}O_{15}$	RA
58	11.311	Soyasaponin I	Neg	942.5145	$C_{48}H_{78}O_{18}$	RA
59	11.422	Methyl tanshinonate	Pos	338.1087	$C_{20}H_{18}O_5$	RSM
60	11.588	Carnosic acid	Neg	332.4311	$C_{20}H_{28}O_4$	RSM
61	11.644	Kaempferol-3-O-glucoside	Neg	448.3752	$C_{21}H_{20}O_{11}$	FC
62	11.699	Hydroxytanshinone IIA	Pos	310.1199	$C_{19}H_{18}O_4$	RSM
63	11.792	3-Butylidene-7-hydroxyphalide	Neg	204.2331	$C_{12}H_{12}O_3$	RCX
64	11.921	Tanshinone II-B	Pos	310.1187	$C_{19}H_{18}O_4$	RSM
65	12.198	Senkyunolide A	Pos	192.2516	$C_{12}H_{16}O_2$	RCX
66	12.975	Salvianolic acid F	Neg	314.0735	$C_{17}H_{14}O_6$	RSM
67	13.196	Kumatakenin	Neg	314.3359	$C_{17}H_{14}O_6$	RA
68	13.233	3-n-Butylphthalide	Pos	190.2356	$C_{12}H_{14}O_2$	RCX
69	13.474	(Z)-ligustilide[a]	Pos	190.2109	$C_{12}H_{14}O_2$	RAS
70	13.483	(E)-ligustilide[a]	Pos	190.2109	$C_{12}H_{14}O_2$	RAS
71	13.917	Trijuganone B	Pos	280.1107	$C_{18}H_{16}O_3$	RSM
72	16.098	Cryptotanshinone[a]	Neg	296.3642	$C_{19}H_{20}O_3$	RSM
73	16.394	Senkyunolide M	Pos	278.1565	$C_{16}H_{22}O_4$	RCX
74	17.503	O-Phthalic anhydride	Pos	148.0207	$C_8H_4O_3$	FC
75	17.614	Chlorogenic acid[a]	Neg	354.3120	$C_{16}H_{18}O_9$	CS
76	18.076	Tanshinone IIA	Pos	294.3430	$C_{19}H_{18}O_3$	RSM
77	18.205	Angelicide	Pos	380.1917	$C_{24}H_{28}O_4$	RCX
78	20.460	Carthamidin	Pos	288.2575	$C_{15}H_{12}O_6$	FC
79	22.078	Linoleic acid	Neg	280.2387	$C_{18}H_{32}O_2$	SP
80	22.659	Acetyl-11-keto-β-boswellic acid	Pos/Neg	512.7458	$C_{32}H_{48}O_5$	FK
81	22.881	Oleanolic acid	Neg	456.3652	$C_{30}H_{48}O_3$	RSM

"a" refers to the component has been verified by standard substance.

Table 3 showed the specific absorption parameters of all of the components. The data indicated that there were a total of 63 chemical compositions (Figure 2) that met the five principles of drug absorption. As shown, 7 glycosides were identified. Although the relative molecular masses of those compounds were greater than 500, they could also be absorbed, because those compounds could be divided into two parts, including aglycones which mainly mediated drug efficacy and sugar chains in the body. So we could import these glycosides' aglycones into PharmMapper to obtain the relevant parameters. The results showed that both of these components were consistent with the five principles of drug absorption, so we considered that these 7 chemical compositions could be absorbed in the body.

3.3. Potential Targets and Pathways.
By importing 63 chemical compositions that were predicted to be absorbable into the PharmMapper database for directional docking,

we obtained a total of 123 targets. We then imported these targets into the Molecule Annotation System and obtained 77 pathways regulated by NXT with highly significant differences, from which we chose the top 40 pathways that met the criterion of $P < 0.01$ (Table 4). A total of 34 targets were related to these top 40 pathways, and HRAS, MAP2K1, and MAPK14 were associated with most of these pathways, so we considered these factors to be the main targets. As shown in Table 4, NFAT and hypertrophy of the heart (transcription in the broken heart) ranked first among these pathways.

In Table 5, these top 40 pathways were classified into 5 categories, which included pathways associated with heart diseases and blood vessels, metabolism, cell cycle (with proliferation and apoptosis), immunity, and other pathways. By classifying these pathways, we accessed and marked the corresponding medicinal materials of NXT (Table 5). In the pathways associated with heart diseases and blood vessels,

TABLE 3: Absorption parameters of the components.

Number	Compounds	MW	nON	nOHNH	miLogP	Results
1	Arginine	174.204	6	7	−3.632	×
2	Valine	117.15	3	3	−1.91	√
3	Proline	115.132	3	2	−1.723	√
4	Malic acid	134.087	5	3	−1.57	√
5	Citric acid	192.123	7	4	−1.983	√
6	D-5-oxoproline	129.115	4	2	−2.402	√
7	L-5-oxoproline	129.115	4	2	−2.402	√
8	Succinic acid	118.088	4	2	−0.655	√
9	ρ-Coumaric acid	164.160	3	2	1.43	√
10	o-Phthalic acid	166.132	4	2	1.034	√
11	Adenosine	267.245	9	5	−0.854	√
12	Leucine	131.175	3	3	−1.382	√
13	Isoleucine	131.175	3	3	−1.41	√
14	Gallic acid[a]	170.120	5	4	0.589	√
15	Phenylalanine	165.192	3	3	−1.231	√
16	Danshensu	198.174	5	4	−0.251	√
17	Palmitic acid	256.43	2	1	7.059	×
18	Senkyunolide B	204.225	3	1	2.81	√
19	Senkyunolide C	204.225	3	1	2.574	√
20	Protocatechuic aldehyde	138.122	3	2	0.759	√
21	Mulberroside A[a]	568.528	14	10	−0.852	√
22	Gallicin	184.147	5	3	0.848	√
23	Hydroxysafflor yellow A	612.54	16	12	−4.12	√
24	7-Hydroxycoumarin	162.144	3	1	1.511	√
25	Vanillic acid	168.148	4	2	1.187	√
26	Benzoic acid	122.123	2	1	1.848	√
27	Epicatechin	290.271	6	5	1.369	√
28	Catechin	290.271	6	5	1.369	√
29	Albiflorin	480.466	11	5	−1.636	×
30	Quercetin-7-O-glucoside	464.379	12	8	−0.104	×
31	Rutin	610.521	16	10	−1.063	√
32	Calycosin[a]	284.267	5	2	2.377	√
33	Calycosin-7-O-glucoside	446.408	10	5	0.59	√
34	Ferulic acid[a]	194.186	4	2	1.249	√
35	Paeoniflorin[a]	480.466	11	5	0.044	×
36	Pentagalloylglucose[a]	940.681	26	15	2.761	√
37	Kaempferol-3-O-rutinoside[a]	594.522	15	9	−0.574	√
38	3,5-Di-O-caffeoylquinic acid[a]	516.455	12	7	1.424	×
39	Dicaffeoylquinic acid	516.46	12	7	1.21	×
40	Z-Butylidenephthalide[a]	188.226	2	0	3.077	√
41	Salvianolic acid A	494.452	10	7	3.014	×
42	4-Hydroxyl-3-butylphthalide	206.241	3	1	3.42	√
43	Salvianolic acid B	718.620	16	9	1.615	×
44	Ononin	430.409	9	4	1.307	√
45	Senkyunolide F	206.24	3	1	1.72	√
46	Salvianolic acid E	718.62	16	10	2.83	×
47	Biochanin A	284.267	5	2	2.804	√
48	(6aR,11aR)-3-Hydroxy-9,10-dimethoxy pterocarpan	300.31	5	1	2.546	√
49	N1-N5-(Z)-N10-(E)-tri-p-coumaroylspermidine	538.68	9	5	4.3	×
50	Benzoylpaeoniflorin	584.574	12	4	2.472	×
51	Pratensein	300.27	6	3	2.09	√

TABLE 3: Continued.

Number	Compounds	MW	nON	nOHNH	miLogP	Results
52	Hydroxyl calendic acid	294.435	3	2	4.93	√
53	Trans-Oxyresveratrol	244.246	4	4	2.723	√
54	Formononetin[a]	268.268	4	1	3.095	√
55	Astragaloside IV	784.98	14	9	1.21	√
56	Senkyunolide H	220.224	4	2	2.314	√
57	Astragaloside II	827.02	15	8	1.91	√
58	Soyasaponin I	943.13	18	11	1.7	×
59	Methyl tanshinonate	338.36	5	0	0.93	√
60	Carnosic acid	332.440	4	3	4.603	√
61	Kaempferol-3-O-glucoside	448.380	11	7	0.125	×
62	Hydroxytanshinone IIA	310.35	4	1	3.24	√
63	3-Butylidene-7-hydroxyphthalide	204.225	3	1	2.81	√
64	Tanshinone II-B	310.35	4	1	2.97	√
65	Senkyunolide A	192.258	2	0	3.521	√
66	Salvianolic acid F	314.29	6	5	2.33	√
67	Kumatakenin	314.29	6	2	2.98	√
68	3-n-Butylphthalide	190.242	2	0	3.483	√
69	(Z)-Ligustilide[a]	190.242	2	0	2.927	√
70	(E)-Ligustilide[a]	190.242	2	0	2.927	√
71	Trijuganone B	280.32	3	1	3.9	√
72	Cryptotanshinone[a]	296.366	3	0	3.83	√
73	Senkyunolide M	278.35	4	1	2.55	√
74	O-Phthalic anhydride	148.12	3	0	0.93	√
75	Chlorogenic acid[a]	354.311	9	6	−0.453	×
76	Tanshinone IIA	294.350	3	0	4.158	√
77	Angelicide	380.48	4	0	5.73	×
78	Carthamidin	288.255	6	4	1.649	√
79	Linoleic acid	280.45	2	1	6.86	×
80	Acetyl-11-keto-β-boswellic acid	512.73	5	1	6.39	×
81	Oleanolic acid	456.71	3	2	6.72	×

Note. "√" means that component could be absorbed; "×" means that component could not be absorbed.
"a" refers to the component has been verified by standard substance.

RCX, RSM, and FC were the most important. In the regulation of metabolism, RA, RSM, and RCX showed diametrical effect. All the herbs except Semen Persicae (SP) were related metabolism pathways due to the current research. RA, RSM, RCX, and FC could regulate the pathways about cell cycle, proliferation, and apoptosis. Some other important pathways were also affected by some herbs like RA, RSM, and RCX, for example, Insulin Signaling Pathway and p38 MAPK Signaling Pathway.

3.4. Pharmacology Network of NXT. Using the Cytoscape software, we constructed a pharmacology network of NXT (Figure 3), which showed us the relationships of the top 40 pathways, targets, and chemical components. We obtained preliminary understanding of the mechanism of NXT through this network.

In this research, we found three major targets of NXT: HRAS, MAP2K1, and MAPK14, which were involved in most regulated pathways. By Figure 4, based on illustration of

the main targets with their corresponding compounds, we found the most effective ingredients of NXT were organic acids, saponins, and tanshinones. The main sources of organic acids were RA, RCX, RAS, and RAB. The saponins were mainly derived from RA. Meanwhile, tanshinones were mainly concentrated in RSM.

4. Discussion

The burden of cardiovascular and circulatory disease is becoming more and more serious, with cerebrovascular disease (CBD) and ischemic heart disease being the most serious [7]. As the causes of cardiovascular disease (CVD) and CBD are complicated, the symptoms of these diseases are also very diverse. NXT is commonly used during clinical treatment of CVD and CBD, and the effect of this drug is remarkable. Although complex traditional Chinese medicine has great significance for the treatment of complex diseases, some questions such as the material basis and the potential mechanisms remain unanswered.

TABLE 4: Top 40 Biocarta pathways regulated by NXT ($P < 0.01$).

Rank	Pathway	Count	P-value	q-value	Gene
1	NFAT and hypertrophy of the heart (transcription in the broken heart)	6	$5.75E - 10$	$3.58E - 09$	HRAS; GSK3B; MAPK14; FKBP1A; F2; MAP2K1
2	Phosphoinositides and their downstream targets	5	$1.39E - 09$	$8.47E - 09$	GSK3B; PDPK1; BTK; RAB5A; EEA1
3	Intrinsic Prothrombin Activation Pathway	4	$8.50E - 08$	$2.82E - 07$	F10; FGG; F11; F2
4	Bioactive Peptide Induced Signaling Pathway	4	$4.08E - 07$	$9.30E - 07$	HRAS; MAPK14; F2; MAP2K1
5	BCR Signaling Pathway	4	$4.88E - 07$	$1.08E - 06$	HRAS; MAPK14; BTK; MAP2K1
6	Estrogen-responsive protein Efp controls cell cycle and breast tumors growth	3	$6.40E - 07$	$1.34E - 06$	CDK2; ESR1; CDK6
7	Nuclear receptors in lipid metabolism and toxicity	4	$8.02E - 07$	$1.58E - 06$	CYP2C9; VDR; NR1H3; PPARA
8	Map kinase inactivation of SMRT corepressor	3	$1.53E - 06$	$2.48E - 06$	THRB; MAPK14; MAP2K1
9	MAP Kinase Signaling Pathway	5	$2.09E - 06$	$3.05E - 06$	HRAS; MAPK10; MAPK14; TGFBR1; MAP2K1
10	Extrinsic Prothrombin Activation Pathway	3	$2.99E - 06$	$4.05E - 06$	F10; FGG; F2
11	amiPathway	3	$5.17E - 06$	$6.40E - 06$	F10; FGG; F2
12	Roles of β-arrestin-dependent recruitment of Src kinases in GPCR signaling	3	$6.57E - 06$	$7.86E - 06$	HRAS; HCK; MAP2K1
13	Aspirin blocks signaling pathway involved in platelet activation	3	$8.19E - 06$	$9.49E - 06$	HRAS; F2; MAP2K1
14	Insulin Signaling Pathway	3	$2.03E - 05$	$2.03E - 05$	HRAS; INSR; MAP2K1
15	IL-2 Signaling Pathway	3	$2.37E - 05$	$2.29E - 05$	HRAS; MAP2K1; LCK
16	Role of ERBB2 in signal transduction and oncology	3	$2.37E - 05$	$2.29E - 05$	HRAS; ESR1; MAP2K1
17	Links between Pyk2 and MAP kinases	3	$2.74E - 05$	$2.45E - 05$	HRAS; MAPK14; MAP2K1
18	NF-κB activation by nontypeable Hemophilus influenzae	3	$2.74E - 05$	$2.45E - 05$	MAPK14; TGFBR1; NR3C1
19	Influence of Ras and Rho proteins on G1 to S transition	3	$3.14E - 05$	$2.82E - 05$	HRAS; CDK2; CDK6
20	fMLP induced chemokine gene expression in HMC-1 cells	3	$3.14E - 05$	$2.82E - 05$	HRAS; MAPK14; MAP2K1
21	Growth Hormone Signaling Pathway	3	$3.14E - 05$	$2.82E - 05$	HRAS; INSR; MAP2K1
22	Cell cycle: G1/S checkpoint	3	$4.06E - 05$	$3.37E - 05$	CDK2; GSK3B; CDK6
23	Fc epsilon receptor I signaling in mast cells	3	$4.58E - 05$	$3.70E - 05$	HRAS; BTK; MAP2K1
24	Signaling of hepatocyte growth factor receptor	3	$6.40E - 05$	$4.89E - 05$	HRAS; MET; MAP2K1
25	p38 MAPK signaling pathway	3	$7.85E - 05$	$5.76E - 05$	HRAS; MAPK14; TGFBR1
26	Keratinocyte differentiation	3	$1.13E - 04$	$7.81E - 05$	HRAS; MAPK14; MAP2K1
27	T cell receptor signaling pathway	3	$1.13E - 04$	$7.81E - 05$	HRAS; MAP2K1; LCK
28	TSP-1 induced apoptosis in microvascular endothelial cell	2	$1.46E - 04$	$9.59E - 05$	CASP3; MAPK14
29	The role of FYVE-finger proteins in vesicle transport	2	$1.46E - 04$	$9.59E - 05$	RAB5A; EEA1
30	Mechanism of gene regulation by peroxisome proliferators via PPARa(alpha)	3	$1.82E - 04$	$1.15E - 04$	HSP90AA1; NR1H3; PPARA
31	Visceral fat deposits and the metabolic syndrome	2	$1.95E - 04$	$1.21E - 04$	HSD11B1; NR3C1
32	RB tumor suppressor/checkpoint signaling in response to DNA damage	2	$2.50E - 04$	$1.44E - 04$	CDK2; CHEK1
33	Platelet Amyloid Precursor Protein Pathway	2	$2.50E - 04$	$1.44E - 04$	F11; F2
34	Fibrinolysis Pathway	2	$3.12E - 04$	$1.77E - 04$	FGG; F2
35	Corticosteroids and cardioprotection	2	$3.12E - 04$	$1.77E - 04$	HSP90AA1; NR3C1
36	Phosphorylation of MEK1 by cdk5/p35 downregulates the MAP kinase pathway	2	$3.81E - 04$	$2.09E - 04$	HRAS; MAP2K1

TABLE 4: Continued.

Rank	Pathway	Count	P-value	q-value	Gene
37	VEGF, hypoxia, and angiogenesis	2	$5.38E-04$	$2.79E-04$	HRAS; KDR
38	How progesterone initiates oocyte membrane	2	$6.27E-04$	$3.17E-04$	HRAS; PGR
39	IL-3 Signaling Pathway	2	$6.27E-04$	$3.17E-04$	HRAS; MAP2K1
40	Sprouty regulation of tyrosine kinase signals	2	$6.27E-04$	$3.17E-04$	HRAS; MAP2K1

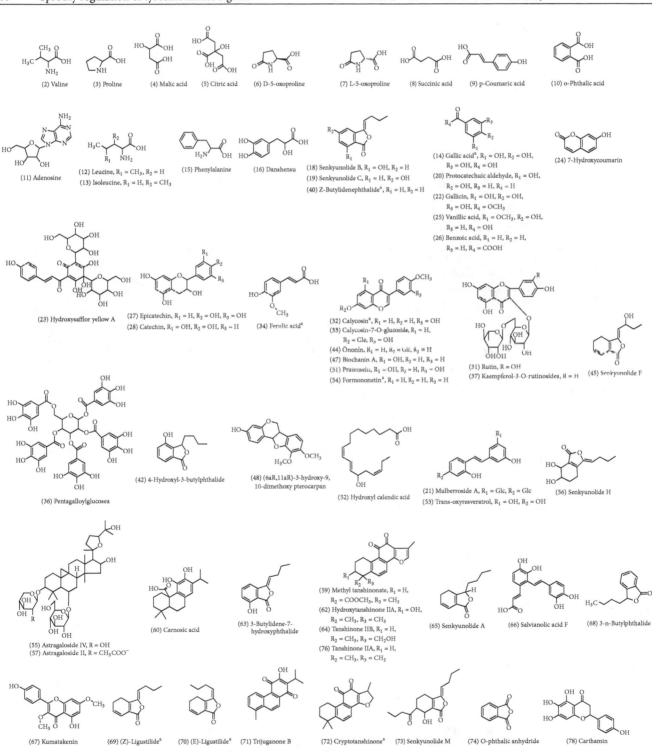

FIGURE 2: Structures of 63 absorbable components.

TABLE 5: The herbs of NXT involved in the top 40 pathways.

Category	Pathway	NXT	RA	RPR	RSM	RAS	RCX	SP	FC	CS	RAB	RC	RM	PT
Pathway associated with heart diseases and blood vessels	NFAT and hypertrophy of the heart (transcription in the broken heart)	1	1	1	1	1	1	0	1	1	1	1	1	1
	Intrinsic Prothrombin Activation Pathway	1	0	1	1	1	1	0	1	0	0	0	1	0
	Extrinsic Prothrombin Activation Pathway	1	0	1	1	1	1	0	1	0	0	0	0	0
	Aspirin blocks signaling pathway involved in platelet activation	1	1	1	1	1	1	0	1	1	1	1	1	1
	TSP-1 induced apoptosis in microvascular endothelial cell	1	1	1	1	1	1	0	1	0	0	0	0	0
	Platelet Amyloid Precursor Protein Pathway	1	0	0	0	0	1	0	1	0	0	0	1	0
	Fibrinolysis Pathway	1	0	1	1	0	1	0	1	0	0	1	0	0
	Corticosteroids and cardioprotection	1	1	0	1	0	1	0	0	0	0	0	1	0
	VEGF, hypoxia, and angiogenesis	1	1	1	1	1	1	1	1	1	1	1	1	1
Pathway associated with metabolism	Nuclear receptors in lipid metabolism and toxicity	1	1	1	1	0	1	1	1	0	1	0	1	0
	Growth Hormone Signaling Pathway	1	1	1	1	1	1	0	1	1	1	1	1	1
	Visceral fat deposits and the metabolic syndrome	1	1	0	1	1	1	0	0	0	0	0	0	0
Pathway associated with immunity	BCR Signaling Pathway	1	1	1	1	1	1	0	1	1	1	1	1	1
	IL-2 Signaling Pathway	1	1	1	1	1	1	0	1	1	1	1	1	1
	fMLP induced chemokine gene expression in HMC-1 cells	1	1	1	1	1	1	0	1	1	1	1	1	1
	T Cell Receptor Signaling Pathway	1	1	1	1	1	1	0	1	1	1	1	1	1
Pathway associated with cell cycle, proliferation, and apoptosis	Phosphoinositides and their downstream targets	1	0	0	1	0	1	0	1	1	0	0	0	0
	Estrogen-responsive protein Efp controls cell cycle and breast tumors growth	1	1	1	1	1	1	0	0	1	0	0	0	0
	Map kinase inactivation of SMRT corepressor	1	1	1	1	1	1	0	1	0	0	0	0	0
	MAP Kinase Signaling Pathway	1	1	1	1	1	1	0	1	1	1	1	1	1
	Roles of β-arrestin-dependent recruitment of Src kinases in GPCR signaling	1	1	1	1	1	1	0	1	1	1	1	1	1
	Role of ERBB2 in signal transduction and oncology	1	1	1	1	1	1	0	1	1	1	1	1	1
	Links between Pyk2 and MAP kinases	1	1	1	1	1	1	0	1	1	1	1	1	1
	NF-κB activation by nontypeable Hemophilus influenzae	1	1	0	1	1	1	0	1	0	0	0	0	0

TABLE 5: Continued.

Category	Pathway	NXT	RA	RPR	RSM	RAS	RCX	SP	FC	CS	RAB	RC	RM	PT
	Influence of Ras and Rho proteins on G1 to S transition	1	1	1	1	1	1	0	1	1	1	1	1	1
	Cell cycle: G1/S checkpoint	1	1	1	1	1	1	0	0	1	0	0	0	0
	Fc epsilon receptor I signaling in mast cells	1	1	1	1	1	1	0	1	1	1	1	1	1
	Signaling of hepatocyte growth factor receptor	1	1	1	1	1	1	0	1	1	1	1	1	1
	Keratinocyte differentiation	1	1	1	1	1	1	0	1	1	1	1	1	1
	RB tumor Suppressor/checkpoint signaling in response to DNA damage	1	1	1	1	1	1	0	0	1	0	0	0	0
	IL-3 Signaling Pathway	1	1	1	1	1	1	0	1	1	1	1	1	1
	Sprouty regulation of tyrosine kinase signals	1	1	1	1	1	1	0	1	1	1	1	1	1
Other pathways	Bioactive Peptide Induced Signaling Pathway	1	1	1	1	1	1	0	1	1	1	1	1	1
	amiPathway	1	0	1	1	1	1	0	1	0	0	0	0	0
	Insulin Signaling Pathway	1	1	1	1	1	1	0	1	1	1	1	1	1
	p38 MAPK Signaling Pathway	1	1	1	1	1	1	0	1	1	1	1	1	1
	The role of FYVE-finger proteins in vesicle transport	1	0	0	0	0	0	0	1	0	0	0	0	0
	Mechanism of gene regulation by peroxisome proliferators via PPARα	1	1	0	1	0	1	0	0	0	0	0	1	0
	Phosphorylation of MEK1 by cdk5/p35 downregulates the MAP kinase pathway	1	1	1	1	1	1	0	1	1	1	1	1	1
	How progesterone initiates oocyte membrane	1	1	1	1	1	1	1	1	1	1	1	1	1

Note. "1" means that the Chinese herbal medicine acts on the pathway while "0" means it does not. The pathways in each category are sorted by the significant differences in P value.

Our study successfully predicted absorbable chemical compositions of NXT. These constituents primarily included ferulic acid, succinic acid, astragaloside IV, and tanshinone IIA. Ferulic acid, which is derived primarily from RA, RCX, RAS, and RAB, is reported to act as an angiogenic agent that augments angiogenesis, which is critical in ischemic diseases, such as myocardial infarction and stroke [8]. Succinic acid has been demonstrated to activate Akt phosphorylation to inhibit apoptosis and necrosis caused by cardiomyocyte hypoxia/reoxygenation [9]. Previous studies demonstrated that astragaloside IV could protect the heart through NO-dependent mechanism [10]. NO has been confirmed to prevent the mitochondrial permeability transition pore from opening [11]. During early reperfusion, it can prevent the heart from reperfusion injury by inhibiting the opening of the mitochondrial permeability transition pore [12]. Tanshinone IIA also has cardioprotective effects, such as protection of cardiomyocytes from oxidative stress-triggered damage [13]. These reports were consistent with our results.

In addition to active ingredients, we also successfully predicted drug targets of NXT. The major targets were HRAS, MAP2K1, and MAPK14. The HRAS gene encodes the GTPase HRas, which is an enzyme known as transforming protein p21 [14]. With the ability to increase the effects of growth factor, HRas plays an important role in regulating the growth, differentiation, and death of endothelial cells [15]. The MAP2K1 gene encodes an enzyme named dual specificity mitogen-activated protein kinase kinase 1, and MAPK14 encodes p38-α. Both of these factors are closely related to inflammation and p38-α is also associated with cardiac hypertrophy via p38 MAPK activity in the heart. In addition, p38-α has been recognized as an isoenzyme of cardiovascular importance [16].

Among the numerous identified pathways, NFAT and hypertrophy of the heart (transcription in the broken heart) were ranked first. Nuclear factor of activated T-cells (NFAT) transcription factors, which have four different isoforms, plays crucial roles in the regulation of gene expression during

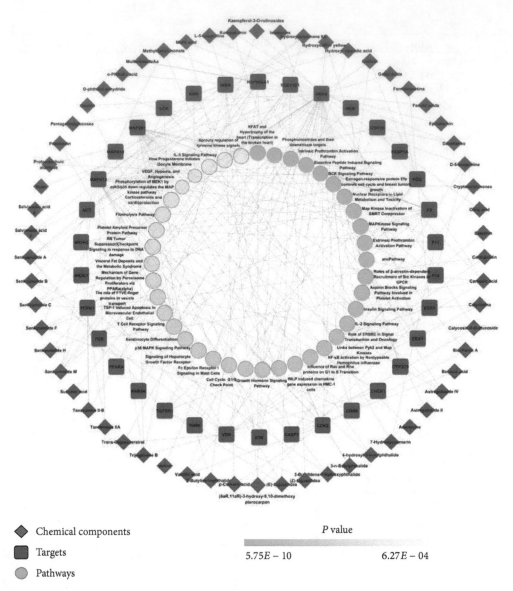

FIGURE 3: Pharmacology network of the "components-targets-pathways" regulated by NXT.

heart development [17]. The isoforms NFATc3 and NFATc4 are involved in hypertrophic development, while NFATc1 plays a key role in cardiac development [18]. The dephosphorylation of NFATs can promote calcineurin regulating immune response genes [19]. Via compensatory hypertrophy, the heart adapts to persistent stress conditions, but, over time, dysfunction and myocardial failure evolve [20]. Like NFAT and hypertrophy of the heart (transcription in the broken heart), most of these pathways are involved in the formation and regulation of cardiovascular disease, such as nuclear receptors in lipid metabolism and toxicity. Nuclear receptors include a superfamily of ligand-dependent transcription factors that regulate genetic networks that control cell growth, development, and metabolism. Regulating nuclear receptors is beneficial for patients with metabolic diseases, such as cardiovascular disease, due to the requirement for balance

among a number of pathways for normal metabolic control [21]. These studies confirmed the validity of our study.

From the above results, we also found the different significances of the total of 16 herbs in NXT. According to Chinese Pharmacopoeia 2015, the content of RA in NXT is 66 g, which is 2-3 times the content of any other herb in the whole prescription. It was reported that RA was the monarch drug of NXT and played a key role in improving the immune system, invigorating blood circulation, and the condition of myocardial ischemia and hypoxia [22]. Our study found that RA contained a lot of effective components, organic acids, and saponins and was critical source of the main active components of NXT. Through the comparison of the herbs involved in the top 40 pathways, RA was also proved to be the most important. In the top 40 pathways regulated by NXT, RA was involved in 33 pathways. Some other herbs, such as

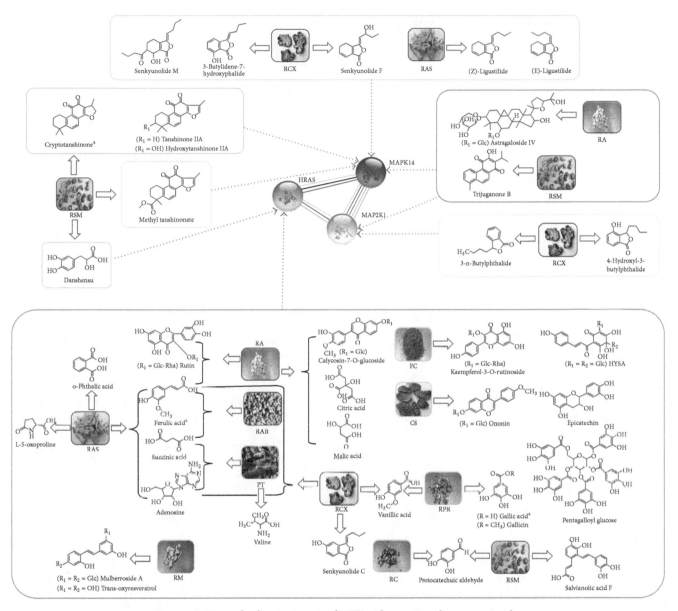

FIGURE 4: Network of major targets of NXT with corresponding compounds.

RSM, RCX, FC, and RAS, were also the important contents in the whole prescription of NXT.

The network pharmacology method used in this study is a novel methodology based on the construction of multilayer networks of disease phenotype-gene-drug to predict drug targets in a holistic manner and promote efficient drug discovery [23]. This method represents a breakthrough in comparison to the traditional herbal medicine research pattern "gene-target-disease" and initiates the new pattern "multiple genes-multiple targets-complex diseases" [24]. By this method, we proved that RA was the critical ingredient mainly involved in the regulation of metabolism and immunity in NXT. RAS was a major herb that regulated cell growth. RSM, RCX, and FC also played important roles in regulation of heart disease, blood vessels, and others. The results indicated that NXT, a complex prescription in the treatment of complex diseases, played a therapeutic effect through multiple targets and multiple pathways. This was the first study to investigate the mechanism of NXT using this method, and we successfully predicted the main targets and pathways, providing a foundation for further research. This method has important value for the study of complex drugs and should be applied in future studies.

5. Conclusion

The main components that mediated the efficacy of NXT were organic acids, saponins, and tanshinones. Radix Astragali was the critical herbal medicine in NXT, which contained more active components than others and regulated more targets and pathways. NXT had a therapeutic effect on the treatment of heart diseases through the pattern "multiple components-multiple targets-multiple pathways."

Abbreviations

ACS:	Acute coronary syndrome
AMI:	Acute myocardial infarction
CBD:	Cerebrovascular disease
CVD:	Cardiovascular disease
ESI:	Electrospray ionization
HRAS:	Harvey rat sarcoma viral oncogene homolog
MAP2K1:	Mitogen-activated protein kinase kinase 1
MAPK14:	Mitogen-activated protein kinase 14
NFAT:	Nuclear factor of activated T cells
NXT:	Naoxintong capsule
TCMs:	Traditional Chinese medicines
UPLC/Q-TOF-MS:	Ultraperformance liquid chromatography/quadrupole time-of-flight mass spectrometry.

Competing Interests

The authors have no conflicting financial interests.

Authors' Contributions

Xianghui Ma and Bin Lv contributed equally to this work.

Acknowledgments

This work was supported by the National Program for Key Basic Research Projects (2012CB518404), the NSFC (81202850 and 81125024), the Ministry of Education of PRC "Program for Innovative Research Team in University" (no. IRT1276), and the Program of International S&T Cooperation Project of China (2015DFA30430).

References

[1] L. Su, Y. Li, B. Lv et al., "Clinical study on Naoxintong capsule for stroke recovery of Qi-deficiency and blood-stasis syndrome," *Zhongguo Zhongyao Zazhi*, vol. 36, no. 11, pp. 1530–1533, 2011.

[2] L.-X. Li, L. Chen, and H.-J. Zhao, "Effect of naoxintong capsule on the vascular endothelial function and the infarct size of patients with acute myocardial infarction," *Chinese Journal of Integrated Traditional And Western Medicine*, vol. 31, no. 12, pp. 1615–1618, 2011.

[3] S.-R. Li, T.-H. Wang, and B.-J. Zhang, "Effects of naoxintong capsule on the inflammation and prognosis in borderline lesion coronary heart disease patients," *Chinese Journal of Integrated Traditional and Western Medicine*, vol. 32, no. 5, pp. 607–611, 2012.

[4] J. Zhao, H. Zhu, S. Wang et al., "Naoxintong protects against atherosclerosis through lipid-lowering and inhibiting maturation of dendritic cells in LDL receptor knockout mice fed a high-fat diet," *Current Pharmaceutical Design*, vol. 19, no. 33, pp. 5891–5896, 2013.

[5] X.-N. Zhong, H.-H. Wang, Z.-Q. Lu et al., "Effects of naoxintong on atherosclerosis and inducible nitric oxide synthase expression in atherosclerotic rabbit," *Chinese Medical Journal*, vol. 126, no. 6, pp. 1166–1170, 2013.

[6] F. Zhang, B. Huang, Y. Zhao et al., "BNC protects H9c2 cardiomyoblasts from H_2O_2-induced oxidative injury through ERK1/2 signaling pathway," *Evidence-based Complementary and Alternative Medicine*, vol. 2013, Article ID 802784, 12 pages, 2013.

[7] J. Liu, Y. Liu, L. Wang et al., "The disease burden of cardiovascular and circulatory diseases in China, 1990 and 2010," *Chinese Journal of Preventive Medicine*, vol. 49, no. 4, pp. 315–320, 2015.

[8] C.-M. Lin, J.-H. Chiu, I.-H. Wu, B.-W. Wang, C.-M. Pan, and Y.-H. Chen, "Ferulic acid augments angiogenesis via VEGF, PDGF and HIF-1α," *Journal of Nutritional Biochemistry*, vol. 21, no. 7, pp. 627–633, 2010.

[9] X.-L. Tang, J.-X. Liu, P. Li et al., "Protective effect of succinic acid on primary cardiomyocyte hypoxia/reoxygenation injury," *China Journal of Chinese Materia Medica*, vol. 38, no. 21, pp. 3742–3746, 2013.

[10] W.-D. Zhang, H. Chen, C. Zhang, R.-H. Liu, H.-L. Li, and H.-Z. Chen, "Astragaloside IV from Astragalus membranaceus shows cardioprotection during myocardial ischemia in vivo and in vitro," *Planta Medica*, vol. 72, no. 1, pp. 4–8, 2006.

[11] G. Wang, D. A. Liem, T. M. Vondriska et al., "Nitric oxide donors protect murine myocardium against infarction via modulation of mitochondrial permeability transition," *American Journal of Physiology—Heart and Circulatory Physiology*, vol. 288, no. 3, pp. H1290–H1295, 2005.

[12] D. J. Hausenloy, M. R. Duchen, and D. M. Yellon, "Inhibiting mitochondrial permeability transition pore opening at reperfusion protects against ischaemia-reperfusion injury," *Cardiovascular Research*, vol. 60, no. 3, pp. 617–625, 2003.

[13] J. Fu, H. Huang, J. Liu, R. Pi, J. Chen, and P. Liu, "Tanshinone IIA protects cardiac myocytes against oxidative stress-triggered damage and apoptosis," *European Journal of Pharmacology*, vol. 568, no. 1–3, pp. 213–221, 2007.

[14] M. W. Russell, D. J. Munroe, E. Bric et al., "A 500-kb physical map and contig from the Harvey ras-1 gene to the 11p telomere," *Genomics*, vol. 35, no. 2, pp. 353–360, 1996.

[15] J. R. Burgoyne, D. J. Haeussler, V. Kumar et al., "Oxidation of HRas cysteine thiols by metabolic stress prevents palmitoylation in vivo and contributes to endothelial cell apoptosis," *The FASEB Journal*, vol. 26, no. 2, pp. 832–841, 2012.

[16] E. D. Martin, G. Felice De Nicola, and M. S. Marber, "New therapeutic targets in cardiology: P38 alpha mitogen-activated protein kinase for ischemic heart disease," *Circulation*, vol. 126, no. 3, pp. 357–368, 2012.

[17] E. van Rooij, P. A. Doevendans, C. C. De Theije, F. A. Babiker, J. D. Molkentin, and L. J. de Windt, "Requirement of nuclear factor of activated T-cells in calcineurin-mediated cardiomyocyte hypertrophy," *The Journal of Biological Chemistry*, vol. 277, no. 50, pp. 48617–48626, 2002.

[18] A. Rinne, N. Kapur, J. D. Molkentin et al., "Isoform- and tissue-specific regulation of the Ca2+-sensitive transcription factor NFAT in cardiac myocytes and heart failure," *American Journal*

of Physiology-Heart and Circulatory Physiology, vol. 298, no. 6, pp. H2001–H2009, 2010.

[19] A. Rao, C. Luo, and P. G. Hogan, "Transcription factors of the NFAT family: regulation and function," *Annual Review of Immunology*, vol. 15, pp. 707–747, 1997.

[20] V. Papademetriou, "From hypertension to heart failure," *Journal of Clinical Hypertension*, vol. 6, no. 10, supplement 2, pp. 14–17, 2004.

[21] I. G. Schulman, "Nuclear receptors as drug targets for metabolic disease," *Advanced Drug Delivery Reviews*, vol. 62, no. 13, pp. 1307–1315, 2010.

[22] M.-W. Huang, H. Wang, W.-J. Zhong, X.-Y. Wu, and H. Chen, "Chinese herbal medicine Naoxintong capsule combined with dual antiplatelet therapy in a rat model of coronary microembolization induced by homologous microthrombi," *Journal of Chinese Integrative Medicine*, vol. 9, no. 1, pp. 38–48, 2011.

[23] Z.-H. Liu and X.-B. Sun, "Network pharmacology: new opportunity for the modernization of traditional Chinese medicine," *Acta Pharmaceutica Sinica*, vol. 47, no. 6, pp. 696–703, 2012.

[24] A. L. Hopkins, "Network pharmacology: the next paradigm in drug discovery," *Nature Chemical Biology*, vol. 4, no. 11, pp. 682–690, 2008.

Ligustrazine for the Treatment of Unstable Angina: A Meta-Analysis of 16 Randomized Controlled Trials

Suman Cao,[1] Wenli Zhao,[1,2] Huaien Bu,[3] Ye Zhao,[4] and Chunquan Yu[5]

[1]Graduate School, Tianjin University of Traditional Chinese Medicine, Tianjin 300193, China
[2]Department of Neurology, Nankai Hospital, Tianjin Academy of Integrative Medicine, Tianjin 300100, China
[3]Department of Chinese Medicine, Tianjin University of Traditional Chinese Medicine, Tianjin 300193, China
[4]Department of Clinical Research, Nankai Hospital, Tianjin Academy of Integrative Medicine, Tianjin 300100, China
[5]Editorial Department, Tianjin University of Traditional Chinese Medicine, Tianjin 300193, China

Correspondence should be addressed to Ye Zhao; zakzy@163.com and Chunquan Yu; ycq-4@163.com

Academic Editor: Stephanie Tjen-A-Looi

Ligustrazine is a principal ingredient of chuanxiong. Concerns regarding the evaluation of the effectiveness of ligustrazine in the treatment of UA have resulted in a meta-analysis combined with recent clinical evidence. Seven computer databases that included the China hospital knowledge database (CHKD), Wanfang Med Online, the Chinese medical journal database (CMJD), PubMed, Cochrane, Embase (Ovid), and Medline (Ovid) were systematically searched. We included randomized controlled trials and quasi-randomized controlled trials. Our systematic review identified 16 RCTs that met our eligibility criteria. Ligustrazine combined with conventional medicine was associated with an increased rate of marked improvement in symptoms and an increased rate of marked improvement of ECG compared with conventional Western medicine alone. Additionally, the use of ligustrazine was associated with significant trends in the reduction of the consumption of nitroglycerin and the level of fibrinogen when compared with conventional Western medicine alone. No firm results were found between the intervention and the control method groups in the reduction of the time of onset or the frequency of acute attack angina due to the high level of heterogeneity. In conclusion, our meta-analysis found that ligustrazine was associated with some benefits for people with unstable angina.

1. Introduction

United Nations member states have agreed to reduce premature cardiovascular disease (CVD) mortality 25% by 2025. However, CVD is the major cause of death worldwide which is almost a third of all deaths globally in 2013 [1]. In low and middle income countries (LMIC), the situation is not optimistic similarly. The greatest burden of CVD is approximately 80% of cardiovascular deaths occurring in LMIC [2]. The most of CVD deaths were from coronary heart disease (CHD) [3]. Unstable angina is a common manifestation of this disease. The three principal presentations of UA include rest angina, new-onset severe angina, and increasing angina [4]. Unstable angina is a crucial phase of coronary heart disease with widely variable symptoms and prognoses [5]. Thoracic pain may mark the onset of acute myocardial infarction. It typically occurs at rest and has a sudden onset, sudden worsening, and stuttering recurrence over days and weeks. Unstable angina which is a potentially life-threatening event is relatively more harmful than stable angina pectoris [6].

The objective of UA treatment is the improvement of symptoms, the relief of the progress of the disease, and the prevention of cardiovascular events, particularly myocardial infarction and death [7, 8]. Recently, conventional medicine has consisted of antiplatelet agents, anticoagulant agents, nitrates, beta-adrenergic blockers, calcium channel blockers, and inhibitors of the renin-angiotensin-aldosterone system [9]. Although these treatments are widely used in the acute relief of secondary angina pectoris and the long-term prophylactic management of angina pectoris, chuanxiong might also be useful for UA and for increased safety. Therefore, we contrasted chuanxiong with conventional medicine in this meta-analysis.

Traditional Chinese Medicine (TCM) is the result of Chinese civilization over 3000 years. The Chinese herb chuanxiong belongs to the Umbelliferae family [10]. A book named Shen Nong Ben Cao Jing, which was published 2000 years ago, has been the original and existing writing record about chuanxiong. Ligustrazine is a principal ingredient of chuanxiong. It has been shown to play a critical role in cardiovascular treatments, mediated by inhibition of Ca^{2+} influx and by the release of intracellular Ca^{2+} [11, 12]. It significantly inhibits L-type calcium current in a concentration-dependent manner to make vasodilatory effect, to improve the situation of myocardium ischemia [13, 14]. It also suppressed calcium transient and contraction in rabbit ventricular myocytes under physiological and pathophysiological conditions [15]. Besides, ligustrazine improves attenuation of oxidative stress. Treatment by ligustrazine decreased reactive oxygen species (ROS) production and enhanced cellular glutathione (GSH) levels [16]. Ligustrazine treatment partially restored superoxide dismutase1 (SOD1) activity [17], increasing in NO production [18]. Recently, the oxidative stress has been shown to play a critical role in atherogenesis (AS). The PPAR signal pathway is involved in the molecular mechanism of ligustrazine in the treatment of AS [19]. Although pharmacology research might indicate the cardiovascular protective effects of ligustrazine, the specific outcomes of the effectiveness of ligustrazine have not been elucidated. Therefore, this meta-analysis combined recent clinical evidence to evaluate the effectiveness of ligustrazine in the treatment of UA.

2. Methods

2.1. Search Strategy.

The group systematically searched seven computer databases that included the China hospital knowledge database (CHKD), Wanfang Med Online, the Chinese medical journal database (CMJD), PubMed, Cochrane, Embase (Ovid), and Medline (Ovid). The index words were the following: chuan*xiong, chuanxiong rhizome, Ligusticum wallichii, ligustilide, cnidilide, cnidiumlactone, sedanolide, senkyunolide, ligustrazine, tetramethylpyrazine, chuan*xiong extract, Senkyunone, unstable angina, randomized, controlled trials, controlled clinical trials, and random.

2.2. Eligibility Criteria

2.2.1. Types of Studies.

We included randomized controlled trials and quasi-randomized controlled trials.

2.2.2. Types of Interventions and Participants.

Types of interventions and participants are as follows: (1) Participants who were diagnosed with UAP according to the American College of Cardiology Foundation/American Heart Association (ACCF/AHA) Guidelines for the Diagnosis and Management of Patients with Unstable Ischemic Heart Disease [20]; (2) the International Society and Federation of Cardiology/World Health Organization (ISFC/WHO) guideline [21]; (3) the Chinese Society of Cardiology (CSC) guidelines [22]; (4) other criteria; (5) the included trials designed to compare the effectiveness and safety of chuanxiong with conventional medicine and conventional medicine alone.

2.2.3. Types of Outcomes Measures.

Cardiovascular events (CEs) including acute myocardial infarction (AMI) and angina pectoris were the outcome measures. The improvement in the angina symptoms (IAS) and electrocardiogram (IECG) results were used as the outcome measures. Moreover, the lack of improvement or worsening of angina symptoms (NIWAS) and the lack of improvement or worsening of ECG (NIWECG) were used as the outcome measures. Angina onset time (AOT), seizure frequency (SF), reduction in nitroglycerin use (RNU), and the level of fibrinogen (FIB) were also included.

2.2.4. Definitions of Improvements of Symptom and ECG.

Compared with the basic improvement in angina symptoms, the improvement of symptom involves that frequency and duration of feeling angina chest pain should be reduced at least 50%. Improvement of ECG should be achieved with at least 0.05 mv at ST segment in ECG compared with basic improvements in ECG [23].

2.2.5. Adverse Events.

Adverse events are death, lifethreatening events, crippling, disabling, teratogenic effects, requiring special events, and hospitalization.

2.3. Data Extraction and Quality Assessment.

The qualities of the data were assessed by two independent researchers. Each trial identified in the search was assessed for gender, age, design, diagnosis, standards for the participants, interventions, and outcome measures. Any disagreement between the researchers regarding each trial was resolved by consulting a third researcher. Duplicate studies and records were excluded by screening the titles and abstracts. All remaining articles were screened by examining the full text. The qualities of the trials included in this study were evaluated by each researcher according to the Systematic Reviews of Interventions on Cochrane Handbook, version 5.1.0 [24].

2.4. Statistical Analysis.

We used RevMan 5.3 (review manager) as provided by the Cochrane collaboration to perform the meta-analyses of the database. Dichotomous data were evaluated with the risk ratios (RRs), and continuous outcomes were evaluated with the mean differences (MDs); for both, the 95% confidence intervals (CIs) and forest plots were applied. The chi-squared test and the I-squared statistic were used to assess the heterogeneity. For the studies that did not report statistical heterogeneity ($P > 0.1$, I-squared < 25%), a fixed-effect model was used to pool the results. In contrast, the heterogeneity was assessed, and the subgroup analyses that produced the heterogeneity were accounted for. If the studies had statistical heterogeneity that did not have clinical heterogeneity, a random-effect model was used. For the studies with extensive heterogeneity or obvious clinical heterogeneity, descriptiveness analyses were used.

3. Results

3.1. Description of the Included Trials. A total of 1591 trials were identified by database searching and other sources. After examination of duplicates, 1179 trials remained. Proceeding, we excluded 1107 trials. Based on reads of the full articles, 16 RCTs were included according to the eligibility criteria and exclusion criteria. All of these studies were published in Chinese. The literature search and a flowchart of the selection are provided in Figure 1.

All 16 of the included trials were RCTs, and all of the trials recruited participants for the treatment of unstable angina pectoris with chuanxiong in combination with conventional medicine versus conventional medicine. The majority of the studies used the improvement of symptoms and ECG as the outcome measures. Among the studies, five mentioned fibrinogen as an outcome. The time of onset and seizure frequency were also reported in three studies. Reductions in nitroglycerin use were reported in two studies. Cardiovascular events were reported in one study. Table 1 summarizes the characteristics of these original studies.

3.2. The Effect of Ligustrazine

3.2.1. The Rate of Cardiovascular Events. A single study showed that ligustrazine was no better or worse at reducing cardiovascular events, including the incidence of angina relapse after four weeks (RR = 0.25, 95% CI (0.06–1.10)) (Figure 2), the incidence of angina relapse after 12 weeks (RR = 0.44, 95% CI (0.15–1.32)) (Figure 3), or the incidence of AMI relapse after 12 weeks (RR = 0.25, 95% CI (0.03–2.13)) (Figure 4). None of the participants relapsed into AMI after four weeks.

3.2.2. Rate of Symptom Improvement. The rates of symptom improvement were reported in 16 RCTs that involved 1356 participants. All of these studies reported improvements in angina symptoms with ligustrazine compared with conventional medicine. Some of these studies reported evidence that ligustrazine improved angina symptoms (RR = 1.24, 95% CI; 1.18, 1.30). There was no heterogeneity among the 16 studies ($P = 0.96$, $I^2 = 0\%$) (Figure 5).

3.2.3. Rates of No Improvement or Worsening of Symptoms. The rates of no improvement or worsening of symptoms were reported in 16 RCTs involving 1356 participants. Some of the evidence indicated that ligustrazine reduced the number of people with rates of no improvement or worsening of symptoms (RR = 0.28, 95% CI (0.21, 0.38)). There was no heterogeneity among the 16 studies ($P = 0.98$, $I^2 = 0\%$) (Figure 6).

3.2.4. Rate of Marked Improvement in ECG. The improvement in ECG was reported in eight RCTs involving 638 participants. All of these studies reported improvements in ECG with ligustrazine compared with conventional medicine. Some evidence indicated that ligustrazine improved ECG

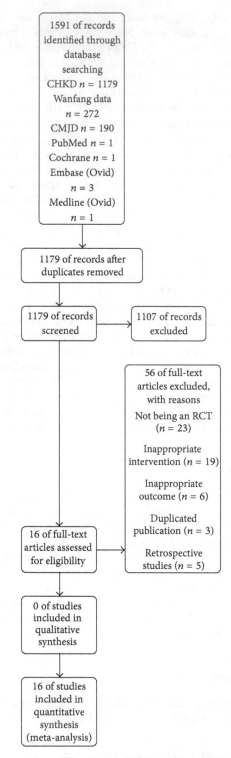

FIGURE 1: Flow diagram of included and excluded studies.

(RR = 1.32, 95% CI (1.21, 1.45)). There was no heterogeneity among these eight studies ($P = 0.33$, $I^2 = 12\%$) (Figure 7).

3.2.5. Rate of No Improvement or Worsening of ECG. The rates of no improvement or worsening of ECG were reported in eight RCTs involving 638 participants. Ligustrazine reduced

TABLE 1: Characteristics of included studies.

Studies	Sample (t/c)	Diagnosis standard	Age	Intervention group	Control group	Course (day)	Outcome measures
Guo 2007 [25]	20/16	ISFC/WHO	59 ± 6.7	Ligustrazine injection, nitrates, aspirin, ACE inhibitor	Nitrates, aspirin, ACE inhibitor	14	IAS, NIWAS, IECG, NIWECG
Liao and Luo 2006 [26]	34/34	ISFC/WHO	46–71	Ligustrazine injection, nitrates, aspirin	Nitrates and aspirin	15	IAS and NIWAS
Da 2008 [27]	38/36	CSC	41–83	Ligustrazine injection, nitrates, aspirin, Low Molecular Weight Heparin (LMWH), beta blockers	Nitroglycerin, aspirin, LMWH, beta blockers	14	IAS, NIWAS, IECG, NIWECG
Rong et al. 2001 [28]	32/32	Other	64.3 ± 7.2	Ligustrazine injection, nitrates, aspirin	Nitrates and aspirin	10	IAS and NIWAS
Peng 2014 [29]	43/42	CSC	61.2 ± 5.94	Ligustrazine injection, nitrates, antiplatelet drugs	Nitrates and antiplatelet drugs	14	IAS, NIWAS, IECG, NIWECG, AOT, SF, RNU, FIB
Wang and Hua 2004 [30]	30/28	ISFC/WHO	Unclear	Ligustrazine injection, beta blockers, aspirin, calcium channel blockers (CCB), LMWH, ACE inhibitor	Beta blockers, aspirin, CCB, LMWH, ACE inhibitor	28	IAS and NIWAS
Wei et al. 2012 [31]	60/60	CSC	48–79	Ligustrazine injection, antiplatelet drugs, nitrates, beta blockers	Antiplatelet drugs, nitrates, beta blockers	14	IAS, NIWAS, AOT, SF, FIB
Wang 2006 [32]	65/65	CSC	67.5 ± 9	Ligustrazine injection, beta blockers, nitrates, aspirin, CCB, ACE inhibitor	Beta blockers, nitrates, aspirin, CCB, ACE inhibitor	14	IAS and NIWAS
Zhou 2008 [33]	78/50	ISFC/WHO	39–89	Ligustrazine injection, nitroglycerin, aspirin, CCB, beta blockers	Nitroglycerin, aspirin, CCB, beta blockers	14	IAS and NIWAS
Li 2010 [34]	38/30	Other	42–76	Ligustrazine injection, nitroglycerin, aspirin, LMWH, beta blockers	Nitroglycerin, aspirin, LMWH, beta blockers	14	IAS and NIWAS
Sun 2007 [35]	48/48	Other	48–80	Ligustrazine injection, nitrates, aspirin, beta blockers, statins, ACE inhibitor	Nitrates, aspirin, beta blockers, statins, ACE inhibitor	21	IAS, NIWAS, IECG, NIWECG, FIB
Wang 2008 [36]	42/42	ISFC/WHO	48–78	Ligustrazine injection, nitrates, aspirin, beta blockers, CCB, statins, ACE inhibitor	Nitrates, aspirin, beta blockers, CCB, statins, ACE inhibitor	14	IAS, NIWAS, IECG, NIWECG
Fan 2014 [37]	63/63	Other	73.5 ± 12.6	Ligustrazine injection, nitrates, aspirin, statins	Nitrates, aspirin, statins, beta blockers	14	IAS, NIWAS, IECG, NIWECG, AOT, SF, RNU
Fu and Lin 2009 [38]	40/41	Other	Unclear	Ligustrazine injection, nitrates, aspirin, statins, LMWH, beta blockers	Nitrates, aspirin, statins, LMWH, beta blockers	14	IAS and NIWAS
Meng et al. 2005 [39]	38/38	ISFC/WHO	68.8 ± 7.8	Ligustrazine injection, nitrates, beta blockers, ACE inhibitor, CCB, LMWH	Nitrates, beta blockers, ACE inhibitor, CCB, LMWH	10	IAS, NIWAS, IECG, NIWECG, FIB, CEs
Wang et al. 2005 [40]	32/30	ISFC/WHO	50–66	Ligustrazine injection, nitrates, aspirin, LMWH, beta blockers	Nitrates, aspirin, LMWH, beta blockers	14	IAS, NIWAS, IECG, NIWECG

| Study or subgroup | Experimental | | Control | | Weight | Risk ratio | Risk ratio |
	Events	Total	Events	Total		M-H, fixed, 95% CI	M-H, fixed, 95% CI
Meng et al. 2005	2	38	8	38	100.0%	0.25 [0.06, 1.10]	
Total (95% CI)		**38**		**38**	**100.0%**	**0.25 [0.06, 1.10]**	
Total events	2		8				
Heterogeneity: not applicable							
Test for overall effect: $Z = 1.83$ ($P = 0.07$)							

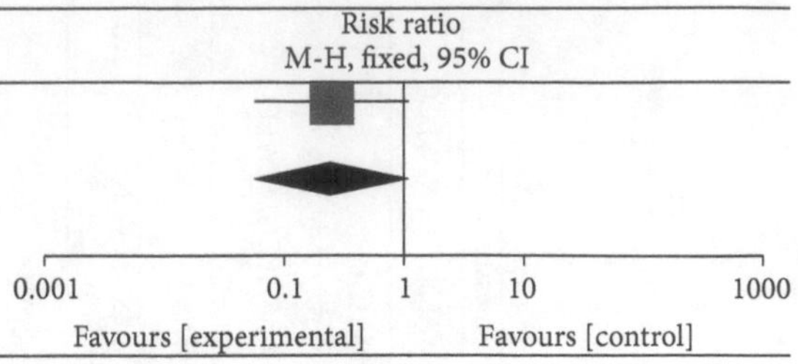

0.001   0.1   1   10   1000
Favours [experimental]   Favours [control]

FIGURE 2: The rate of cardiovascular events and the incidence of angina relapse after 4 weeks.

| Study or subgroup | Experimental | | Control | | Weight | Risk ratio | Risk ratio |
	Events	Total	Events	Total		M-H, fixed, 95% CI	M-H, fixed, 95% CI
Meng et al. 2005	4	38	9	38	100.0%	0.44 [0.15, 1.32]	
Total (95% CI)		**38**		**38**	**100.0%**	**0.44 [0.15, 1.32]**	
Total events	4		9				
Heterogeneity: not applicable							
Test for overall effect: $Z = 1.46$ ($P = 0.14$)							

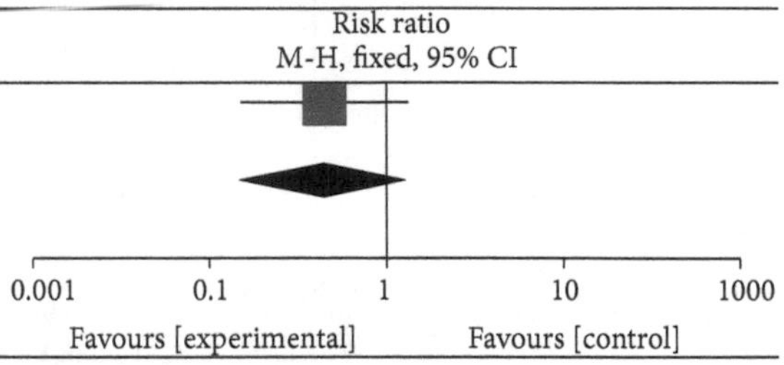

0.001   0.1   1   10   1000
Favours [experimental]   Favours [control]

FIGURE 3: The incidence of angina relapse after 12 weeks.

| Study or subgroup | Experimental | | Control | | Weight | Risk ratio | Risk ratio |
	Events	Total	Events	Total		M-H, fixed, 95% CI	M-H, fixed, 95% CI
Meng et al. 2005	1	38	4	38	100.0%	0.25 [0.03, 2.13]	
Total (95% CI)		**38**		**38**	**100.0%**	**0.25 [0.03, 2.13]**	
Total events	1		4				
Heterogeneity: not applicable							
Test for overall effect: $Z = 1.27$ ($P = 0.21$)							

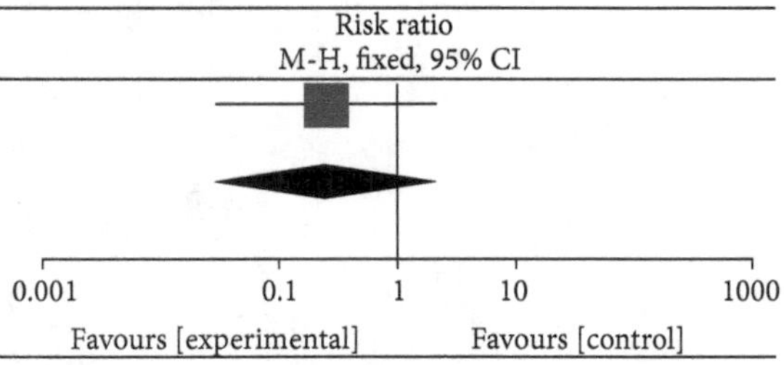

0.001   0.1   1   10   1000
Favours [experimental]   Favours [control]

FIGURE 4: The incidence of AMI relapse after 12 weeks.

| Study or subgroup | Experimental | | Control | | Weight | Risk ratio | Risk ratio |
	Events	Total	Events	Total		M-H, fixed, 95% CI	M-H, fixed, 95% CI
Da 2008	34	38	25	36	5.1%	1.29 [1.01, 1.64]	
Fan 2014	58	63	51	63	10.1%	1.14 [0.99, 1.31]	
Fu and Lin 2009	38	40	29	41	5.7%	1.34 [1.09, 1.66]	
Guo 2007	17	20	10	16	2.2%	1.36 [0.89, 2.07]	
Li 2010	33	38	22	30	4.9%	1.18 [0.92, 1.52]	
Liao and Luo 2006	33	34	28	34	5.6%	1.18 [1.00, 1.39]	
Meng et al. 2005	34	38	29	38	5.8%	1.17 [0.95, 1.44]	
Peng 2014	41	43	32	42	6.4%	1.25 [1.04, 1.50]	
Rong et al. 2001	30	32	22	32	4.4%	1.36 [1.06, 1.75]	
Sun 2007	44	48	33	48	6.6%	1.33 [1.08, 1.64]	
Wang and Hua 2004	29	30	20	28	4.1%	1.35 [1.06, 1.73]	
Wang et al. 2005	31	32	26	30	5.3%	1.12 [0.96, 1.30]	
Wang 2006	59	65	47	65	9.3%	1.26 [1.06, 1.49]	
Wang 2008	39	42	30	42	6.0%	1.30 [1.05, 1.60]	
Wei et al. 2012	55	60	45	60	8.9%	1.22 [1.04, 1.44]	
Zhou 2008	76	78	40	50	9.7%	1.22 [1.06, 1.41]	
Total (95% CI)		**701**		**655**	**100.0%**	**1.24 [1.18, 1.30]**	
Total events	651		489				
Heterogeneity: $\chi^2 = 6.73$, df = 15 ($P = 0.96$); $I^2 = 0\%$							
Test for overall effect: $Z = 8.67$ ($P < 0.00001$)							

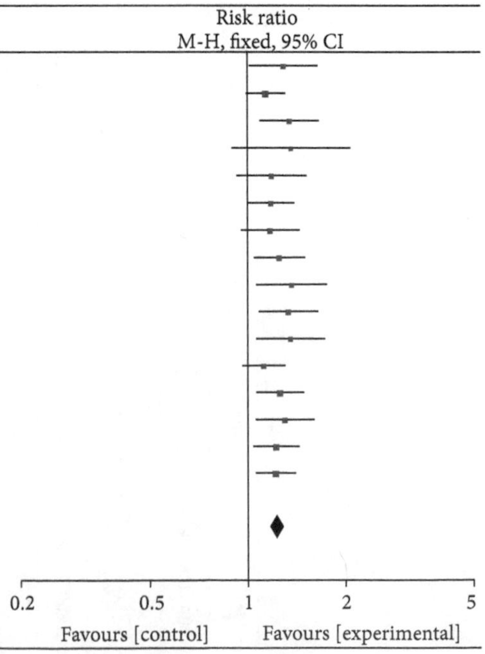

0.2   0.5   1   2   5
Favours [control]   Favours [experimental]

FIGURE 5: Rate of marked improvement of symptoms.

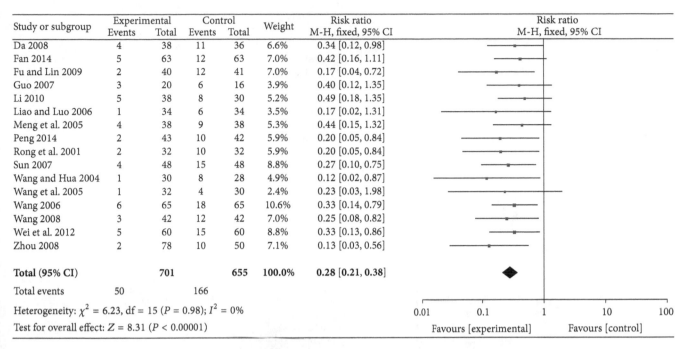

Study or subgroup	Experimental Events	Experimental Total	Control Events	Control Total	Weight	Risk ratio M-H, fixed, 95% CI
Da 2008	4	38	11	36	6.6%	0.34 [0.12, 0.98]
Fan 2014	5	63	12	63	7.0%	0.42 [0.16, 1.11]
Fu and Lin 2009	2	40	12	41	7.0%	0.17 [0.04, 0.72]
Guo 2007	3	20	6	16	3.9%	0.40 [0.12, 1.35]
Li 2010	5	38	8	30	5.2%	0.49 [0.18, 1.35]
Liao and Luo 2006	1	34	6	34	3.5%	0.17 [0.02, 1.31]
Meng et al. 2005	4	38	9	38	5.3%	0.44 [0.15, 1.32]
Peng 2014	2	43	10	42	5.9%	0.20 [0.05, 0.84]
Rong et al. 2001	2	32	10	32	5.9%	0.20 [0.05, 0.84]
Sun 2007	4	48	15	48	8.8%	0.27 [0.10, 0.75]
Wang and Hua 2004	1	30	8	28	4.9%	0.12 [0.02, 0.87]
Wang et al. 2005	1	32	4	30	2.4%	0.23 [0.03, 1.98]
Wang 2006	6	65	18	65	10.6%	0.33 [0.14, 0.79]
Wang 2008	3	42	12	42	7.0%	0.25 [0.08, 0.82]
Wei et al. 2012	5	60	15	60	8.8%	0.33 [0.13, 0.86]
Zhou 2008	2	78	10	50	7.1%	0.13 [0.03, 0.56]
Total (95% CI)		**701**		**655**	**100.0%**	**0.28 [0.21, 0.38]**
Total events	50		166			

Heterogeneity: $\chi^2 = 6.23$, df = 15 ($P = 0.98$); $I^2 = 0\%$
Test for overall effect: $Z = 8.31$ ($P < 0.00001$)

FIGURE 6: Rate of no improvement or worsening of symptoms.

Study or subgroup	Experimental Events	Experimental Total	Control Events	Control Total	Weight	Risk ratio M-H, fixed, 95% CI
Da 2008	27	38	14	36	7.0%	1.83 [1.16, 2.89]
Fan 2014	56	63	50	63	24.2%	1.12 [0.96, 1.31]
Guo 2007	14	20	7	16	3.8%	1.60 [0.86, 2.99]
Meng et al. 2005	35	38	25	38	12.1%	1.40 [1.09, 1.79]
Peng 2014	39	42	30	42	14.5%	1.30 [1.05, 1.60]
Sun 2007	40	48	30	48	14.5%	1.33 [1.04, 1.72]
Wang et al. 2005	28	32	18	30	9.0%	1.46 [1.06, 2.01]
Wang 2008	38	42	31	42	15.0%	1.23 [1.00, 1.50]
Total (95% CI)		**323**		**315**	**100.0%**	**1.32 [1.21, 1.45]**
Total events	277		205			

Heterogeneity: $\chi^2 = 7.98$, df = 7 ($P = 0.33$); $I^2 = 12\%$
Test for overall effect: $Z = 6.08$ ($P < 0.00001$)

FIGURE 7: Rate of marked improvement of ECG.

the number of people who exhibited no improvement or worsening of ECG (RR = 0.44, 95% CI (0.32, 0.60)). There was no heterogeneity among these eight studies ($P = 0.87$, $I^2 = 0\%$) (Figure 8).

3.2.6. Time of Onset.
The time of onset was reported in three RCTs involving 331 participants. All of these studies reported the times of onset for the comparisons of ligustrazine with conventional medicine (MD = −1.68, 95% CI (−3.27, −0.08)). There was a high level of heterogeneity among these three studies ($P < 0.00001$, $I^2 = 98\%$) (Figure 9).

3.2.7. Frequency of Acute Attack Angina.
The frequency of acute attack angina was reported in three RCTs involving 331 participants, and these studies compared the frequency

of acute attack angina between ligustrazine and conventional medicine (MD = −0.53, 95% CI (−1.08, −0.03)). There was heterogeneity ($P = 0.002$, $I^2 = 84\%$) (Figure 10).

3.2.8. Consumption of Nitroglycerine.
Consumption of nitroglycerine was reported in two RCTs involving 211 participants, and these studies reported the comparisons of nitroglycerine consumption between ligustrazine and conventional medicine. Strong evidence revealed that ligustrazine reduced the consumption of nitroglycerine (MD = −0.14, 95% CI 95% (−0.20, −0.08)). There was no heterogeneity ($P = 0.83$, $I^2 = 0\%$) (Figure 11).

3.2.9. Level of Fibrinogen.
The level of fibrinogen was reported in five RCTs involving 437 participants, and all of

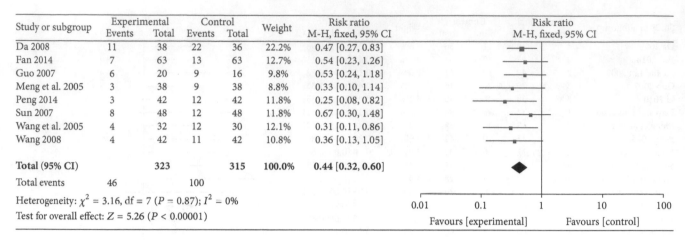

Study or subgroup	Experimental		Control		Weight	Risk ratio M-H, fixed, 95% CI
	Events	Total	Events	Total		
Da 2008	11	38	22	36	22.2%	0.47 [0.27, 0.83]
Fan 2014	7	63	13	63	12.7%	0.54 [0.23, 1.26]
Guo 2007	6	20	9	16	9.8%	0.53 [0.24, 1.18]
Meng et al. 2005	3	38	9	38	8.8%	0.33 [0.10, 1.14]
Peng 2014	3	42	12	42	11.8%	0.25 [0.08, 0.82]
Sun 2007	8	48	12	48	11.8%	0.67 [0.30, 1.48]
Wang et al. 2005	4	32	12	30	12.1%	0.31 [0.11, 0.86]
Wang 2008	4	42	11	42	10.8%	0.36 [0.13, 1.05]
Total (95% CI)		323		315	100.0%	0.44 [0.32, 0.60]
Total events	46		100			

Heterogeneity: $\chi^2 = 3.16$, df = 7 ($P = 0.87$); $I^2 = 0\%$
Test for overall effect: $Z = 5.26$ ($P < 0.00001$)

FIGURE 8: Rate of no improvement or worsening of ECG.

Study or subgroup	Experimental			Control			Weight	Mean difference IV, random, 95% CI
	Mean	SD	Total	Mean	SD	Total		
Fan 2014	3.72	1.58	63	5.69	2.15	63	32.4%	−1.97 [−2.63, −1.31]
Peng 2014	4.75	0.21	43	5.19	0.35	42	34.3%	−0.44 [−0.56, −0.32]
Wei et al. 2012	3.06	1.32	60	5.72	1.36	60	33.3%	−2.66 [−3.14, −2.18]
Total (95% CI)			166			165	100.0%	−1.68 [−3.27, −0.08]

Heterogeneity: $\tau^2 = 1.93$, $\chi^2 = 93.86$, df = 2 ($P < 0.00001$); $I^2 = 98\%$
Test for overall effect: $Z = 2.06$ ($P = 0.04$)

FIGURE 9: Time of onset.

Study or subgroup	Experimental			Control			Weight	Mean difference IV, random, 95% CI
	Mean	SD	Total	Mean	SD	Total		
Fan 2014	1.82	1.06	63	2.36	1.72	63	30.8%	−0.54 [−1.04, −0.04]
Peng 2014	0.32	0.12	43	0.46	0.17	42	40.9%	−0.14 [−0.20, −0.08]
Wei et al. 2012	2.78	1.52	60	3.86	1.72	60	28.3%	−1.08 [−1.66, −0.50]
Total (95% CI)			166			165	100.0%	−0.53 [−1.08, −0.03]

Heterogeneity: $\tau^2 = 0.19$, $\chi^2 = 12.25$, df = 2 ($P = 0.002$); $I^2 = 84\%$
Test for overall effect: $Z = 1.87$ ($P = 0.06$)

FIGURE 10: Frequency of acute attack angina.

these studies reported the levels of fibrinogen comparing ligustrazine with conventional medicine. Some evidence revealed that ligustrazine reduced the level of fibrinogen (MD = −0.68, 95% CI (−0.9, −0.46)). There was heterogeneity among these five studies ($P = 0.03$, $I^2 = 64\%$). We rejected one study for high levels of heterogeneity. The results revealed that ligustrazine reduced level of fibrinogen (MD = −0.78 95% CI (−0.91, −0.65)). There was no heterogeneity among the four included studies ($P = 0.44$, $I^2 = 0\%$) (Figure 12).

3.2.10. Adverse Events.
There were no recorded severe adverse events.

3.3. Methodological Qualities of the Included Trials.
The risks of seven biases among the 16 trials were evaluated, including random sequence generation, allocation concealment, blinding of participants and personnel, blinding of outcome assessment, incomplete outcome data, selective reporting, and other biases according to the criteria in the Cochrane Handbook for Systematic Reviews [24]. All of the studies described correct randomization methods. There was only one trial with blinding of participants and personnel and blinding of outcome assessment, and nearly all of the trials failed to mention allocation concealment, the blinding of the participants and personnel, and the blinding of outcome assessments. The methodological qualities of the included trials are summarized in Table 2.

3.4. Funnel Plot of Publication Bias.
The research team used a funnel plot to evaluate the publication biases of all of the included studies, and this plot is summarized in Figure 13. The outcome suggests that there was little publication bias.

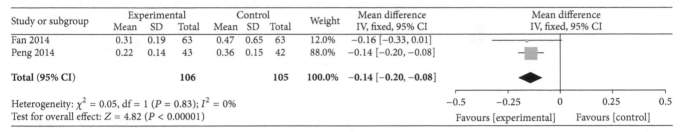

Study or subgroup	Experimental			Control			Weight	Mean difference IV, fixed, 95% CI
	Mean	SD	Total	Mean	SD	Total		
Fan 2014	0.31	0.19	63	0.47	0.65	63	12.0%	−0.16 [−0.33, 0.01]
Peng 2014	0.22	0.14	43	0.36	0.15	42	88.0%	−0.14 [−0.20, −0.08]
Total (95% CI)			**106**			**105**	**100.0%**	**−0.14 [−0.20, −0.08]**

Heterogeneity: $\chi^2 = 0.05$, df $= 1$ $(P = 0.83)$; $I^2 = 0\%$
Test for overall effect: $Z = 4.82$ $(P < 0.00001)$

FIGURE 11: Consumption of nitroglycerine.

Study or subgroup	Experimental			Control			Weight	Mean difference IV, fixed, 95% CI
	Mean	SD	Total	Mean	SD	Total		
Meng et al. 2005	2.11	0.73	38	2.89	0.84	38	13.4%	−0.78 [−1.13, −0.43]
Sun 2007	3.54	0.71	60	4.27	0.69	60	26.7%	−0.73 [−0.98, −0.48]
Peng 2014	3.2	0.45	43	3.86	0.65	42	29.6%	−0.66 [−0.90, −0.42]
Wei et al. 2012	3.15	0.59	60	4.08	0.72	60	30.3%	−0.93 [−1.17, −0.69]
Total (95% CI)			**201**			**200**	**100.0%**	**−0.78 [−0.91, −0.65]**

Heterogeneity: $\chi^2 = 2.68$, df $= 3$ $(P = 0.44)$; $I^2 = 0\%$
Test for overall effect: $Z = 11.75$ $(P < 0.00001)$

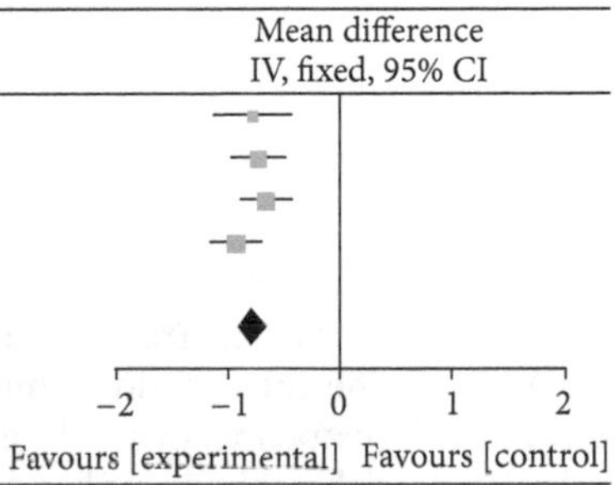

FIGURE 12: Level of fibrinogen.

TABLE 2: Methodological quality of the included studies.

Studies	Random sequence generation	Allocation concealment	Blinding of participants and personnel	Blinding of outcome assessment	Incomplete outcome data	Selective reporting	Other bias
Guo 2007 [25]	Low risk	Unclear	Low risk	Low risk	Low risk	Low risk	Low risk
Liao and Luo 2006 [26]	Low risk	Unclear	Unclear	Unclear	Low risk	Low risk	Low risk
Da 2008 [27]	Low risk	Unclear	Unclear	Unclear	Low risk	Low risk	Low risk
Rong et al. 2001 [28]	Low risk	Unclear	Unclear	Unclear	Low risk	Low risk	Low risk
Peng 2014 [29]	Low risk	Unclear	Unclear	Unclear	Low risk	Low risk	Low risk
Wang and Hua 2004 [30]	Low risk	Unclear	Unclear	Unclear	Low risk	Low risk	Low risk
Wei et al. 2012 [31]	Low risk	Unclear	Unclear	Unclear	Low risk	Low risk	Low risk
Wang 2006 [32]	Low risk	Unclear	Unclear	Unclear	Low risk	Low risk	Low risk
Zhou 2008 [33]	Low risk	Unclear	Unclear	Unclear	Low risk	Low risk	Low risk
Li 2010 [34]	Low risk	Unclear	Unclear	Unclear	Low risk	Low risk	Low risk
Sun 2007 [35]	Low risk	Unclear	Unclear	Unclear	Low risk	Low risk	Low risk
Wang 2008 [36]	Low risk	Unclear	Unclear	Unclear	Low risk	Low risk	Low risk
Fan 2014 [37]	Low risk	Unclear	Unclear	Unclear	Low risk	Low risk	Low risk
Fu and Lin 2009 [38]	Low risk	Unclear	Unclear	Unclear	Low risk	Low risk	Low risk
Meng et al. 2005 [39]	Low risk	Unclear	Unclear	Unclear	Low risk	Low risk	Low risk
Wang et al. 2005 [40]	Low risk	Unclear	Unclear	Unclear	Low risk	Low risk	Low risk

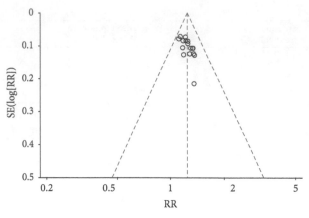

FIGURE 13: Funnel plots.

3.5. Dosage and Purity of Ligustrazine. Ligustrazine is one natural extract of ligustrazine. Ligustrazine hydrochloride was used in the intervention group of these 16 RCTs. The dosage of ligustrazine hydrochloride is 80 mg once daily. Calculated on the anhydrous basis, the purity of ligustrazine hydrochloride must not be any less than 99.0% [41]. Therefore, the strict pharmaceutical standardization makes the usage of ligustrazine evaluable.

4. Discussion

Ischaemic diseases can be improved by the so-called complementary medicine in some report [42]. Nevertheless, few relevant articles on ligustrazine for UA have been published in the English medical journals, and the situation reduces the evaluation of ligustrazine. Our study was designed to compare the efficacy and safety of ligustrazine preparations and conventional medicine by including 16 RCTs and 1356 participants. As shown above, there was a single study that mentioned the rate of cardiovascular events. Therefore, we were unable to summarize the effects of the routine use of antiangina treatment with ligustrazine on the reduction in incidence of acute myocardial infarction.

Nevertheless, the pooled analyses revealed that ligustrazine combined with conventional medicine appeared to have some benefits, such as increasing the rate of marked improvement of symptoms (RR = 1.24, 95% CI (1.18, 1.30)) and the rate of marked improvement of ECG (RR = 1.32, 95% CI (1.21, 1.45)) when compared with conventional Western medicine alone. Additionally, the use of ligustrazine was associated with significant trends in the reduction of the consumption of nitroglycerin (MD = −0.14, 95% CI (−0.20, −0.08)) and the level of fibrinogen (MD = −0.78, 95% CI (−0.91, −0.65)) when compared with conventional Western medicine alone. Furthermore, in the meta-analysis of these four outcomes, no statistical heterogeneity was noted among the comparisons (all I^2s = 0%). The outcomes of the time of the onset and the frequency of acute attack angina exhibited heterogeneity. Therefore, we should be careful in drawing conclusions about the efficiency of ligustrazine in the

reduction of the time of onset or frequency of acute attack angina. There were no serious recorded adverse effects.

Although ligustrazine and conventional antiangina treatments that include ligustrazine exhibited some benefit, there are a number of limitations to this review. (1) The majority of the studies had small samples. (2) We only found and included Chinese studies. (3) The included studies were of low methodological quality and used neither blinding nor allocation concealment. (4) The duration of treatment was insufficient in the majority of the studies (14 days). Limitations still contribute enlightenment to future studies. Researchers can improve the methodology, such as allocation concealment, blinding method, treatment duration, and long-term follow-up. Well-designed trials of ligustrazine in UA management will promote its application correctly and our paper may stimulate appropriate evaluation on ligustrazine historically.

5. Conclusion

The addition of ligustrazine to conventional medicine possibly benefits unstable angina. However, quality evidence is needed to further assess its efficacy and safety.

Disclosure

The funders had no role in study design and data collection and analysis, decision to publish, or preparation of the paper.

Competing Interests

The authors declare that there is no conflict of interests regarding the publication of this paper.

Authors' Contributions

Suman Cao and Wenli Zhao contributed equally to this study.

Acknowledgments

The authors thank Mr. Yueshen Ma for assistance with data extraction. This project was supported by the National Basic Research Program of China (973 Program 2014CB542902, http://program.most.gov.cn/).

References

[1] GBD 2013 Mortality and Causes of Death Collaborators, "Global, regional, and national age–sex specific all-cause and cause-specific mortality for 240 causes of death, 1990–2013: a systematic analysis for the Global Burden of Disease Study 2013," *The Lancet*, vol. 385, no. 9963, pp. 117–171, 2015.

[2] P. Bovet and F. Paccaud, "Cardiovascular disease and the changing face of global public health: a focus on low and middle income countries," *Public Health Reviews*, vol. 33, no. 2, pp. 397–415, 2012.

[3] P. Bhatnagar, K. Wickramasinghe, J. Williams, M. Rayner, and N. Townsend, "The epidemiology of cardiovascular disease in the UK 2014," *Heart*, vol. 101, no. 15, pp. 1182–1189, 2015.

[4] J. L. Anderson, C. D. Adams, E. M. Antman et al., "ACC/AHA 2007 guidelines for the management of patients with unstable angina/non-ST-Elevation myocardial infarction: a report of the American College of Cardiology/American Heart Association Task Force on Practice Guidelines (Writing Committee to Revise the 2002 Guidelines for the Management of Patients With Unstable Angina/Non-ST-Elevation Myocardial Infarction) developed in collaboration with the American College of Emergency Physicians, the Society for Cardiovascular Angiography and Interventions, and the Society of Thoracic Surgeons endorsed by the American Association of Cardiovascular and Pulmonary Rehabilitation and the Society for Academic Emergency Medicine," *Journal of the American College of Cardiology*, vol. 50, no. 7, pp. e1–e157, 2007.

[5] C. W. Hamm and E. Braunwald, "A classification of unstable angina revisited," *Circulation*, vol. 102, no. 1, pp. 118–122, 2000.

[6] A. P. Schroeder and E. Falk, "Vulnerable and dangerous coronary plaques," *Atherosclerosis*, vol. 118, pp. S141–S149, 1995.

[7] E. Braunwald, D. B. Mark, R. H. Jones et al., *Unstable angina: diagnosis and management. Clinical practice guideline number 10. AHCPR Publication No. 94-0602. Rockville (MD): Agency for Health Care Policy and Research and the National Heart, Lung, and Blood Institute*, vol. 154 of *Public Health Service, US Department of Health and Human Services*, 1994.

[8] Institute for Clinical Systems Improvement (ICSI), *Health Care Guideline: Diagnosis and Treatment of Chest Pain and Acute Coronary Syndrome (ACS)*, Institute for Clinical Systems Improvement, Bloomington, Minn, USA, 2012, https://www.icsi.org/_asset/ydv4b3/ACS-Interactive1112b.pdf.

[9] J. T. Anderson, C. D. Adams, E. M. Antman et al., "2011 ACCF/AHA focused update incorporated into the ACC/AHA 2007 guidelines for the management of patients with unstable angina/non-ST-elevation myocardial infarction a report of the American College of Cardiology Foundation/American Heart Association Task Force on Practice Guidelines," *Circulation*, vol. 123, no. 18, pp. e426–e579, 2011.

[10] The State Pharmacopoeia Commission of the People's Republic of China, *Chinese Pharmacopoeia*, vol. 1, Chemical Industry Press, Beijing, China, 2010.

[11] C. Y. Kwan, E. E. Daniel, and M. C. Chen, "Inhibition of vasoconstriction by tetramethylpyrazine: does it act by blocking the voltage-dependent Ca channel?" *Journal of Cardiovascular Pharmacology*, vol. 15, no. 1, pp. 157–162, 1990.

[12] K.-L. Wong, P. Chan, W.-C. Huang et al., "Effect of tetramethylpyrazine on potassium channels to lower calcium concentration in cultured aortic smooth muscle cells," *Clinical and Experimental Pharmacology and Physiology*, vol. 30, no. 10, pp. 793–798, 2003.

[13] C.-Y. Kwan, "Plant-derived drugs acting on cellular Ca^{2+} mobilization in vascular smooth muscle: tetramethylpyrazine and tetrandrine," *Stem Cells*, vol. 12, no. 1, pp. 64–67, 1994.

[14] A. L. S. Au, Y. W. Kwan, C. C. Kwok, R.-Z. Zhang, and G.-W. He, "Mechanisms responsible for the in vitro relaxation of ligustrazine on porcine left anterior descending coronary artery," *European Journal of Pharmacology*, vol. 468, no. 3, pp. 199–207, 2003.

[15] Z. Ren, J. Ma, P. Zhang et al., "The effect of ligustrazine on L-type calcium current, calcium transient and contractility in rabbit ventricular myocytes," *Journal of Ethnopharmacology*, vol. 144, no. 3, pp. 555–561, 2012.

[16] X. Gong, V. N. Ivanov, M. M. Davidson, and T. K. Hei, "Tetramethylpyrazine (TMP) protects against sodium arsenite-induced nephrotoxicity by suppressing ROS production, mitochondrial dysfunction, pro-inflammatory signaling pathways and programed cell death," *Archives of Toxicology*, vol. 89, no. 7, pp. 1057–1070, 2014.

[17] F. Jiang, J. Qian, S. Chen, W. Zhang, and C. Liu, "Ligustrazine improves atherosclerosis in rat via attenuation of oxidative stress," *Pharmaceutical Biology*, vol. 49, no. 8, pp. 856–863, 2011.

[18] L. Lv, S.-S. Jiang, J. Xu, J.-B. Gong, and Y. Cheng, "Protective effect of ligustrazine against myocardial ischaemia reperfusion in rats: the role of endothelial nitric oxide synthase," *Clinical and Experimental Pharmacology and Physiology*, vol. 39, no. 1, pp. 20–27, 2012.

[19] R. Fu, Y. Zhang, Y. Guo, Y. Zhang, Y. Xu, and F. Chen, "Digital gene expression analysis of the pathogenesis and therapeutic mechanisms of ligustrazine and puerarin in rat atherosclerosis," *Gene*, vol. 552, no. 1, pp. 75–80, 2014.

[20] E. Braunwald, E. M. Antman, J. W. Beasley et al., "ACC/AHA Guidelines for the management of patients with unstable angina and non–ST-segment elevation myocardial infarction: executive summary and recommendations a report of the American College Of Cardiology/American Heart Association Task Force on Practice Guidelines (committee on the management of patients with unstable angina)," *Circulation*, vol. 102, no. 10, pp. 1193–1209, 2000.

[21] E. Rapaport, "Nomenclature and criteria for diagnosis of ischemic heart disease. Report of the Joint International Society and Federation of Cardiology/World Health Organization task force on standardization of clinical nomenclature," *Circulation*, vol. 59, no. 3, pp. 607–609, 1979.

[22] Chinese Society of Cardiology, "Recommendations for the diagnosis and treatment of unstable angina pectoris," *Chinese Journal of Cardiology*, vol. 28, no. 6, pp. 409–412, 2000.

[23] R. J. Gibbons, K. Chatterjee, J. Daley et al., "ACC/AHA/ACP-ASIM guidelines for the management of patients with chronic stable angina1: a report of the American College of Cardiology/American Heart Association Task Force on Practice Guidelines (Committee on Management of Patients With Chronic Stable Angina)," *Journal of the American College of Cardiology*, vol. 33, no. 7, pp. 2092–2197, 1999.

[24] J. P. T. Higgins and S. Green, *Cochrane Handbook for Systematic Reviews of Interventions*, Version 5.1.0, 2011, http://handbook.cochrane.org/.

[25] H. Guo, "Clinical observation of Ligustrazine on unstable angina," *Modern Journal of Integrated Traditional Chinese and Western Medicine*, vol. 16, no. 29, pp. 4294–4295, 2007.

[26] J.-Q. Liao and X.-W. Luo, "Efficacy of Ligustrazine on unstable angina," *Medical Information*, vol. 19, no. 7, pp. 1242–1243, 2006.

[27] M.-F. Da, "Clinical observation of Ligustrazine on unstable angina," *Qinghai Medical Journal*, vol. 38, no. 10, pp. 69–70, 2008.

[28] W.-M. Rong, W.-Z. Li, and Y.-H. Chen, "Effect of ligustrazine on serum C-reactive protein concentration of patients with unstable angina pectoris," *Lingnan Journal of Emergency Medicine*, vol. 6, no. 2, pp. 87–93, 2001.

[29] L. Peng, "Adjuvant treatment of Ligustrazine injection clinical observation on unstable angina," *Modern Journal of Integrated Traditional Chinese and Western Medicine*, vol. 23, no. 10, pp. 1108–1110, 2014.

[30] Z.-Z. Wang and J.-P. Hua, "Clinical observation of Ligustrazine injection and conventional medicine on unstable angina," *Clinical Journal of Traditional Chinese Medicine*, vol. 16, no. 5, article 426, 2004.

[31] X.-M. Wei, Y. Wen, and M.-F. Ren, "The concentration of vascular endothelial growth factor and clinical observation of ligustrazine injection on unstable angina," *Chinese Journal of Cardiovascular Research*, vol. 10, no. 3, pp. 181–183, 2012.

[32] X.-F. Wang, "Clinical evaluation on the effects of Ligustrazine injection in 65 cases aged with UAP," *Research and Practice of Chinese Medicines*, vol. 20, no. 3, pp. 56–57, 2006.

[33] J.-H. Zhou, "78 cases of high-dose Ligustrazine treatment of unstable angina clinical observation," *Journal of Emergency in Traditional Chinese Medicine*, vol. 17, no. 11, pp. 1504–1505, 2008.

[34] Y. Li, "Evaluation of the clinical diagnosis and treatment of unstable angina medicine," *Chinese Journal of Modern Drug Application*, vol. 4, no. 9, pp. 113–114, 2010.

[35] D.-N. Sun, "Analysis of therapeutic effect of Ligustrazine injection in curing unstable angina," *Journal of Practical Medical Techniques*, vol. 14, no. 11, pp. 1431–1432, 2007.

[36] Q.-Z. Wang, "Clinical research of Ligustrazine injection on unstable angina," *Chinese Remedies & Clinics*, vol. 5, no. 32, pp. 29–30, 2008.

[37] B. Fan, "Efficacy analysis of Ligustrazine injection on elderly unstable angina," *Medical Information*, vol. 27, no. 3, pp. 484–485, 2014.

[38] W.-H. Fu and H. Lin, "Integrative clinical observation of medicine treatment on unstable angina," *Chinese Journal of Clinical Rational Drug Use*, vol. 2, no. 15, pp. 54–55, 2009.

[39] H.-H. Meng, M.-J. Ma, and X. Lin, "Combined low-molecular-weight heparins calcium injection with Ligustrazine injection for 76 cases of unstable angina," *Clinical Journal of Traditional Chinese Medicine*, vol. 17, no. 3, pp. 255–256, 2005.

[40] F. Wang, W.-Q. Gu, and J. Bai, "The clinical observation of combined nitroglycerin with Ligustrazine injection for 32 cases on unstable angina," *Chinese Journal of Integrative Medicine on Cardiovascular Disease*, vol. 3, no. 1, article 78, 2005.

[41] The State Pharmacopoeia Commission of the People's Republic of China, *Chinese Pharmacopoeia*, vol. 2, Chemical Industry Press, Beijing, China, 2015.

[42] F. K.-H. Sze, F. F. Yeung, E. Wong, and J. Lau, "Does Danshen improve disability after acute ischaemic stroke?" *Acta Neurologica Scandinavica*, vol. 111, no. 2, pp. 118–125, 2005.

Permissions

The contributors of this book come from diverse backgrounds, making this book a truly international effort. This book will bring forth new frontiers with its revolutionizing research information and detailed analysis of the nascent developments around the world.

We would like to thank all the contributing authors for lending their expertise to make the book truly unique. They have played a crucial role in the development of this book. Without their invaluable contributions this book wouldn't have been possible. They have made vital efforts to compile up to date information on the varied aspects of this subject to make this book a valuable addition to the collection of many professionals and students.

This book was conceptualized with the vision of imparting up-to-date information and advanced data in this field. To ensure the same, a matchless editorial board was set up. Every individual on the board went through rigorous rounds of assessment to prove their worth. After which they invested a large part of their time researching and compiling the most relevant data for our readers.

The editorial board has been involved in producing this book since its inception. They have spent rigorous hours researching and exploring the diverse topics which have resulted in the successful publishing of this book. They have passed on their knowledge of decades through this book. To expedite this challenging task, the publisher supported the team at every step. A small team of assistant editors was also appointed to further simplify the editing procedure and attain best results for the readers.

Apart from the editorial board, the designing team has also invested a significant amount of their time in understanding the subject and creating the most relevant covers. They scrutinized every image to scout for the most suitable representation of the subject and create an appropriate cover for the book.

The publishing team has been an ardent support to the editorial, designing and production team. Their endless efforts to recruit the best for this project, has resulted in the accomplishment of this book. They are a veteran in the field of academics and their pool of knowledge is as vast as their experience in printing. Their expertise and guidance has proved useful at every step. Their uncompromising quality standards have made this book an exceptional effort. Their encouragement from time to time has been an inspiration for everyone.

The publisher and the editorial board hope that this book will prove to be a valuable piece of knowledge for researchers, students, practitioners and scholars across the globe.

List of Contributors

V. P. Bagla, V. Z. Lubisi, T. Ndiitwani,M. P.Mokgotho, L.Mampuru and V. Mbazima
Department of Biochemistry, Microbiology and Biotechnology, Faculty of Science and Agriculture, University of Limpopo, Turfloop Campus, Private Bag X1106, Sovenga, Limpopo 0727, South Africa

Xin Li, Qing-qing Xiao, Fu-lun Li, Rong Xu, Bin Fan, Min-feng Wu, Min Zhou, Su Li, Jie Chen and Bin Li
Department of Dermatology, Yueyang Hospital of Integrated Traditional Chinese and Western Medicine Shanghai University of Traditional Chinese Medicine, Shanghai 200437, China
Institute of Dermatology, Shanghai Academy of Traditional Chinese Medicine, Shanghai 201203, China

Shi-guang Peng
Department of Dermatology, Beijing Chao-Yang Hospital, Capital Medical University, Beijing 100020, China

Jinbong Park, Yunu Jung, Dong-Hyun Youn, JongWook Kang and Daeyeon Yoon
Department of Pharmacology, Graduate School, Kyung Hee University, 26 Kyungheedae-ro, Dongdaemun-gu, Seoul 02447, Republic of Korea

Yong-Deok Jeon, Dae-Seung Kim, Yo-Han Han and Seung-Heon Hong
Center for Metabolic Function Regulation,Wonkwang University, 460 Iksandae-ro, Iksan, Jeonbuk 54538, Republic of Korea

Hye-Lin Kim and Junhee Lee
College of Korean Medicine, Kyung Hee University, 26, Kyungheedae-ro, Dongdaemun-gu, Seoul 02447, Republic of Korea

Mi-Young Jeong
Center for Metabolic Function Regulation, Wonkwang University, 460 Iksandae-ro, Iksan, Jeonbuk 54538, Republic of Korea
College of Korean Medicine, Kyung Hee University, 26, Kyungheedae-ro, Dongdaemun-gu, Seoul 02447, Republic of Korea

Jong- Hyun Lee
College of Pharmacy, Dongduk Women's University, 60 Hwarang-ro 13-gil, Seongbuk-gu, Seoul 02748, Republic of Korea

Jae-Young Um
Department of Pharmacology, Graduate School, Kyung Hee University, 26 Kyungheedae-ro, Dongdaemun-gu, Seoul 02447, Republic of Korea3College of Korean Medicine, Kyung Hee University, 26, Kyungheedae-ro, Dongdaemun-gu, Seoul 02447, Republic of Korea

Jianling Liu, Tianli Pei and Jiexin Mu
College of Life Science, Northwest University, Xi'an, Shaanxi 710069, China
Center of Bioinformatics, College of Life Science, Northwest A&F University, Yangling, Shaanxi 712100, China

Chunli Zheng, Xuetong Chen, Chao Huang, Yingxue Fu and Yonghua Wang
Center of Bioinformatics, College of Life Science, Northwest A&F University, Yangling, Shaanxi 712100, China

Zongsuo Liang
College of Life Science, Zhejiang Sci-Tech University, Hangzhou, Zhejiang 310000, China

Mei-hong Shen
The Second Clinical College, Nanjing University of Chinese Medicine, Nanjing, Jiangsu 210046, China

Chun-bing Zhang
College of Basic Medicine, Nanjing University of Chinese Medicine, Nanjing, Jiangsu 210046, China
Department of Clinical Laboratory, Jiangsu Province Hospital of Traditional Chinese Medicine, Affiliated Hospital of Nanjing University of Chinese Medicine, Nanjing, Jiangsu 210029, China

Jia-hui Zhang
College of Basic Medicine, Nanjing University of Chinese Medicine, Nanjing, Jiangsu 210046, China

Peng-fei Li
Department of Clinical Laboratory, Jiangsu
Province Hospital of Traditional Chinese Medicine,
Affiliated Hospital of Nanjing University of Chinese
Medicine, Nanjing, Jiangsu 210029, China

**Khaled K. Al-Qattan, Martha Thomson, Divya
Jayasree and Muslim Ali**
Department of Biological Sciences, Faculty of
Science, Kuwait University, P.O. Box 5969, 13060
Safat, Kuwait

Lolita Rapolienė
Klaipeda Seamen's Health Care Center, Taikos
Street 46, LT-91213 Klaipėda, Lithuania
Department of Nursing of Klaipeda University, H.
Manto Street 84, LT-92294 Klaipėda, Lithuania

Artūras Razbadauskas
Klaipeda Seamen's Hospital, Liepojos Street 45, LT-
92288 Klaipėda, Lithuania
Faculty of Health Science, Klaipėda University, H.
Manto Street 84, LT-92294 Klaipėda, Lithuania

Jonas Sdlyga
Department of Nursing of Klaipeda University, H.
Manto Street 84, LT-92294 Klaipėda, Lithuania
Klaipeda Seamen's Hospital, Liepojos Street 45, LT-
92288 Klaipėda, Lithuania

Arvydas Martinkėnas
Department of Statistics, Klaipėda University, H.
Manto Street 84, LT-92294 Klaipėda, Lithuania

ShudongWang, Zheng Wang and Wenya Liu
Department of Pharmaceutics, Jinling Hospital,
Nanjing University School of Medicine, Nanjing
210002, China

**Tao Li, Wei Qu, Xin Li, Shaoxin Ma and Shanshan
and Hou**
China Pharmaceutical University, Nanjing 211198,
China

Jihua Fu
Department of Physiology, China Pharmaceutical
University, 639 Long Mian Road, Nanjing, Jiangsu
211198, China

Marcin Ozarowski
Department of Pharmaceutical Botany and Plant
Biotechnology, Poznan University of Medical
Sciences, Sw. Marii Magdaleny 14, 61-861 Poznan,
Poland

Department of Pharmacology and Phytochemistry,
Institute of Natural Fibres and Medicinal Plants,
Wojska Polskiego 71b, 60-630 Poznan, Poland

Przemyslaw L. Mikolajczak
Department of Pharmacology and Phytochemistry,
Institute of Natural Fibres and Medicinal Plants,
Wojska Polskiego 71b, 60-630 Poznan, Poland
Department of Pharmacology, University of Medical
Sciences, Rokietnicka 5a, 60-806 Poznan, Poland

Anna Piasecka and Piotr Kachlicki
Department of Pathogen Genetics and Plant
Resistance, Metabolomics Team, Institute of
Plant Genetics of the Polish Academy of Science,
Strzeszynska 34, 60-479 Poznan, Poland

**Radoslaw Kujawski, Agnieszka Gryszczynska,
Bogna Opala and Zdzislaw Lowicki**
Department of Pharmacology and Phytochemistry,
Institute of Natural Fibres and Medicinal Plants,
Wojska Polskiego 71b, 60-630 Poznan, Poland

Anna Bogacz
Laboratory of Experimental Pharmacogenetics,
Department of Clinical Pharmacy and Biopharmacy,
University ofMedical Sciences, 14 Sw. Marii
Magdaleny, 61-861 Poznan, Poland
Department of Stem Cells and Regenerative
Medicine, Institute of Natural Fibres and Medicinal
Plants, Wojska Polskiego 71b, 60-630 Poznan, Poland

Joanna Bartkowiak-Wieczorek
Laboratory of Experimental Pharmacogenetics,
Department of Clinical Pharmacy and Biopharmacy,
University ofMedical Sciences, 14 Sw. Marii
Magdaleny, 61-861 Poznan, Poland

Michal Szulc and Ewa Kaminska
Department of Pharmacology, University of Medical
Sciences, Rokietnicka 5a, 60-806 Poznan, Poland

**Malgorzata Kujawska and Jadwiga Jodynis-
Liebert**
Department of Toxicology, Poznan University of
Medical Sciences, Dojazd 30, 60-631 Poznan, Poland

Agnieszka Seremak-Mrozikiewicz
Department of Pharmacology and Phytochemistry,
Institute of Natural Fibres and Medicinal Plants,
Wojska Polskiego 71b, 60-630 Poznan, Poland
Division of Perinatology and Women's Diseases,
Poznan University of Medical Sciences, Polna 33,
60-535 Poznan, Poland

Laboratory of Molecular Biology, Poznan University of Medical Sciences, Polna 33, 60-535 Poznan, Poland

Boguslaw Czerny
Department of Stem Cells and Regenerative Medicine, Institute of Natural Fibres and Medicinal Plants, Wojska Polskiego 71b, 60-630 Poznan, Poland
Department of General Pharmacology and Pharmacoeconomics, Pomeranian Medical University, Zolnierska 48, 70-204 Szczecin, Poland

Ning Wang, Hor Yue Tan, Ming Hong, Sha Li and Yibin Feng
School of Chinese Medicine, Li Ka Shing Faculty of Medicine,The University of Hong Kong, Pokfulam, Hong Kong

Qihe Xu
Centre for Integrative Chinese Medicine and Department of Renal Medicine, Faculty of Life Sciences and Medicine, King's College London, London SE5 9NU, UK

Man-Fung Yuen
Division of Gastroenterology and Hepatology, Queen Mary Hospital and Department of Medicine, Li Ka Shing Faculty of Medicine,The University of Hong Kong, Pokfulam, Hong Kong

Jingfen Zhu, Tian Shen and Yi Feng
Department of Community Health and Family Medicine, School of Public Health, Shanghai Jiao Tong University, Shanghai 200025, China

Rong Shi
School of Public Health, Shanghai University of TCM, Shanghai 201203, China

Su Chen
Si-Tang Community Health Service Center of Shanghai, Shanghai 200431, China

Lihua Dai
Department of Emergency Medicine, Xin Hua Hospital Affiliated to Shanghai Jiao Tong University School of Medicine, Shanghai 200092, China

Pingping Gu
Southern California Kaiser Sunset, 4867 Sunset Boulevard, Los Angeles, CA 90027, USA

Mina Shariff and Tuong Nguyen
Department of Research, DRM Resources, 1683 Sunflower Avenue, Costa Mesa, CA 92626, USA

Yeats Ye
Maryland Population Research Center, University of Maryland, College Park, MD 20742, USA

Jianyu Rao
Department of Pathology and Laboratory Medicine, David Geffen School of Medicine, University of California at Los Angeles, Los Angeles, CA 90095, USA

Guoqiang Xing
Imaging Institute of Rehabilitation and Development of Brain Function, North Sichuan Medical University, Nanchong Central Hospital, Nanchong 637000, China
Lotus Biotech.com LLC, John Hopkins University-MCC, 9601 Medical Center Drive, Rockville, MD 20850, USA

Dong-Seon Kim
KM Convergence Research Division, Korea Institute of Oriental Medicine, 1672 Yuseong-daero, Yuseong-gu, Daejeon 305-811, Republic of Korea

Seung-Hyung Kim
Institute of Traditional Medicine and Bioscience, Daejeon University, Daejeon 300-716, Republic of Korea

Jimin Cha
Department ofMicrobiology, Faculty ofNatural Science, DankookUniversity, Cheonan, Chungnam 330-714, Republic of Korea

Qian Zhang, Hao Yang, Jing An, Rui Zhang and Bo Chen
Translational Medicine Center, Hong Hui Hospital, Xi'an Jiaotong University College of Medicine, Xi'an 710054, China

Ding-Jun Hao
Department of Spine Surgery, Hong Hui Hospital, Xi'an Jiaotong University College of Medicine, Xi'an, China

Xianghui Ma, Bin Lv, Pan Li, Xiaoqing Jiang, Qian Zhou and Xiumei Gao
State Key Laboratory of Modern Chinese Medicine, Tianjin University of Traditional Chinese Medicine, Tianjin 300193, China

Xiaoying Wang
State Key Laboratory of Modern Chinese Medicine, Tianjin University of Traditional Chinese Medicine, Tianjin 300193, China
College of Traditional Chinese Medicine, Tianjin University of Traditional Chinese Medicine, Tianjin 300193, China

Suman Cao
Graduate School, Tianjin University of Traditional Chinese Medicine, Tianjin 300193, China

Wenli Zhao
Graduate School, Tianjin University of Traditional Chinese Medicine, Tianjin 300193, China
Department of Neurology, Nankai Hospital, Tianjin Academy of Integrative Medicine, Tianjin 300100, China

Huaien Bu
Department of Chinese Medicine, Tianjin University of Traditional Chinese Medicine, Tianjin 300193, China

Ye Zhao
Department of Clinical Research, Nankai Hospital, Tianjin Academy of Integrative Medicine, Tianjin 300100, China

Chunquan Yu
Editorial Department, Tianjin University of Traditional Chinese Medicine, Tianjin 300193, China

Index

A

Acetylthiocholine Iodide (atch), 102
Adipocyte Differentiation, 23, 26, 28, 31-32
Akt And P38 Pathways, 87
Alzheimer's Disease, 99, 109, 111-114, 129, 136-141, 156, 161, 167
Ameliorative Actions, 66-67
Antigen-presenting Cells (apcs), 11
Antimetastatic Potential, 1, 3, 5, 7, 9
Associated Pathogens, 1

B

Balneotherapy, 77-81, 83-86
Berberine Inhibition, 115, 117, 119, 121, 123, 125
Blood Pressure Implications, 66
Blood-heat Syndrome, 11-13, 17-21
Brainwater Content, 52, 54

C

Cerebral Ischemia, 51, 53, 55, 57-65, 110, 113-114, 161
Cervical Cancer Cells, 1, 3, 5, 7, 9
China Hospital Knowledge Database (chkd), 198
Chinese Medical Journal Database (cmjd), 198
Chuanxiong, 156, 159, 168, 184, 198-200
Cognitive Function, 77, 81, 83, 99, 109, 127, 137
Combined Plant Extracts, 142-143, 145, 149
Confidence Interval (ci), 80
Consumption of Nitroglycerin, 198, 206
Cynanchum Paniculatum (cp), 88, 95
Cytoplasmic Lipid Chaperones, 23

D

Data Extraction, 12, 199
Dietary Supplement, 126-127, 129, 131, 133-135, 137, 139, 141, 157
Diminish Stress, 77
Diospyros Lycioides Extract, 1, 3, 5, 7, 9
Drug Targeting, 34-37, 47

E

Embase (ovid), 198-200
Excretion (adme) Screening, 34

F

Fatigue Management, 77, 79, 81, 83, 85
Fetal Bovine Serum (fbs), 3, 23
Fibrogenesis, 115, 117, 119, 121, 123-125

G

General Symptoms Distress Scale (gsds), 80
Glutathione (gsh), 53, 155, 199

H

Hammer Blow, 87-88
Heart Diseases, 183-184, 187, 192, 196
Hemorrhagic Stroke (hs), 51
Hepatic Manifestation, 171
High-salinity Geothermal Mineral Water, 77-78

I

Ih Ethanol Extracts Spray, 87
Illicium Henryi (ih), 87, 95
Immune Signatures, 13, 17, 19, 21
Immune-mediated Skin Disease, 11
Immunological Serum Markers, 11-12, 18
In Vivo and In Vitro, 22, 163, 196
Integrating Absorption, 34
Intervention Effects, 171, 173, 175, 177, 179, 181
Isobutylmethylxanthine (ibmx), 23

J

Jervine Prevent Adipogenesis, 22-23, 25, 27, 29, 31, 33

L

Ligustrazine, 153-156, 159, 168, 198-200, 203-208
þÿ Lkb1 - ampkØ5Þü - acc Axis, 22, 26
Long-term Memory, 98-99, 101, 107, 109-111, 113, 127

M

Medicinal Plants, 1, 9-10, 98-99, 112-114
Medline (ovid), 199-200
Middle Cerebral Artery Occlusion, 51-55, 57, 59, 61, 63, 65
Middle Cerebral Artery Occlusion (mcao), 51
Molecule Annotation System, 183, 187
Multiple Components, 35, 183, 185, 187, 189, 191, 193, 196-197

Multiple Pathways, 183, 185, 187, 189, 191, 193, 196-197

Multiple Targets, 35, 183, 185, 187, 189, 191, 193, 197

N

Network Pharmacology, 35, 48, 183-184, 197

Neurodegenerative Disorders, 99, 141

Nonalcoholic Fatty Liver Disease (nafld), 171

P

Pathophysiological Events, 153-154

Pathway Analysis, 34, 47

Phyllostachys Pubescens Leaf Extract, 142

Polymerase Chain Reaction, 89

Polyvinylidene Difluoride (pvdf), 25

Pooled Analyses, 11, 206

Porphyromonas Gingivalis, 1

Psoriasis Vulgaris, 11-13, 17-21

R

Rawgarlic Aqueous Extract (ge), 66

Renal Clearance, 66, 72-74

Renin-angiotensin System (ras), 66

Reperfusion Injury, 32, 51, 53, 55, 57, 59, 61, 63-65, 96, 110, 114, 167-170, 193, 196

Reverse Transcription, 53, 89, 102

S

Scopolamine Animal Model, 98-99, 101, 107, 109, 111, 113

Scopolamine Hydrobromide Trihydrate, 99

Scutellaria Baicalensis Root Extract, 142, 149-150

Short-time Randomized Controlled Trial, 77, 79, 81, 83, 85

Soft-tissue Injury (sti), 87-88

Streptozotocin, 66-67, 69, 71, 73-76, 110

Stress Management, 81, 83-84

Supplementary Treatment, 153, 164

Suppressing Activations, 87, 94

Surgical Procedures, 153-154

Systems Pharmacology, 35-37, 39, 41, 43, 45, 47-49

T

Therapeutic Effects, 47, 99, 129, 153, 155, 157, 159, 161, 163, 165, 167, 169, 171-173, 178, 183

Traditional Chinese Medicine (tcm), 11, 34, 153, 199

Transmission Electron Microscopy (tem), 53

Treatment of Unstable Angina, 198-200, 203, 205, 207-208

Turmeric Extract, 171, 173, 175, 177, 179, 181

U

Untargeted Metabolomics, 171, 173, 175, 177, 179, 181

V

Viral Hemorrhagic Fevers (vhf), 34

X

Xiangqing Anodyne Spray (xqas), 87-88, 96